AF833520

M. Aebi · J.S. Thalgott · J.K. Webb, AO ASIF Principles in Spine Surgery

Springer-Verlag Berlin Heidelberg GmbH

M. Aebi · J.S. Thalgott · J.K. Webb

AO ASIF Principles in Spine Surgery

With Contributions by
M. Goytan, B. Jeanneret, F. Magerl,
and M. B. Williamson, Jr.

With 296 Figures in 869 Parts

Springer

Prof. Dr. Max Aebi, FRCS(C)
Division of Orthopaedic Surgery
Mc Gill University
Royal Victoria/Montreal General Hospital
687 Pine Avenue West
Montreal, Quebec H3A 1A1/Canada

John S. Thalgott, M.D.
International Spinal Development & Research Foundation
500 South Rancho Drive, Suite 8 A
Las Vegas, NV 89106-4806/USA

John K. Webb, FRCS
Queens Medical Centre
Centre of Spinal Studies and Surgery
Nottingham NG7 2UH/U.K.

Contributors:
Michael Goytan, M.D., FRCS(C)
University of Manitoba, Health Sciences Center
820 Sherbrook St., Winnipeg, Manitoba R3A 1R9

Bernard Jeanneret, Docent
Orthopaedic Clinic of the University
Felix-Platter-Spital, CH-4012 Basel

Prof. Dr. Friedrich Magerl
Clinic Rosenberg
Rorschacherstr. 150, CH-9006 St. Gallen

Mark B. Williamson, Jr., M.D.
Carolina Specialty Care
124 Sunset Hill Road, Statesville, North Carolina 28625/USA

ISBN 978-3-642-63746-9

Cataloging-in-Publication Data applied for

Die Deutsche Bibliothek – CIP-Einheitsaufnahme
AO ASIF principles in spine surgery: with tables / M. Aebi ; John S. Thalgott ; John K. Webb. – Berlin ; Heidelberg ; New York ; Barcelona ; Budapest ; Hong Kong ; London ; Milan ; Paris ; Santa Clara ; Singapore ; Tokyo : Springer.
ISBN 978-3-642-63746-9 ISBN 978-3-642-58824-2 (eBook)
DOI 10.1007/978-3-642-58824-2

This work is subject to copyright. All rights are reserved, whether the whole or part of the material is concerned, specifically the rights of translation, reprinting, reuse of illustrations, recitation, broadcasting, reproduction on microfilm or in any other way, and storage in data banks. Duplication of this publication or parts thereof is permitted only under the provisions of the German Copyright Law of September 9, 1965, in its current version, and permission for use must always be obtained from Springer-Verlag. Violations are liable for prosecution under the German Copyright Law.

© Springer-Verlag Berlin Heidelberg 1998
Originally published by Springer-Verlag Berlin Heidelberg New York in 1998
Softcover reprint of the hardcover 1st edition 1998

The use of general descriptive names, registered names, trademarks, etc. in this publication does not imply, even in the absence of a specific statement, that such names are exempt from the relevant protective laws and regulations and therefore free for general use.
Product liability: The publishers cannot guarantee the accuracy of any information about the application of operative techniques and medications contained in this book. In every individual case the user must check such information by consulting the relevant literature.

Cover design: design & production GmbH, D-69121 Heidelberg
Typesetting: FotoSatz Pfeifer GmbH, D-82166 Gräfelfing
24/3111 – 10 9 8 7 6 – Printed on acid-free paper SPIN 11011422

Preface

This book has become necessary as a consequence of the rapid expansion of the surgical procedures and implants available for spinal surgery within the "AO Group". We have not attempted to write an in-depth book on spinal surgery, but one which will help the surgeon in the use of AO concepts and implants. We consider the practical courses held all over the world essential for the teaching of sound techniques so that technical complications and poor results can be avoided for both the surgeon and, in particular the patient. This book is a practical manual and an outline of what is taught in the courses. It is intended to help the young spinal surgeon to understand the correct use of AO implants. The indications given will aid the correct use of each procedure.

It must be strongly emphasized that surgery of the spine is technically demanding. The techniques described in this book should only be undertaken by surgeons who are trained and experienced in spinal surgery.

Certain techniques, in particular pedicle screw fixation and cages, have not yet been fully approved by the FDA in the United States. However, throughout the rest of the world, the use of pedicle screws has become a standard technique for the spine surgeon, since it has been shown to improve fixation techniques and allow segmental correction of the spine. The use of cages has become more and more popular, specifically as a tool of minimally invasive spinal surgery. The descriptions of these techniques will provide the surgeon with useful guidelines for their use.

Table of Contents

CHAPTER 1

Aims and Principles

1.1 Introduction

AO implants were primarily developed for internal fixation of fractures using the philosophy of the AO Group. This philosophy was developed some years ago (Müller et al. 1984) and its goals of internal fixation still apply:

1. Stable internal fixation designed to fulfill the local biomechanical demands
2. Preservation of blood supply by means of atraumatic surgery and soft tissue preservation
3. Anatomical alignment – particularly in regard to the sagittal plane
4. Early active pain-free movement of muscles and joints

1.2 Stable Internal Fixation

Stable internal fixation is designed to fulfill the local biomechanical demands. In the spine the understanding of this very basic principle needs to be widened to consider multiarticular coupled spinal units, where not only internal fixation is done but it is combined with fusion in order to achieve the required stability. This applies regardless of whether the problem is limited to one or two mobile segments (fracture, tumor, degenerative disease, spondylolisthesis) or several segments (deformities). The concepts of internal fixation may change accordingly. However, the functions of the implants are always the same: tension banding, buttressing, neutralization, lag screw principle and correction. The goal of all these methods is to provide adequate stability to maintain not only the integrity of a mobile segment and make it fuse, but also to maintain the balance and the physiologic three-dimensional form of a whole spine area.

1.3 Preservation of Blood Supply

The preservation of blood supply is an important principle of the AO techniques. The surgical approaches to the spine need basic training and understanding of general surgical principles, specifically when it comes to anterior approaches to the spine. Posterior surgery needs meticulous subperiosteal muscle dissection in order to prevent denervation and devascularization of the paraspinal muscles. The preservation of blood supply is important both anteriorly and posteriorly, leaving segmental vessels to the spine undisturbed. This is extremely important when dealing with the segmental arteries close to the spinal cord.

1.4 Anatomical Alignment

Anatomical alignment has been a fundamental goal in the management of fractures. The principles, however, also remain true for the management of all spinal disorders. *Preservation of the sagittal plane alignment is a key issue:* the prevention of kyphosis in lumbar and cervical spine surgery is essential. It is common to see iatrogenic flat backs or kyphotic cervical spines. Every malalignment in a particular area of the spine may cause a secondary compensatory deformity in the adjacent spine. This may be the source of persistent pain rather than the deformity itself. *Awareness of the sagittal plane is essential in any reconstructive procedure.*

1.5 Early Pain-Free Mobilization

The principle of early pain-free mobilization has stood the test of time. The goals of internal fixation should allow the patient to get out of bed and walk preferably without external support as soon as possible. A number of pathophysiological events occur after major surgery or trauma which have been shown to be related to the treatment modalities. If the human body spends an extended period of time in the unphysiological supine position, this can lead to cardiorespiratory disturbances. Patients should be able to stand and walk within 24–48 h after major surgery to the spine. The design and application of implants allow this goal to be achieved.

CHAPTER 2

Biomechanics of the Spine and Spinal Instrumentation

Mark B. Williamson, Jr. and M. Aebi

2.1 Introduction

The musculoskeletal system and its functions can be defined using the basic laws of mechanics. The field of biomechanics explores the effects of energy and forces on biological systems. The spinal column and its associated vertebrae and contiguous soft-tissue structures can be better appreciated with an understanding of these principles. In evaluating the spine, forces, moments and motion must be separated into individual entities. This separation allows understanding of normal as well as abnormal conditions such as fractures, deformities and degenerative conditions. The function and purpose of surgical restoration of normal spinal alignment must respect the laws of mechanics and their biomechanical principles. Achieving an understanding of these principles, including force analysis, kinematics, static and dynamic loading, modes of spinal failure and implant failure, allows one to critically evaluate his work. Understanding these mechanical and biomechanical principles would then allow one to plan and apply spinal instrumentation from a sound scientific perspective.

2.2 Mechanical Principles

Vectors and forces are illustrated with the use of arrows and are two-dimensional quantities. The arrow's direction represents the direction of the force; the arrow's length represents the degree of magnitude. The importance of direction is easily illustrated when describing forces which are applied to the front or the back of the head. The resultant injury will directly depend upon the direction and magnitude of the force which is applied.

Forces may be linear or circular. A circular force is called a *moment.* A force moment creates a rotational vector around an axis. The magnitude of a force moment is a *torque.* As an example, inserting a screw through a pedicle creates a force moment onto the vertebra. The magnitude of the moment about the axis is equal to the magnitude of the force multiplied by the perpendicular distance from the axis. Moment forces exist whenever a force occurs to a point which is not located along its line of action. Torque forces can be *coupled.* This occurs when two non-collinear forces act about the same axis. The resultant force moment about the axis is made up of the sum of the individual forces. Using a thumb and an index finger to tighten a screw with a screwdriver is an example of force coupling.

Holding a weighted object away from the body creates a compressive force upon the spinal column equal to the magnitude of the weight multiplied by the distance of the weight from the spinal column. The effect of this weight creates a force moment onto the spine which must be offset by (coupled with) an extensor-muscle force which is supplied by the erector spinal muscles. This force moment equals the magnitude of the extensor muscle force multiplied

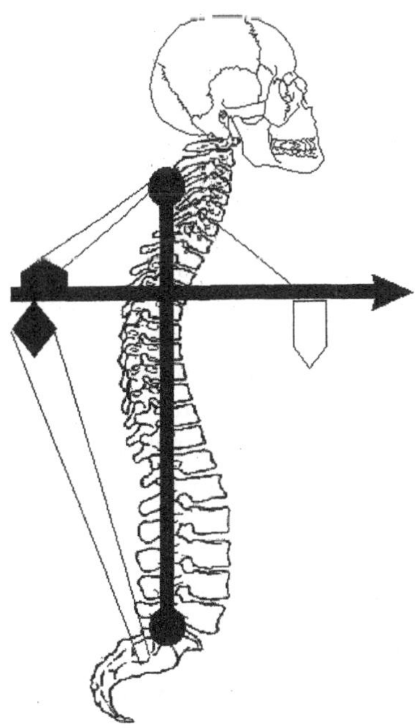

Fig. 2.1 Classic representation of muscle forces on the spine

by the distance from the spinal column. When the sum of all forces acting upon the spine is zero and the sum of all moments acting upon the spine is also zero, the spinal column is in equilibrium. No linear or angular acceleration occurs. The inability to *force couple* would prevent an individual from lifting an object away from the body. For instance, the T-6 paraplegic patient is unable to reach for a plate of food with both hands. Without extensor muscles, he topples forward, causing him to lose his upright position (Fig. 2.1).

Work-place reeducation courses (back schools) train the manual laborer in techniques which reduce both the distance and the weight of the object intended to be lifted, thereby, causing dramatic reduction in the magnitude of the forces acting upon the spine.

2.3 Mechanical Properties of Materials

Thus far, all discussion has been related to forces applied to an object. The resultant effect of this force application upon the object may be to place the object in equilibrium to cause acceleration or to maintain constant velocity. All materials respond to force application by undergoing deformation which is a change in its shape or size. The amount of deformation may be minuscule. Alternatively, it may occur to such a degree that it extends beyond the yield point (breaking point) of the material. Such an example is the osteoporotic vertebral compression fracture resulting from lifting a milk jug from a low countertop. The muscular forces remain constant regardless of the strength of the bone. The material (bone) attempts to resist the forces applied; however, because of material weakness, collapse occurs leading to fracture. The study of *deformation* allows one to understand modes of failure under various conditions, such as vertebral body fractures, posterior ligamentous disruption or implant failures.

Deformation occurs due to *stress* and *strain* produced within the object as a direct result of forces and moments acting upon that object. Objects vary in degree of deformation. The amount or degree of deformation depends upon the shape and size of the object as well as its intrinsic material properties. The combination of shape, size and intrinsic properties forms the basis for an object's deformational response to a force. This deformational response is a *structural property* of the material. Intrinsic material properties are independent of an object's shape and size.

A rod 1.0 cm in diameter would be four times stiffer than a rod 0.5 cm in diameter, assuming that both were made of the same material. The structural stiffness of each rod is dependent upon its cross-sectional area ($A = \pi r^2$). The study of intrinsic material properties of bone or spinal implants requires that the effect of the object's geometry (shape and size) are eliminated.

In evaluating the deformation of an object based on the load applied, a stress/strain analysis of the intrinsic material properties of the object is required. Stress equals the force or load applied to the object divided by its cross-sectional area. Strain equals the elongation of the original object divided by the original length of the object. For metallic implants, the change in length or strain is generally insignificant. This stress/strain behavior of the object describes its intrinsic material response. All physical quantities or values obtained from the stress/strain response of an object are characteristics of its intrinsic material properties.

Objects that have intrinsic material properties independent of the direction of loading are termed *isotropic*. Metal, plastic and glass are examples of isotropic materials. Materials that have intrinsic material properties dependent on the direction of loading are considered *anisotropic*. Examples include wood fiber-reinforced composite materials and musculoskeletal tissue, including bone, ligament, tendon, cartilage and intervertebral disc. Isotropic materials have a randomly dispersed internal structure, whereas anisotropic materials are characterized by an observable orderly internal structural arrangement.

Load deformation analysis defines the deformation of an object which occurs as a result of a force vector. Such a force applied to an object generally causes a change in both the X and the Y direction.

Compressive forces applied to an intervertebral disc decrease its height (Y axis) while allowing the disc to bulge (increase in the X axis). Force applied to an object over a fixed area is an example of applied stress to the object. Materials which are stressed by a deforming force undergo a change in length. This represents its *strain*. The relationship of stress or force and strain or deformation defines a material's *stiffness*.

Elastic deformation occurs whenever strain on a material is totally recovered when the stress is removed. *Plastic deformation* occurs at the point where stress is no longer proportional to strain. The point at which elastic deformation becomes plastic deformation is known as the *yield point*. The *ultimate tensile strength* or *ultimate tensile point* is the point at which the object fails (i.e., the point at which the plate breaks, the vertebra fractures, etc.). The maximum stress which a material can sustain is known as its *strength*. This point coincides with the area under the stress/strain curve to the point of its ultimate tensile strength. The ultimate tensile strength of cortical bone is 130 MPa, steel is 600 MPa and titanium is 650 MPa. The ultimate tensile strength of trabecular bone is 50 MPa.For instance, correction of a scoliotic deformity using rigid implants occurs due to elastic deformation of the spinal deformity. Loss of correction over time is occasionally seen following corrective surgery for scoliosis. This is a result of stress relaxation which is a time-dependent return of the deformity.

Iatrogenically created events may cause failure. Such an example is stress concentration to a longitudinal member of a spinal implant in a region of delayed union, which may ultimately result in failure due to the local material's ultimate strength being exceeded. Implant failure may result as a direct response to instantaneous overload or as a result of cyclical loading. Fatigue fracture or failure depends upon the intrinsic material properties of the implant as well as exposure to repetitive force (stress). Other causes of stress concentration include structural imperfections, sudden changes in cross-sectional area, material cracks, drill holes and surface irregularities noted on the implanted device.

Finite element analysis utilizes the principles discussed previously and attempts to apply them to the clinical situation. Various factors, such as variable loading conditions, geometric shape and design, material properties of both bone and implanted device, and inherent biologic properties are all considered. Principles of fixation, contact points and forces applied during implantation or utilization are analyzed. Such complex problems require separation into smaller units which can be individually analyzed and progressively combined through computer technology. This biomechanical and laboratory testing is then used as a basis for clinical study.

Materials with properties that allow permanent deformation before failure are considered *ductile*, whereas those that fail without permanent deformation are considered *brittle*. Metals such as stainless steel or titanium undergo elastic deformation until their yield point is reached, whereupon conversion to plastic deformation occurs until ultimate failure. Unlike metal, bone undergoes fracture without permanent deformation. Its yield point equals the ultimate failure point.

The area under the stress/strain curve represents the energy absorbed prior to failure. This defines the material's *toughness* during elastic deformation. The energy expended in creating such a deformation can be recovered by removal of the stress applied. The energy expended up to the yield point is a measure of the material's *resilience*.

Fatigue failure occurs as a result of repetitive loading because of cumulative damage. Although the individual load should be below the ultimate failure point, the accumulation of stress causes cumulative micro-injury to the implant until the material fails. The average spine cycles approximately three million times per year. Fatigue failure of rods and screws occurs when metals fail prior to solid fusion. While higher stresses cause fatigue failure after fewer cycles, all materials will ultimately fail in the absence of solid fusion, regardless of the amount of stress applied, if cyclical loading occurs.

Fatigue fracture occurs through the process of *crack initiation* followed by *crack propagation*. Intrinsic factors which increase resistance to fatigue failure include manufacturing and/or mechanical methods to limit crack initiation, and increasing the intrinsic material toughness, thereby, preventing crack propagation.

Material hardness is a measure of the mechanical surface properties of a material. Those materials that resist plastic deformation at their surface address issues of crack initiation. Hardness can be enhanced by application of various surface coatings.

2.4 Implant Materials

Commonly used spinal implant materials include stainless steel, commercially pure titanium and titanium-aluminium-vanadium alloy. Standardization of alloys is regulated by the American Society for Testing and Materials (ASTM). Whereas trade names vary per manufacturer, standard alloys must have set specifications of composition. Manufacture and implant properties are based on ASTM standards. Of the 50 or more alloys of commercially available stainless steel , only two (ASTMF-55 and ASTMF-56) are used extensively in the orthopedic implant industry. ASTMF-55 and ASTMF-56 alloys are also known as grade 316 and grade 316L stainless steel. These alloys are made up of chromium, which provides a corrosion-resistant oxide-film, nickel which also provides corrosion resistance, and molybdenum, which resists corrosion due to pitting. This alloy contains some carbon, an undesirable component due to its unique manufacturing properties causing segregation and encouraging corrosion.

Crevice corrosion occurs at the junction of two similar metals. Fluid located within the gap between the materials contains a lower dissolved oxygen concentration. This phenomenon creates a *voltage cell* due to the difference in oxygen concentration between adjacent fluids, allowing local corrosion to occur. This concept becomes important in rod/screw or plate/screw devices which arc unconstrained (semi-rigid).

Commercially purc titanium (ASTMF-67) and titanium-aluminium-vanadium alloy (ASTMF-136) have greater biocompatability and corrosion resistance than that of stainless steel. Pitting corrosion and crevice corrosion appear less significant. Titanium-aluminium-vanadium alloy has approximately 6% aluminium and 4% vanadium and is commonly known as Ti6A14V. Unique characteristics include high strength-to-weight ratio, enhanced ductility, and increased fatigue life. Its only drawback involves increased *notch sensitivity*. Notch sensitivity refers to crack initiation due to stress concentration at a specific point along the longitudinal member. Notch sensitivity can be decreased by changes in manufacturing methods as well as by appropriate surgical technique and handling.

Stainless steel has a modulus of elasticity which is 12 times that of bone, whereas titanium and its alloys have a modulus of elasticity six times that of bone. Because of the greater approximation of elastic modulus by titanium to bone, many believe that it is a superior implant for spinal fixation when compared with stainless steel. It is critical to minimize fatigue sensitivity caused by notching of the implant. This is most significant on long constructs, such as those for scoliosis or kyphosis. Failure of implants is predominantly the result of fatigue fracture due to loads occurring about the spine that exceed the endurance limit of the implants. Meticulous surgical technique with satisfactory fusion must occur prior to fatigue failure of the device. Correct manufacturing standards and quality control issues have resulted in minimizing intrinsic material failure. Despite this, failure remains a function of intrinsically or iatrogenically created defects. Resistance to fatigue failure becomes important in cases of delayed union or nonunion. It is imperative that these conditions are recognized early and are appropriately addressed, surgically, via augmentation of fusion and exchange of implant devices to increase the fatigue life of the construct.

2.5 Principles of Surgical Stabilization

The application of metallic implants about the spine must follow narrowly prescribed principles for optimum results. Clinical examples provided throughout this text will be following the general principles which are described in the next few paragraphs.

2.5.1 Buttressing Principle

Buttressing principles are designed to prevent axial deformity. Forces which can cause axial deformity may be directly related to axial loading or may be secondary to bending or shear forces. Spinal instrumentation applied for purposes of buttressing is placed on the side of load application and is applied to the area of the spine requiring support. Buttress plates function to minimize compression and shear forces and also act to minimize torque forces. Maximum surface contact requires careful contouring of the implant and preparation of the bony surface. Screw insertion is begun closest to the area of greatest potential motion with the remaining screws being placed in an orderly fashion towards the ends of the plate. Buttressing examples include anterior cervical locking-plate systems and anterior thoracolumbar locking-plate systems (Fig. 2.2).

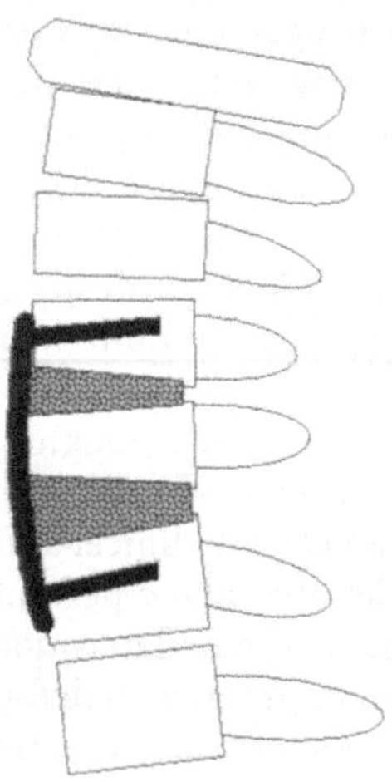

Fig. 2.2 Anterior cervical plate as an example of a buttressing implant

2.5.2 Neutralization principle

Neutralization systems are applied for purposes of stress shielding and minimization of torsional bending, shearing and axial loading forces. Such application allows for an increasing stability of these constructs, thereby, providing opportunities for earlier functional restoration of movement. Examples include simple posterior, lateral and anterior stabilization using plates or rods with multiple screws inserted for protection of neural structures and stabilization while fusion occurs (Fig. 2.3).

2.5.3 Tension Band Principle

The use of an implant to provide a posterior tension band requires intact compressive load-bearing ability by the spinal column. The tension band concept resists tensile forces and bending moments. The tension band principle allows dynamic compression through the weight-bearing column, thereby, encouraging fusion. Common examples include posterior single level fixation with cervical hook plates or posterior wire fixation (Fig. 2.4)

2.5.4 Bridge Fixation Principle

If the weight-bearing column is unable to sustain the compressive forces, posterior fixation requires a device which is sufficiently strong to function as a bridge across the weakened segment to maintain length, alignment, and stability. A construct may be developed which is used to *bridge* a segment of the spine. This requires an implant construct which is both stiff and strong. It functions to support the spine until the natural regenerative processes occur (fusion). Classic examples include the use of the fixator interne inserted for thoracolumbar fractures of either the burst or compressive variety. The implant serves to bridge the fracture as long as the anterior column is healing and regaining its structural strength. Over time, following the initial healing period, load sharing occurs If there is no chance that the anterior column may participate in load sharing, such as due to the presence of an anterior defect, then an anterior support system must be surgically placed, either in the form of a cortical cancellous graft or other prosthetic device, such as a *cage* packed with bone to avoid failure of the posterior implant. In the long run, a posterior fusion with instrumentation cannot compensate for a defect of the anterior column.The implant construct must endure three million loading cycles to survive for 1

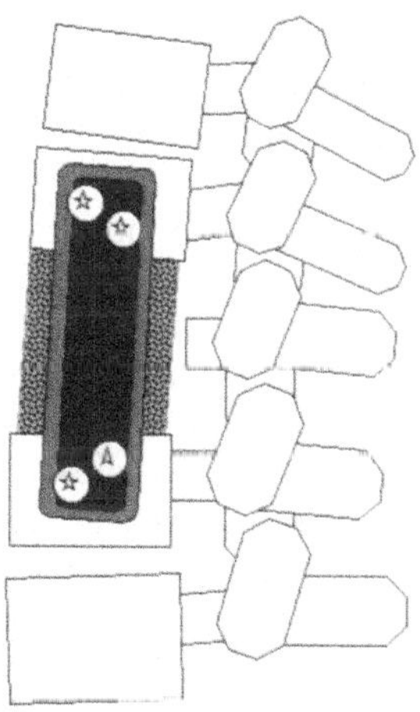

Fig. 2.3 The thoracolumbar locking plate is an example of a neutralization or protection implant

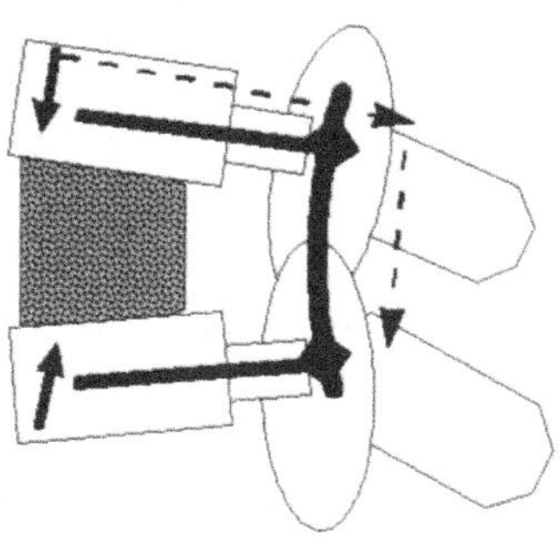

Fig. 2.4 Example of tension band implant allowing dynamic compression through the load bearing column

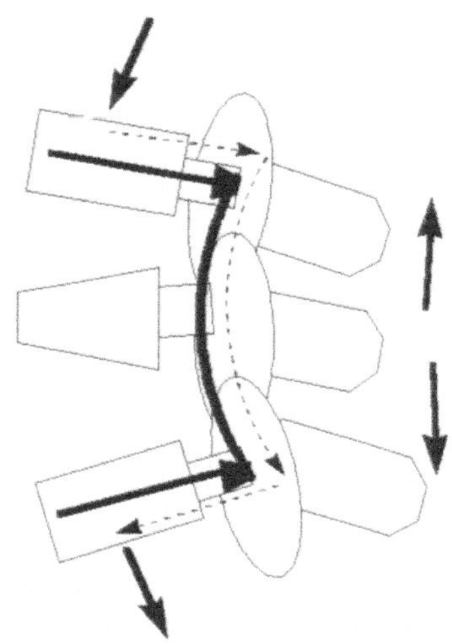

Fig. 2.5 A bridge construct may be used to support the spine during anterior column healing

year after insertion. Therefore, fusion and anterior column restoration must occur quite rapidly to minimize the risk of failure. In bridge constructs, multiple fixation points along the spinal column allow an increased opportunity for stress transfer and act to minimise fatigue failure (Fig. 2.5).

2.6 Instrumentation Application

Spinal instrumentation is designed to maximize preservation of neurological function, maintain overall alignment or reduce a deformity (as in scoliosis and kyphosis), provide mechanical stability to allow early return to function and provide security to the spine until fusion occurs. Instrumentation to the spine involves the use of plates, rods, screws, hooks and wires. Use of these implants requires an understanding of biomechanical principles of both the normal and the pathological spine. Additionally, familiarity with the nuances of each instrumentation system or each style of fixation will help to maximize success and minimize the potential for problems or complications.

Recognition of the difference between constrained and unconstrained devices and their application to particular spinal pathological conditions will allow one to select the appropriate device for use. *Constrained systems* are based upon a rigid lokking mechanism between the individual components, i.e., plate and screw or rod and screw. Maximum rigidity is achieved by segmental fixation of each vertebra to a constrained system. The classic example of a non-segmental, unconstrained implant is the Harrington rod, which spans several motion segments and attaches to the end vertebra with hooks, one of which is not constrained to the longitudinal member. This device was very successful when used under the appropriate conditions and represents an important milestone in implant development.

2.7 Cervical Spinal Instrumentation

Occipital-cervical or C1-C2 ligamentous injuries, in the absence of fracture, require fusion for long-term stability. While in-situ fusion with halo-application is a viable option, issues of head or chest trauma, compliance issues and the surgeon's preference may influence the decision toward internal fixation for stabilization. Occipital-cervical fixation is most commonly in the form of a posterior plate or rod system which attaches to the occiput and the posterior cervical elements via screws or wires. Flexion, extension and rotational forces are substantial and are best minimized by constrained implants with multiple-fixation points to the cranium and to each individual vertebra.

Ligamentous injuries isolated to the C1-C2 region involve weak flexion and extension forces with more significant rotational forces. Posterior wire orablefixation is most commonly employed. Posterior wire fixation corrects the instability of the C1-C2 segment; however, fusion in this condition will obviously eliminate rotational and flexion-extension motion between C1 and C2. Greater rigidity can be achieved through C2-C1 transarticular screw fixation. This demanding technique is appropriate in primary surgery in cases of pseudoarthrosis, following previously attempted posterior fusion procedures of C1-C2, and in cases of C1 ring fracture in association with ligamentous disruption or congenital absence of the continuity at the C1 ring in association with ligamentous insufficiency. These screws are inserted as positioning screws, not placed in a *lag-screw* technique to minimize iatrogenic posterior displacement of the atlas on the axis.

Displaced type II odontoid fractures may be treated with halo-application, fixation of C1-C2 by posterior wire technique or C2-C1 transarticular screw fixation technique or anterior odontoid lag-screw fixation. Halo-application in these conditions has a 30% incidence of non-union and requires extended immoblilization of the entire cervical spine during the period of time that the halo is worn. Anterior odontoid lag screw fixation directly addresses the fracture. Biomechanical and histological literature is sufficient to support single screw placement, although the double screw technique has become the standard following some clinical failures with single screw placement (Fig 2.6).

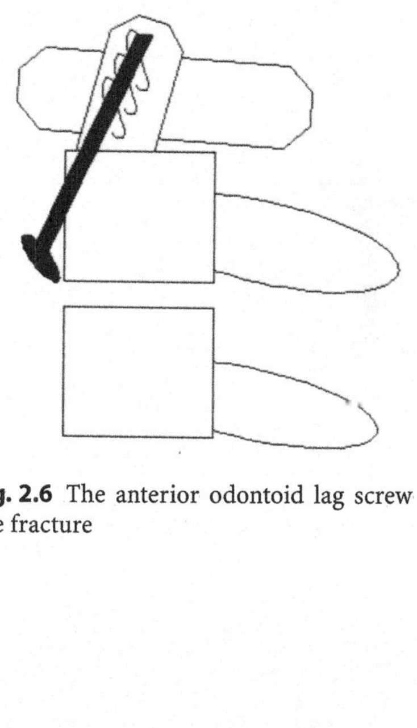

Fig. 2.6 The anterior odontoid lag screw directly addresses the fracture

Middle and lower cervical spine-fixation methods use all previously described principles: Posterior plates may be used as a tension-band system, as a buttress system or as a neutralization system. Wires can be used exclusively as tension-band systems; however they may create a retrolistthesis due to the lack of sagittal axis control with wires. Anterior plating may satisfy the needs for buttressing alone (constrained anterior cervical plate systems, CSLP) or may be used as a tension band system against an interpositional solid graft, thus putting the graft under compression. In this second scenario, the anterior plates cannot be used with locking screws, but must be used with regular cortical screws which are positioned eccentrically to apply a dynamic compression plating effect.

To emphasize the principles of biomechanics, wire fixation is primarily designed for use when tension-band principles are appropriate. Wire fixation provides poor torsional control, poorly resists anterior translation and sacrifices significant rigidity when compared with screw-rod or screw-plate constructs. External cervical immobilization is highly recommended under these circumstances until fusion occurs (Fig. 2.7).

The use of hooks in the cervical spine has significant disadvantages. These devices are inherently small and have the potential for dislodgement due to weakened bone and excessive torque forces. Additionally, dislodgement due to extension moments combined with torsion can occur when the hook is not rigidly fixed to the bone. Application to the lamina causes some degree of spinal encroachment and is not indicated in patients with any preexisting element of stenosis, whether congenital or degenerative in etiology. For these reasons, these devices are seldom indicated.

Constrained anterior cervical plate systems provide equal rigidity to posterior wire fixation techniques with regards to torsion, lateral bending and extension because of their multiple-fixation points and rigid design.. Because these systems are used in a buttress fashion, they do not resist flexion moments well. However, short constructs (including corpectomy for fracture, tumor or infection), with fusion and instrumentation across two motion segments, have been adequately stabilized by anterior plate fixation (Fig 2.8).

Posterior cervical fixation, utilizing screws with plates or rods, allows segmental fixation with increased rigidity in torsion, lateral bending, flexion and extension, when compared with posterior wire techniques. Fixation to either the pedicles or the lateral masses is possible.

2.8 Lumbar and Thoracolumbar Spinal Instrumentation

The thoracolumbar junction is essentially a straight segment of the spine. Restoration of this normal sagittal alignment provides the most physiological outcome. Preservation of canal patency and biomechanical support with early mobility, along with preservation of as many motion segments as possible are the basic principles to be followed.

Anterior decompression of the canal allows a direct approach to compressive fragments and affords the ability to lift the fragment off the dura without causing additional compression to the spinal cord. Following decompression, reconstruction of the anterior column with restoration of sagittal alignment needs to be performed with a cortico-cancellous bone graft or prosthetic device filled with bone. Stabilization with a constrained segmental-fixation device allows control of rotation, torsion, flexion, extension and lateral bending moments. Fixation can be limited to the vertebral body above and below

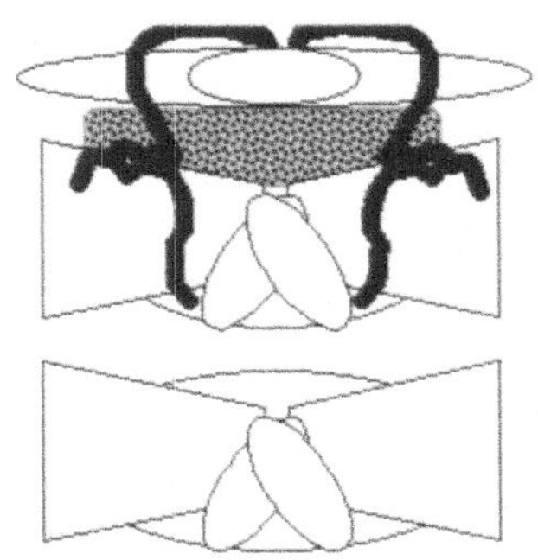

Fig. 2.7 A posterior wire construct does not provide rigid support and may require external immobilization

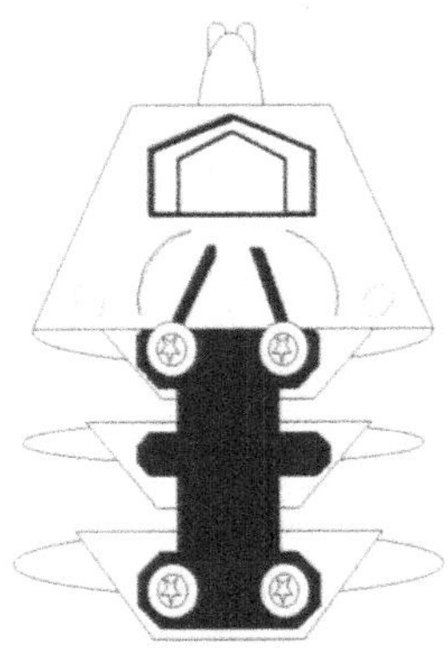

Fig. 2.8 This constrained system with locking screws allows unicortical purchase

that which is fractured. An unconstrained system such as a single rod anterior USS system can be applied initially. Following decompression and anterior column reconstruction, the system can be converted from an unconstrained into a constrained system during surgery, utilizing either a rigid-plate screw system (ATLP) or a double rod and screw system (USS Ventrofix). This allows compression of the graft, thus enhancing the bony incorporation and fusion.

Posterior spinal surgical approaches for the thoracolumbar area require the application of an implant system that is sufficiently strong to serve as a buttress system and that directs forces from the anterior column to the posterior instrumentation construct and back to the anterior columns as the anterior defect is *bridged*. This system needs a stable-angle construct between the pedicle screws and the vertical bars, as realized in the internal fixator module of the USS. The regular USS does not provide the same angular stability. It can still be used, however, providing that an anterior strut is placed under compression with a short posterior USS construct, applied as a tension-band system.

The use of nonsegmental unconstrained systems, such as Harrington rods with sublaminar wire fixation requires extension of fixation to several segments above and below the fracture. Torsional and rotational control is weakly resisted by this system. Shorter constructs with rotational and torsional control include use of the internal fixator with cross-linking devices. Because this is a bridge construct, tremendous forces are placed across the Schanz screws during the bending moment. The system will fail unless *anterior column* reconstitution with appropriate healing via fusion occurs to relieve the implant device of stress. While preservation of motion segments is provided by this technique, torsion and shear may occur due to the combined instability caused by the trauma and posterior decompression. It is, therefore, strongly recommended to crosslink the short-fixation system to resist these torsional and/or shear forces. If anterior column support is combined with posterior instrumentation, then the mechanical forces are quite different. The posterior device then acts solely as a tension-band system, being relieved of stress by the anterior surgery (Fig. 2.9).

2.9 Spinal Deformity

Surgery for correction of spinal deformity such as scoliosis and kyphosis is predicated upon restoration of mechanical alignment. Multisegmental fixation is currently the state of the art in these multisegmental pathologies Unconstrained systems that use sublaminar wires provide satisfactory results; however, they are associated with inherent risks noted during wire passage. Individually placed pedicle hooks with fixation – utilizing pedicle-hook screws – allow rigid segmental fixation of the spine when constrained to a longitudinal bar.

While individual surgical preferences vary with respect to the steps of deformity correction, it is universally accepted that in order to minimize neurological problems, distraction across a deformity should not occur. Translational forces effectively bring the deformity to match the correctly contoured longitudinal bar. It is not uncommon to see some lengthening of the spinal column during this

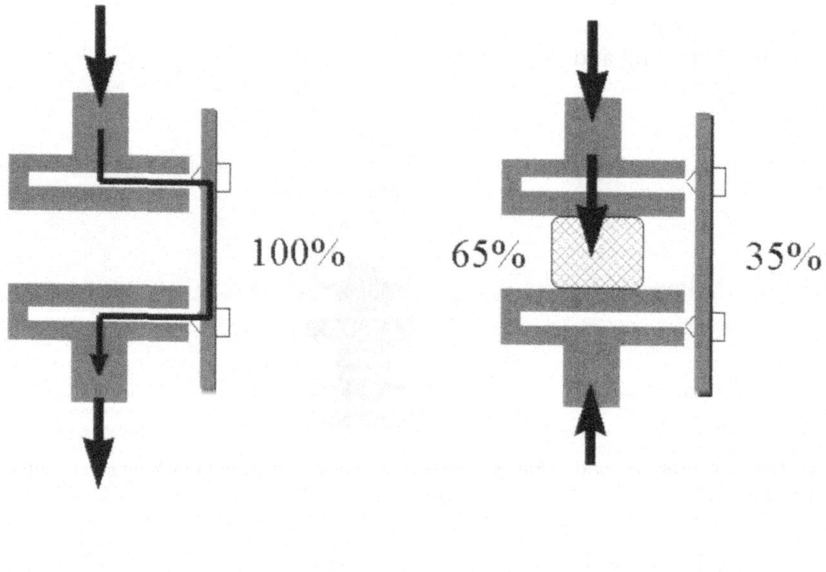

Fig. 2.9 Without anterior column integrity, the posterior bridge construct bears 100 % of the load (left). With anterior column support, in the form of a weight-bearing graft, the posterior implant bears only a fraction of the load (right)

maneuver. Therefore, the longitudinal bar must be fixed at only one point, either cephelad or caudad, such that the spine remains mobile during the translational maneuver. Once translation occurs, additional compression may be applied to further enhance bony union.

Sublaminar wire instrumentation is contraindicated in conditions of spinal stenosis because of increased canal compromise, and in correction of kyphotic deformities because of laminar fracture and cutout or dislodgement of the wires.

2.10 Lumbar Reconstruction

Instrumentation in lumbar degenerative disease, for purposes of stabilization in the absence of deformity, can be performed via a translaminar facet-screw technique. This construct provides resistance against flexion; however, it only weakly resists lateral bending and torsion and does not resist extension. In the face of degenerative disc disease, for one- and two-level constructs, this technique is sufficient to allow enhancement of fusion. A lag-screw technique is not appropriate in this condition because the lamina will be preferentially torqued toward the side of insertion of the first screw.

Segmental fixation utilizing screw and rod or screw and plate instrumentation systems provide increased rigidity due to their multisegmental design and fixation of both the anterior and posterior columns.

Degenerative lumbar scoliosis is best treated by segmental fixation, again because of the strong lateral bending forces and the need for anterior column control. Correction can be from an anterior or posterior direction and on occasion may also be performed from both approaches.

2.11 Spondylolysis

Posterior-element incompetency defects most commonly occur in the region of the *pars interarticularis*. This is not always the case, however. Etiologies such as trauma, iatrogenic causes and pathological causes with tumor invasion account for acquired posterior element defects and may localize to other areas of the posterior elements. In the younger population, without concomitant spondylolisthesis, this developmental condition may or may not require intervention. In the symptomatic patient, without response to conservative treatment, direct repair of the spondylolytic defect is appropriate. In contrast to the adult patient, the spine has not yet acquired secondary changes of posterior-element hypertrophy, *ligamentum flavum* redundancy or disc bulging with spondylophytic production and resultant foraminal narrowing. Whereas direct repair of the *pars* defect can occur with lag-screw or compression-screw systems, this construct generally places the screw in the exact location where bony fusion is desired. Many surgeons prefer a tension-band compression system, such as a simple figure-of-eight wire loop passing from the transverse process, behind the spinous process, to the contralateral transverse process. Alternatively, a pedicle-screw construct with a short linking rod attached to lamina hooks, immobilizing the ipsilateral lamina in a compression mode, can be performed.

Whereas direct repair is biomechanically appropriate in the young patient with simple spondylolysis, without concomitant spondylolisthesis, factors are much different when considering the patient with a forward luxation. The degree of slippage and the patient's skeletal immaturity determine, to a large extent, the potential for progression of deformity. As the weight-bearing axis is shifted anteriorly, the sacrum and pelvis attempt to accomodate by tilting into a vertical posture with secondary bony changes occurring as a result. These changes are less extreme in the adult population and may not be present in many patients with skeletal maturity. Whereas from a biomechanical point of view, normalization of anatomy is the intended goal, the surgeon must remain cognisant of the potential for nerve injury due to excessive traction from overzealous retraction or nerve compression due to incomplete posterior element decompression.

2.12 Implant Failure – Biomechanics

Recognizing that the spine cycles roughly three million to five million cycles per year allows one to understand the failure of implants. Constrained systems fail due to fatigue fracture and unconstrained systems fail as a result of loosening. Utilizing an anterior constrained implant device, one level above and below an unstable motion segment, is equivalent in stiffness to a posterior pedicle-screw instrumentation system which spans two levels above and below the motion segment. Issues of low profile, ease of access and insertion, risk factors associated with surgical exposure and the surgeon's preference must also be considered.

References

Allgower M (1991) In: (Manual of internal fixation, 3rd edn, Springer, New York
Bailey RW (1983) The cervical spine. In: (The cevical spine Research Society. Lippincott, St. Louis
Bridwell KH, Dewald RL (1997) In: (The textbook of spinal surgery, vol I, II, 2nd edition, Lippincott, New York
Bullough MB, Boachie-Adjei O (1988) In: (Atlas of spinal diseases. Lippincott, Philadelphia
Simon SR (1994) In: Orthopaedic Basic Science, AAOS
White AH (1995) In: Spine care vol.II, Mosby, St. Louis

CHAPTER 3

Biology of Spinal Fusions

M. Goytan and M. Aebi

3.1 Introduction

Surgical fusion of the spine dates back to 1911, when the procedure was described by Albee [1], who provided mechanical support to vertebrae involved with tuberculosis, and by Hibbs [2], who treated the progression of scoliosis by spinal fusion. Since this time several techniques of fusion have been described and advocated with and without the use of instrumentation. Frequently the success of spinal surgery is dependent upon a solid fusion between selected intervertebral segments. The bony union which takes place is dependent upon several factors related to the host locally and systemically. Many of these factors have been elucidated, providing further information to enhance the rate of spinal fusion. However, there are certainly many facets of arthrodesis which are incompletely understood or not identified, for which further research is required. The rate of nonunion in the spine ranges from 5% to 35% [3, 4]; the improvement of these figures will be by the determination of the biology involved in achieving a successful fusion.

The goal of this chapter is to review local and systemic factors affecting fusion, the biology of bone graft materials, and the effects of instrumentation on fusion.

Table 3.1 Local factors affecting fusion rates

Positive variables	Negative variables
Large surface area	Scarred tissues
Healthy blood supply	Previous radiation
Pluripotential stem cells	Osteoporosis
Inflammatory cells	Marrow infiltrative diseases
Electrical stimulation?	Infection
Local growth factors	Foreign material
Insulin-like growth factor	i.e., bone wax
Platelet-derived growth factor	Tumor
Fibroblast growth factor	
Transforming growth factor	
beta-Bone morphogenic protein	

3.2 Local Host Factors

3.2.1 Host Soft Tissue Bed

The incorporation of bone graft and the development of a fusion mass is dependent upon the qualities of the soft tissue bed. The local soft tissues must be able to support the influx of inflammatory and osteoprogenitor cells as well as osteoblasts when autograft is used. This vascular supply in turn is critical for: this cell recruitment, the nutrition of these cells, the endocrine pathway which promotes fusion, and the inhibition of infection. This has been previously demonstrated in canines by Hurley [5], where the overlying soft tissues were shown to provide a source of nutrition and growth factors to the graft site.

Hence, the effect of traumatized soft tissues is to lessen the physiologic supportive function to the fusion mass. This negative effect can also be seen in irradiated tissues [6], where the vascular supply of the host bed is altered by an intense vasculitis and inhibition of angiogenesis, and later these effects are manifested as osteonecrosis.

3.2.2 Host Graft Recipient Site

The physiologic integrity of a recipient site and healthy soft tissues are paramount to the success of a fusion. The graft recipient site will be detrimentally affected by infiltrative processes such as Paget's disease, local or metastatic tumor, as well as osteoporosis. These entities as well as previously irradiated bone are biologically inferior [7] to normal bone and may be structurally weaker.

The preparation of the host surface can affect the success of fusion as generally the larger the surface area decorticated, the larger the area available to osteoprogenitor cells and the greater a contact area to support a bony bridge and carry a mechanical load. Care must be taken when decorticating with high-speed burrs, that thermal necrosis is not induced. This can be lessened by the use of copious irrigation and gentle pressure on the underlying bone.

3.2.3 Growth Factors

The tropism, differentiation, and the biologic activity of potential bone-forming mesenchymal cells is known to be positively influenced by several local growth factors. These growth factors are a group of proteins that participate in the modulation of cell growth and division.

Transforming growth factor type beta (TGF-β) is one of a number of transforming growth factors and is one of the most important growth factors in the musculoskeletal system because its effect is to direct mesenchymal cells to divide [8]. One of the most widely investigated of these TGF-βs is bone morphogenic protein (BMP). This is a low molecular weight hydrophobic glycoprotein which has been shown to induce bone formation ectopically. BMP acts in an osteoinductive capacity by initiating tissue transformation by causing a phenotypic change of local mesenchymal tissue into osteoblasts [9, 10].

3.2.4 Electrical Stimulation

Several animal and clinical studies have concluded there is a beneficial use of direct current stimulation and pulsed electromagnetic fields (PEMFs) on spine fusions. Kahanovitch has found that the use of PEMFs can enhance a fusion mass early in the healing process [11] and with the use of direct current stimulation can provide a more advanced histologic and radiographic fusion at 12 weeks in dogs [12].

In 1974, the first clinical use of direct current stimulation in spine fusions was reported by Dwyer and Wickham [13] and they concluded that an earlier, less mature fusion was promoted. Kane [14] revealed a study in 1984 where a randomized prospective study of 59 patients who were at risk for nonunion demonstrated a 54 % radiographic fusion rate in the control group and an 81 % fusion rate in the stimulated patients.

The use of PEMFs clinically has not gained the popularity as seen with direct current methods. Simmons [15] reported on the use of PEMFs to treat failed posterior lumbar interbody fusions, where an increase in bone formation was seen in 85 % of the patients and a solid fusion was obtained over a 4-month treatment period in 10 of 13 patients. Mooney [16] in 1990 revealed in a randomized double-blind prospective study a 92 % fusion rate in a group of 98 patients who were treated with a PEMF stimulator versus a 65 % fusion rate in a placebo group of 97 patients.

Although there are animal and clinical studies advocating the use of electrical stimulation to enhance spine fusions, the conclusions are not definitive. Past studies are limited by mixed diagnoses, different fusion types and a poor evaluation of those cases which improved clinically. Therefore, further clinical investigations are required before electrical stimulation can be advocated as a valid method for spine fusions.

3.3 Systemic Host Factors

3.3.1 Hormones

Hormones are chemical messengers that have a direct and indirect effect upon bone healing in a positive or negative fashion. Considerable insights into their effects have been gained in the last 10 years.

Growth hormone stimulates bone healing through somatomedins [17], which increase the intestinal absorption of calcium and raise the rate of bone formation and mineralization [18]. Thyroid hormone acts synergistically with growth hormone; thyroid hormone is required for the hepatic synthesis of somatomedins [19]. Somatomedins have a stimulatory effect on bone healing as they have a directly positive effect on cartilage growth and maturation [20, 21].

Table 3.2 Systemic factors affecting fusion rates

Positive variables	Negative variables
Insulin	Smoking
Insulin-like growth factor	Corticosteroids
Testosterone	Castration
Estrogen	Nonsteroidal antiinflammatory drugs
Growth hormone	Vitamin A intoxication
Thyroxine	Vitamin D intoxication
Vitamin A	Vitamin D deficiency
Vitamin D	Cancer chemotherapy
Calcitonin	Sepsis
Anabolic steroids	Immune deficiency disorders
Parathyroid homone	

It is accepted that estrogens and androgens are important in the prevention of bone mass loss in the aging population and for skeletal maturation in growing individuals. The effect of sex hormones on bone healing is controversial; they are found to enhance bone formation in some studies [22] but, this effect is refuted in most of the literature [23, 24].

Corticosteroids (endogenous and exogenous) have been shown to have deleterious effects on fusion rates and bone healing as they decrease bone formation and increase bone resorption [25]. The inhibition and promotion of the differentiation of osteoblasts from mesenchymal cells [26, 27] and the inhibition of the rates of synthesis of the components of bone matrix required for osseous healing [28] have been demonstrated in cell culture experiments.

3.3.2 Host Nutrition and Homeostasis

In orthopedic patients the general health and nutritional status has been shown to affect bone and wound healing [29, 30]. There are several known variables to assess the nutrition and health of orthopedic patients; these include serum albumin and transferrin levels, total lymphocyte count, nitrogen balance studies, skin antigen testing and anthropometric studies (height, weight, and lean muscle mass). The aforementioned studies are useful in the assessment of the need for nutritional support in surgical patients to optimize fusion rates.

The availability and number of osteoprogenitor cells in the bone marrow can be compromised by a number of hematologic disorders such as sickle cell disease, thalassemias, and myelofibrosis. These conditions can decrease the osteogenic potential of the bone marrow by the selective overgrowth of hematopoietic cells at the expense of osteoprogenitor elements [31]. Anemia and cardiovascular and cardiopulmonary disease all diminish the oxygen-carrying capacity in the blood and subsequently the tissue perfusion of oxygen and nutrients. This will in turn diminish the rates of fusion and increase the time to and quality of fusion [32].

Smoking and excessive alcohol use cause skeletal bone loss by the inhibition of bone metabolism and formation. Tobacco extracts have been experimentally shown to induce calcitonin resistance [33], interfere with osteablastic function [34], and increase bone resorption at fracture ends [35]. Several studies have shown that the nonunion rate is significantly higher in smokers who have undergone a spinal fusion [36, 37].

3.4 Bone Graft Materials

3.4.1 Properties of Graft Material

The outcome of a spine fusion is not only dependent upon host and local factors but also on the type of bone graft material which is selected. The manner in which bone graft behaves when placed into a recipient bed is largely dependent on the properties inherent in the graft material. These properties may permit the direct production of bone (osteogenesis), the lattice work, which is conductive to bone formation (osteoconduction), and the propensity to provoke and stimulate osteoprogenitor cells to differentiate into osteogenic cells (osteoinduction).

Osteogenesis is a characteristic only found in fresh autogenous bone and bone marrow cells. These graft materials contain viable cells capable of forming bone or the ability of these cells to differentiate into bone-forming cells.

Osteoconduction is present in autogenous and allograft bone, bone matrix, and calcium phosphate ceramic spheres. This physical property of graft material allows for the ingress of neovasculature and osteoprogenitor cells.

Osteoinduction is the capability of a substance to influence an undetermined osteoprogenitor cell to differentiate into an osteogenic cell type. Osteoinductive properties thus far have been demonstrated by auto- and allograft, demineralized bone matrix, and BMP. There is some potential for the manufacture of BMP via recombinant DNA techniques to allow widespread clinical use of this protein.

The ideal bone graft material possesses all of the above characteristics and in some clinical applications a fourth property is provided, a mechanical load-bearing structural support. This property is observed with cortical strut grafts used for an interbody fusion in both auto- and allograft types. The autograft will maintain this function until and after biologic incorporation has taken place. The allo-

Table 3.3 Properties of graft materials

Graft type	Osteo-inductive	Osteo-conductive	Osteogenic
Autograft	Yes	Yes	Yes
Allograft	Yes	Yes	No
Xenograft	No	No	No
Synthetic bone	No	Yes	No

Table 3.4 Factors affecting fusion rates

A) Local	B) Systemic
1. Host soft tissue bed	1. Hormones
2. Growth factors	2. Smoking
3. Electrical stimulation?	3. Nutrition
	4. General health: anemia, cardiopulmonary disease, hemoglobinopathies
C) Graft material	D) Instrumentation
1. Autograft, GOLD standard	1. Anterior, posterior or combined
2. Allograft	2. Compression/ distraction, unisegmental fixation
3. Synthetic bone	

graft will lose its mechanical strength as it is incorporated as the bone resorption takes place with an ensuing loss of load-bearing capacity of the graft.

3.5 Types of Graft Materials

3.5.1 Autograft

The gold standard of bone graft materials is autograft. This type of graft is the most successful biologic material available for achieving a spine fusion. All of the desirable transplant properties are inherent in autograft: osteogenesis, osteoinduction, osteoconduction, and structural support. Autogenous cortical bone is the graft which provides optimal structural support; however, in comparison to cancellous bone there are fewer osteogenic cells and osteoinductive substances. Cortical bone is more resistant to ingrowth of vasculature with subsequent remodeling; hence cortical autografts remain a blend of necrotic and viable bone.

The major downfall in the use of autograft is graft harvest complications, which can occur in up to 25% of patients [38]. Problems associated with autograft procurement are: chronic donor site pain, increased surgical time, increased blood loss, and insufficient quantity of bone for long fusions.

3.5.2 Allograft

Allograft has been popularized in many countries as a direct result of improved methods of harvesting, preparation, and storage of this graft material. This combined with the morbidity of donor site complications has made allograft an attractive alternative to autograft. There is a wide range of applications for allograft in orthopedic surgery; however, the ability to obtain a successful fusion [39] and the possibility of infection [40] places a dubious light on the usefulness of this graft substance in spine surgery. The cost of donor screening, graft processing, and preservation coupled with the risk of HIV transmission and the decreased osteoconductive and inductive capabilities make autograft a superior graft substance despite donor site morbidity.

3.5.3 Xenograft

Bone obtained from a different species is known as xenograft or heterograft. Previously in orthopedic surgery, xenografts had been used extensively and have included ivory, and bovine bone and horn. Xenografts provoke an immune response in spite of adequate processing, this resulting in a graft which becomes encapsulated and walled off from the graft bed. This resistance to incorporation into host bone prevents xenograft from being used successfully for spinal fusions alone [41].

3.5.4 Synthetic Bone Graft Substitutes

The problems of donor site morbidity, limited autograft quantity, the cost of allograft processing and preservation, and the risk of disease transmission, have pushed investigators to develop synthetic bone graft substitutes. There are two graft types which are commercially available and are experiencing a progressive increase in clinical use; these bone graft substitutes are ceramic spheres and coral. These synthetic substances are useful in vivo because of the following properties: biocompatability with surrounding tissues, chemical stability in body fluids, the ability to be shaped into various functional forms, the ability to be sterilized, and a cost effective, quality reassured method of manufacturing.

Synthetic bone has only osteoconductive properties when used alone, and has osteoinductive potential when combined with autograft. There is no structural integrity imparted to this graft material; hence internal fixation must be supplemented if a rigid mechanical environment is required.

Calcium phosphate ceramics have been widely used in orthopedic surgery in the form of hydroxyapatite and tricalcium phosphate (TCP). These materials are brittle with a low fracture resistance and variability in their chemical and crystalline composition. The method of preparation accounts for the differences in crystalline structure, influencing whether or not the material will be porous or dense. The greater density and crystal formation impart a greater mechanical strength with resistance to dissolution and a longer-lasting stability. The contrast is a larger porosity structure with an increased surface area for bony ingrowth and biodegradation of the implant. TCP is generally resorbed 6 weeks after implantation [42], whereas hydroxyapatite is very slowly resorbed [43].

The three-dimensional structure of coral is identical to that of bone. It is this property that is important in the biology of bony ingrowth and allows for the interconnections between lacunae in bone [44]. The large amount of protein and a calcium carbonate crystalline structure limit the usefulness of coral. This is overcome by two processes: depyrogenation, the removal of all proteins from the coral during processing rendering the coral nonimmunogenic, and the conversion of calcium carbonate into hydroxyapatite using a replentiform process while still maintaining the three-dimensional crystalline form. The pore size of the coral is dependent on the species used, currently 200- and 500-µm pore sizes are available. The Pro Osteon 200 implant (200-µm pore size) is biologically similar to cancellous bone and mechanically has a compressive strength similar to that of cortical bone [45]. The Pro Osteon 500 (500-µm pore size) is biologically and mechanically similar to cancellous bone. Clinical use of this bone graft substitute has been promising in the cervical and thoracolumbar spine combined with internal fixation. Future development of this bone substitute will be a combination of osteoinductive proteins and the use of coral as a carrier, and will in turn provide a structural lattice for immediate stability [46].

3.5.5 Effect of Instrumentation on the Biology of Spine Fusions

The stability of the motion segments of the spine to be fused is known to directly affect the rate and quality of fusion [47]. It is widely published in the literature that higher fusion rates occur when instrumentation is used in the spine [48] and a nonunion will likely occur when there is radiographic evidence of hardware loosening [49].

Animal experiments in the past have shed some light on the relationship between instrumentation and fusion. Nagel demonstrated in the sheep model that motion was a major determinant in the outcome of fusion. He determined that in six of seven sheep, nonunions developed at the L6–S1 interspace and all levels were fused cephalad to this. Subsequent in vivo flexion and extension radiographs in nonfused sheep and ex vivo displacement transducers revealed that the lumbosacral junction has a markedly increased magnitude of motion. This provided the evidence that fusion was more difficult to obtain at the lumbosacral junction in sheep [50].

McAfee has shown in canine models that the volumetric density of bone (as assessed by histomorphometry) was lower for fused versus unfused spines and that the rigidity of the instrumentation led to device-related osteoporosis. However, it was noted that the use of instrumentation significantly improved the probability of achieving fusion and this far outweighed the risks of device-related osteoporosis. The term "device-related osteoporosis" is a misnomer and is more accurately replaced by "device-related osteopenia." Stress shielding implies a weakening of the bone, cartilage, and ligamentous complex, as demonstrated by the use of rigid internal fixation in long bones. Biomechanical testing of spine fusions implementing Harrington, Luque, or Cotrel-Dubousset instrumentation showed they were more rigid than spines treated solely with posterolateral bone grafting [51].

3.6 Conclusion

According to animal and clinical studies the gold standard for spinal fusions is the use of autograft combined with instrumentation. Several studies had to be undertaken in order to draw this conclusion, and unfortunately several more studies will be required to determine all the biologic variables and histological sequences that compose a successful fusion. From this future work, surgeons will be able to obtain a rapid, reliable and biomechanically sound fusion in a more predictable fashion.

References

1. Albee FH (1911) Transplantation of a portion of the tibia into the spine for Pott's disease. JAMA 57: 885–886
2. Hibbs RA (1911) An operation for progressive spinal deformities. A preliminary report of three cases from the service of the Orthopedic Hospital. NY State J Med 93: 1013–1016
3. DePalma AF, Rothman RH (1968) The nature of pseudoarthrosis. Clin Orthop 59: 113–118
4. Steinmann JC, Herkowitz HN (1992) Pseudoarthrosis of the spine. Clin Orthop 284: 80–90
5. Hurley LA, Stinchfield FE, Bassett AL, Lyon WH (1959) The role of soft tissues in osteogenesis: an experimental study of canine spine fusions. J Bone Joint Surg 41A: 1243–1254
6. Craven PL, Urist MR (1971) Osteogenesis by radioisotope labelled cell populations in implants of bone matrix under the influence of ionizing radiation. Clin Orthop 76: 231–243
7. Bouchard JA, Koka A, Bensusan JS, et al. (1994) Effect of radiation on posterior spinal fusions: a rabbit model. Spine 19: 1836–1841
8. Joyce ME, Terik RM, Jingushi S, et al. (1990) Role of transforming growth factor-beta in fracture repair. Ann NY Acad Sci 593: 107–123
9. Mohan S, Baylink DJ (1991) Bone growth factors. Clin Orthop 263: 30–48
10. Canalis E (1985) Effect of growth factors on bone cell replication and differentiation. Clin Orthop 193: 246–263
11. Kahanovitz N, Arnoczky SP, Hulse D, Shires A (1994) The effect of electromagnetic pulsing on posterior lumbar spinal fusion in dogs. Spine 19: 705–709
12. Kahanovitz N, Arnoozky SP (1990) The efficacy of direct current electrical stimulation to enhance canine spinal fusions. Clin Orthop 251: 295–299
13. Dwyer AF, Wickham GG (1974) Direct current stimulation in spinal fusions. Med J Aust 1: 73–75
14. Kane WJ (1988) Direct current electrical bone growth stimulation for spinal fusion. Spine 13: 363–365
15. Simmons JW (1985) Treatment of failed posterior lumber interbody fusion (PLIF) of the spine with pulsing electromagnetic fields. Clin Othop 193: 127–132
16. Mooney V (1990) A randomized double blind prospective study of the efficacy of pulsed electromagnetic fields for interbody lumbar fusion. Spine 15: 708–712
17. Phillips LS, Vassilopoulou-Sellin R (1980) Somatomedins – part I and part II. N Engl J Med 302: 371–380, 438–446
18. Misol S, Samaan N, Ponśeti IV (1971) Growth hormone in delayed fracture union. Clin Orthop 74: 206–208
19. Schalch OS, Heinrich UE, Draznin B, et al. (1979) Role of the liver in regulating somatomedin activity: hormonal effects on the synthesis and release of insulin-like growth factor and its carrier protein by the isolated perfused rat liver. Endocrinology 104: 1143–1151
20. Udupa KN, Gupta LP (1965) The effects of growth hormone and thyroxine in the healing of fractures. Ind J Med Res 53: 623–628
21. Burch WM, Lebovitz HE (1982) Triidothyroxine stimulation of in vivo growth and maturation of embryonic chick cartilage. Endocrinology 111: 462–468
22. Baran DT, Bergfeld MA, Teitelbaum SL, Avioli LV (1978) Effect of testosterone therapy on bone formation in an osteoporotic hypogonadal male. Calcif Tissue Int 26: 103–106
23. Lafferty FW, Spencer GE, Pearson OH (1964) Effects of androgens, estrogens, and high calcium intakes on bone formation and resorption in osteoporosis. Am J Ned 36: 514–528
24. Riggs BL, Jowsey J, Goldsmith RS, et al. (1972) Short and long term effects of estrogen and synthetic anabolic hormone in postmenopausal osteoporosis. J Clin Invest 51: 1659–1663
25. Hahn TJ (1978) Corticosteroid-induced osteopenia. Arch Intern Med 138: 882–885
26. Aronow MA, Gerstenfeld LC, Owen TA, et al. (1990) Factors that promote progressive development of the osteoblast phenotype in cultured rat calvarial cells. J Cell Physiol 143: 213–221
27. Simmons DJ, Kunin AS (1967) Autoradiographic and biochemical investigations on the effect of cortisone on the bones of the rat. Clin Orthop 55: 201–215
28. Cruess RL, Sakai T (1972) Effect of cortisone upon synthesis rates of some components of rat bone matrix. Clin Orthop 86: 253–259
29. Einhorn TA, Bonnarens F, Burstein AH (1986) The contribution of dietary protein and mineral to the healing of experimental fractures: a biomechanical study. J Bone Joint Surg 68A: 1389–139S
30. Jensen JE, Jensen TG, Smith TX et al. (1982) Nutrition in orthopedic surgery. J Bone Joint Surg 64: 1263–1272
31. Wyngaarden JB, Smith LH, Bennett JC (eds) (1992) Cecil textbook of medicine, 19th edn., part XII Hematologic diseases. WB Saunders, Philadelphia, pp 817–1017
32. Rothman RH, Klemik JS, Toton JJ (1971) The effect of iron deficiency anemia on fracture healing. Clin Orthop 77: 276–283
33. Hollo I, Gergely I, Boross M (1977) Smoking results in calcitonin resistance. JAMA 237: 2470
34. de Vernejoul MC, Bielakoff J, Herve M, et al. (1983) Evidence for defective osteoblastic function: a role for alcohol and tobacco consumption in osteoporosis in middle aged men. Clin Orthop 179: 107–115
35. Lau GC, Luck JV, Marshall GJ, Griffith G (1989) The effect of cigarette smoking on fracture healing: an animal model. Clin Res 37: 132A
36. Brown CW, Orme TJ, Richardson HD (1986) The rate of pseudoarthrosis (surgical nonunion) in patients who are smokers and patients who are non smokers: a comparison study. Spine 11: 942–943
37. Zdeblick TA (1993) A prospective randomized study of lumbar fusion: preliminary results. Spine 18: 983–991
38. Younger EM, Chapman MW (1989) Morbidity at bone graft donor sites. J Orthop Trauma 3: 192–195
39. McCarthy RE, Peek RD, Morrissy RT, Hough AJ (1986) Allograft bone in spinal fusion for paralytic scoliosis. JBJS 68A: 370–375
40. Buck BE, Malinin TI, Brown MD (1989) Bone transplantation and human immunodeficiency virus. Clin Orthop 240: 129–136
41. Salama R (1983) Xenogeneic bone grafting in humans. Clin Orthop 174: 113–121
42. Jarcho M (1981) Calcium phosphate ceramics as hard tissue prosthetics. Clin Orthop 157: 259–278
43. Hoogendoorn HA, Renooij W, Akkermans LMA, et al. (1984) Long term study of large ceramic implants (porous hydroxyspatite) in dog femora. Clin Orthop 187: 281–288
44. Ripamonti U (1991) The morphogenesis of bone in replicas of hydroxyspatite obtained from conversion of calcium carbonate exoskeletons of coral. JBJS 73A: 692–703

45. White E, Shors EC (1986) Biomaterial material aspects of Interpore-200 porous hydroxyspatite. Dental Clinic North Amer 30: 49–67
46. Thalgott J, Aebi M (eds) (1996) Manual of internal fixation of the spine, Chap. 22. Lippincott-Raven, New York, pp 285–295
47. Gurr KR, McAfee PC, Warden KE, Shih C (1989) Roentographic and biomechanical analysis of lumbar fusions: a canine model. J Orthop Res 7: 838–848
48. Bridwell KH, Sedgewick TA, O'Brien MF, et al. (1993) The role of fusion and instrumentation in the treatment of degenerative spondylolisthesis with spinal stenosis. J Spinal Disorders 6: 461–472
49. Aurori BF, Weierman RJ, Lowell HA, et al. (1985) Pseudoarthrosis after spinal fusion for scoliosis: a comparison of autogeneic and allogeneic bone grafts. Clin Orthop 199: 153–158
50. Nagel DA, Kramers PC, Rahn BA, et al. (1991) A paradigm of delayed union and nonunion in the lumbosacral joint: a study of motion and bone grafting of the lumbosacral spine in sheep. Spine 16: 553–559
51. McAfee PC, Farey ID, Sutterlin CE, et al. (1989) Device related osteoporosis with spinal instrumentation. Spine 14: 919–926

CHAPTER 4

A Comprehensive Classification of Thoracic and Lumbar Injuries

F. Magerl and M. Aebi

4.1 Introduction

A classification should allow the identification of any injury by means of a simple algorithm based on easily recognizable and consistent radiographic and clinical characteristics. In addition, it should provide a concise and descriptive terminology, information regarding the severity of the injury, and guidance as to the choice of treatment and should serve as a useful tool for future studies.

Although fractures of the spine have been classified for over 50 years [3], it was not until 1949 that Nicoll [33] identified two basic groups of injury: stable and unstable fractures. Holdsworth [21, 22] recognized the importance of the mechanism of injury and thus classified the various patterns of injuries into five categories. He also pointed out the significance of the posterior ligament complex for the stability of the spine. Whitesides [46] reorganized the mechanistic classification and in principle defined the two-column concept by comparing the spine to a construction crane: the pressure-resistant vertebral bodies and disks (anterior column) correspond to the boom, while the posterior vertebral elements and ligaments (posterior column) with their tensile strength are similar to the guy ropes. In classifying spinal injuries, Lob [27] took prognostic aspects into consideration in terms of later deformity and nonunions, based on extensive studies on cadaver spines. The advent of the lap belt in the early 1960s resulted in greater awareness of another category of injuries, the flexion-distraction lesions [5, 10, 11, 16–18, 20, 23, 35, 43]. Some of these injuries were described even earlier by Böhler [3].

Louis [28] established a morphological classification system using a concept of three columns consisting of the vertebral bodies and the two rows of the articular masses. In addition, he differentiated between transient osseous instability and chronic instability following discoligamentous injuries.

Concern regarding the relationship of the vertebral injury to the contents of the spinal canal was expressed by Roy-Camille [36, 37], who described the "segment moyen," referring to the neural ring. He related injury of the segment moyen to instability. Denis [9–11] considered the posterior part of the anterior column to be the key structure as regards instability, at least in flexion. He consequently divided the original anterior column into two by introducing a middle column, stating that "the third column is represented by the structures that have to be torn in addition to the posterior ligament complex in order to create acute instability." McAfee and coworkers [31] combined the individual merits of Denis' classification and that proposed by White and Panjabi [45]. Using computed tomography (CT) interpretation, they formulated a simplified classification according to the type of failure of the middle column. Ferguson and Allen [15] based their classification primarily on the mechanism of injury.

Each of these classifications has added to the knowledge and understanding of spinal injuries. However, none can be considered all-encompassing in the light of recent developments and the aforementioned criteria. As a consequence, a more comprehensive classification has been developed from the analysis of 1445 cases and is presented here.

4.2 Concept of the Classification

This classification is primarily based upon the pathomorphological characteristics of the injuries. Categories are formed according to pathomorphological uniformity. The three main categories, *the types*, have a typical fundamental injury pattern which is defined by a few easily recognizable radiological criteria. Since this pattern clearly reflects the effect of forces or moments, three simple mechanisms can be identified as common denominators of the types: (1) compressive force, which causes compression and burst injuries; (2) tensile force, which causes injuries with transverse disruption; and (3) axial torque, which causes rotational injuries.

Morphological criteria are used to classify each main type further into distinct *groups*. By using more detailed morphological findings, identification of *subgroups* and even further specification is possible, providing an accurate description of almost any injury.

In order to provide a simple grid for the classification, the one used for the AO fracture classification [32] has been adopted here. This grid consists of three types with three groups, each of which contains three subgroups and further specifications (Tables 4.1–4.3). Within this classification the injuries are hierarchically ranked according to progressive severity. Thus, severity progresses from type A to type C, and similarly within each type, group, and further subdivision. Ranking of the injuries was primarily determined by the degree of instability. Prognostic aspects were taken into consideration as far as possible.

Remarks. The term 'column' used in the following text refers to the two-column concept as described by Whitesides [46]. Isolated transverse or spinous process fractures are not considered in this classification.

Table 4.1 Type A injuries: groups, subgroups, and specifications

Type A. Vertebral body compression
A1 Impaction fractures
A1.1 End plate impaction
A1.2 Wedge impaction features
1 Supirior wedge impaction fracture
2 Lateral wedge impaction fracture
3 Inferior wedge impaction fracture
A1.3 Vertebral body collapse
A2 Split fractures
A2.1 Sagittal split fracture
A2.2 Coronal split fracture
A2.3 Pincer fracture
A3 Burst fractures
A3.1 Incomplete burst fracture
1 Superior incomplete burst fracture
2 Lateral incomplete burst fracture
3 Inferior incomplete burst fracture
A3.2 Burst-split fracture
1 Superior burst-split fracture
2 Lateral burst-split fracture
3 Inferior burst-split fracture
A3.3 Complete split fracture
1 Pincer burst fracture
2 Complete flexion burst fracture
3 Complete axial burst fracture

Table 4.2 Type B injuries: groups, subgroups, and specifications

Type B. Anterior and posterior element injury with distraction
B1 Posterior disruption predominantly ligamentous (flexion-distraction injury)
B1.1 With transvers disruption of the disk
1 Flexion-subluxation
2 Antirior dislocation
3 Flexion-subluxation/anterior dislocation with fracture of the articular processes
B1.2 With type A fracture of the vertebral body
1 Flexion-subluxation + type A fracture
2 Antirior dislocation + type A fracture
3 Flexion-subluxation/anterior dislocation with fracture of the articular processes + type A fracture
B2 Posterior disruption predominantly ossenous (flexion-distraction injury)
B2.1 Transverse bicolumn fracture
B2.2 With disruption of the disk
1 Disruption through the pedicle and disk
2 Disruption through the pars interarticularis and disk (flexion-spondylolysis)
B2.3 With type A fracture of the vertebral body
1 Fracture through the pedicle + type A body
2 Fraction through the pars interarticularis (flexion-spondylolysis) + type A fracture
B3 Anterior disruption through the disk (hypertension-shear injury)
B3.1 Hyperextension-subluxations
1 Without injury of the posterior coumn
2 With injury of the posterior coumn
B3.2 Hyperextension-spondylolysis
B3.3 Posterior dislocation

Table 4.3 Type C injuries: groups, subgroups, and specifications

Type C. Anterior and posterior element injury with rotation
C1 Type A injuries with rotation (compression injuries with rotation)
C1.1 Rotational wedge fracture
C1.2 Rotational split fractures
1 Rotational sagittal split fracture
2 Rotational coronal split fracture
3 Rotational pincer split fracture
4 Vertebral body seperation
C2 Type B injuries with rotation
C1.1–B.1 injuries with rotation flexion-distraction injuries with rotation)
1 Rotational flexional subluxation
2 Rotational flexional subluxation with unilateral articular process fracture
3 Unilateral dislocation
4 Rotational anterior dislocation without/with fracture of articular processes

(Table 43 cont.)

- 5 Rotational flexional subluxation without/with unilateral articular process fracture + type A fracture
- 6 Unilateral dislocation + type A fracture
- 7 Rotational anterior dislocation without/with fracture of articular processes + type A fracture

C2.2 – B.2 injuries with rotation (flexion-distraction injuries with rotation)

- 1 Rotational transverse bicolumn fracture
- 2 Unilateral flexion-spondylysis with disruption of the disk
- 3 Unilateral flexion-spondylysis + type A fracture

C2.3 – B.3 injuries with rotation (hyperextension-shear injuries with rotation)

- 1 Rotational hyperextension-sublaxation without/ with fracture of posterior vertebral elements
- 2 Unilateral hyperextension-spondylsysis
- 3 Posterior dislocation with rotation

C3 *Rotational-shear injuries*

- C3.1 Slice fracture
- C3.2 Oblique fracture

4.3 Classification of Thoracic and Lumbar Injuries

Common Characteristics of the Types (Fig. 4.1). Type A injuries focus on fractures of the vertebral body. The posterior column is, if at all, only insignificantly injured. Type B injuries describe transverse disruptions with elongation of the distance between the posterior (B1, B2) or anterior (B3) vertebral elements. In addition, B1 and B2 injuries are subgrouped depending on the type of anterior injury. This may be a rupture of the disk or a type A fracture of the vertebra. These type B injuries are diagnosed by the posterior injury but are further subdivided by a description of the anterior lesion. Type C focuses on injury patterns resulting from axial torque which is most often superimposed on either type A or type B lesions. Type A and type B injuries therefore form the basis for further subgrouping of most of the type C injuries. In addition, shearing injuries associated with torsion are described in the type C category. Type A lesions only affect the anterior column, whereas type B and C lesions represent injuries to both columns.

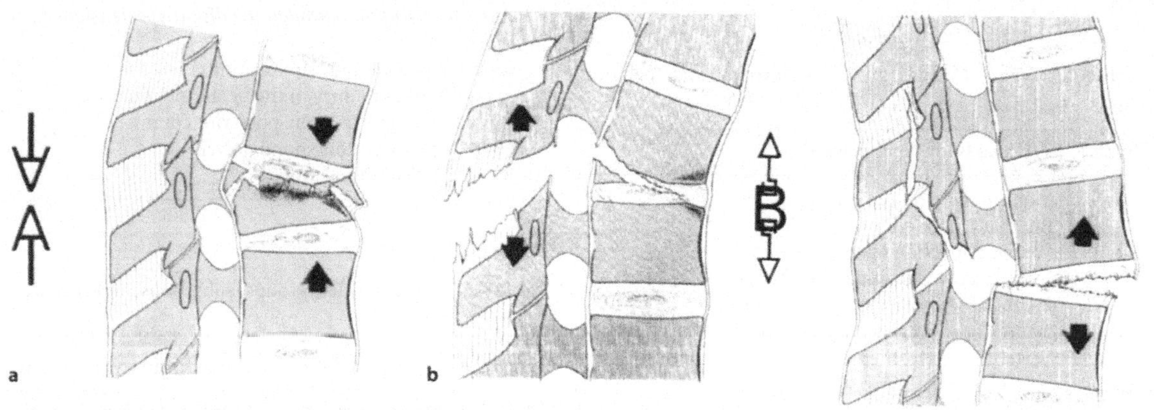

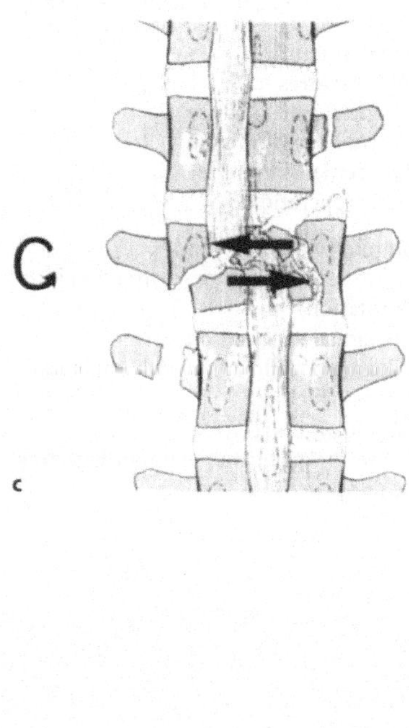

Fig. 4.1 Essential characteristics of the three injury types
a Type A, compression injury of the anterior column
b Type B, two-column injury with either posterior or anterior transverse disruption
c Type C, two-column injury with rotation

4.3.1 Type A: Vertebral Body Compression

Common Characteristics. The injuries are caused by axial compression with or without flexion and affect almost exclusively the vertebral body. The height of the vertebral body is reduced, and the posterior ligamentous complex is intact. Translation in the sagittal plane does not occur.

4.3.1.1 Group A1: Impaction Fractures

Common Characteristics. The deformation of the vertebral body is due to compression of the cancellous bone rather than to fragmentation. The posterior column is intact. Narrowing of the spinal canal does not occur. The injuries are stable, and neurological deficit is very rare (Table 4.5).

A. 1.1: End Plate Impaction (Fig. 4.2). The end plate often has the shape of an hourglass. Minor wedging of up to 5° may be present. The posterior wall of the vertebral body is intact. The injury is most often seen in juvenile and osteoporotic spines.

A. 1.2: Wedge Impaction Fracture (Fig. 4.3). The loss of anterior vertebral height results in an angulation of more than 5°. The posterior wall of the vertebral body remains intact. The loss of height may occur in the upper part of the vertebral body (superior wedge fracture), in the inferior pelt of the vertebral body (inferior wedge fracture), or anterolaterally (lateral wedge fracture). The last is associated with a scoliotic deformity.

A. 1.3: Vertebral Body Collapse (Fig. 4.4). This injury is usually observed in osteoporotic spines. There is symmetrical loss of vertebral body height without significant extrusion of fragments. The spinal canal is not violated. When combined with pronounced impaction of the end plates, the vertebral body has the shape of a 'fish vertebra.' Severe compression of the vertebral body may be associated with extrusion of fragments into the spinal canal and thus with injury to the spinal cord or cauda equine [1, 30, 39, 41]. Since those fractures show characteristics of burst fractures, they should be classified accordingly.

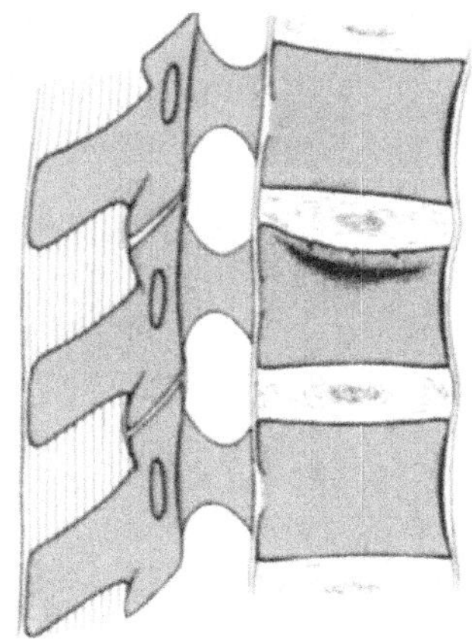

Fig. 4.2 End plate impaction (A1.1)

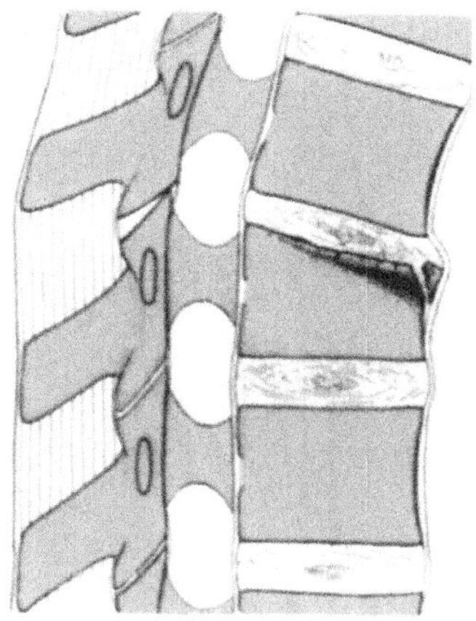

Fig. 4.3 Superior wedge fracture (A1.2.1)

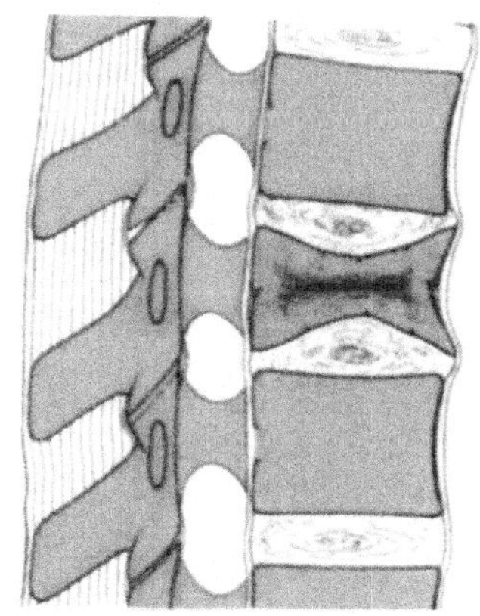

Fig. 4.4 Vertebral body collapse (A1.3)

4.3.1.2 Group A2: Split Fractures

Common Characteristics. As described by Roy-Camille et al. [37], the vertebral body is split in the coronal or sagittal plane with a variable degree of dislocation of the main fragments. When the main fragments are significantly dislocated, the gap is

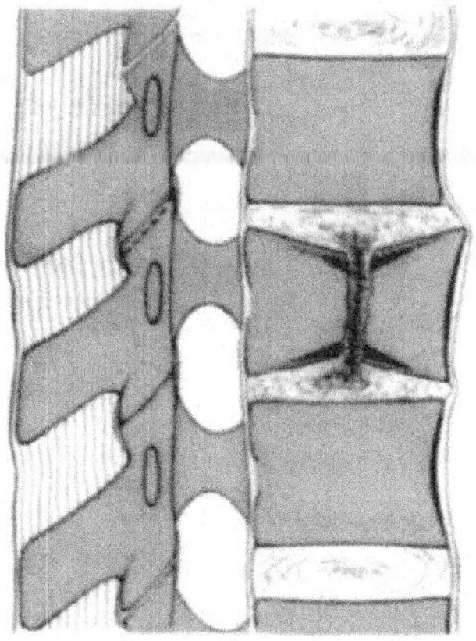

Fig. 4.5 Coronal split fracture (A2.2)

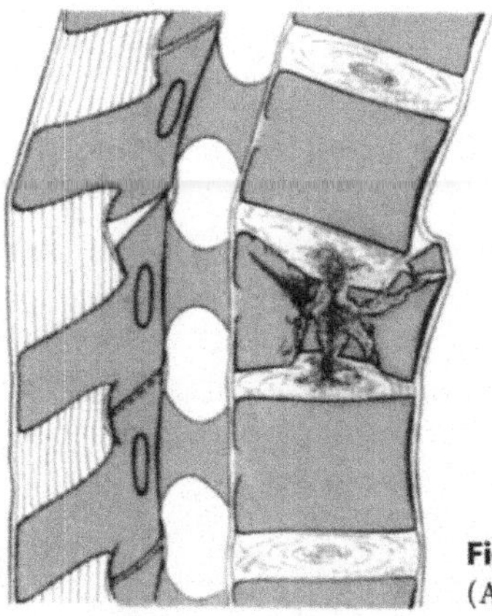

Fig. 4.6 Pincer fracture (A2.3)

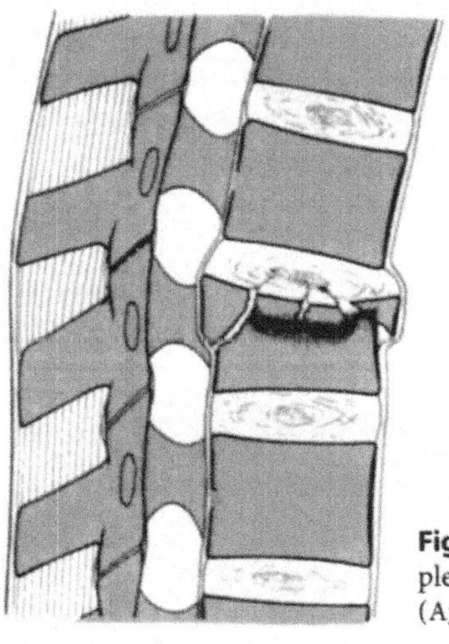

Fig. 4.7 Superior incomplete burst fracture (A3.1.1)

filled with disk material which may result in a nonunion [24, 37]. Neurological deficit is uncommon (Table 4.5). The posterior column is not affected.

A 2.1: Sagittal Split Fracture. These fractures are extremely rare in the thoracolumbar spine. They usually occur as an accompanying lesion of rotational burst fractures.

A 2.2: Coronal Split Fracture (Fig. 4.5). The smooth coronal fracture gap is narrow. The posterior vertebral body wall remains intact, and the injury is stable.

A 2.3: Pincer Fracture (Fig. 4.6). The central past of the vertebral body is crushed and filled with disk material. The anterior main fragment is markedly dislocated anteriorly. The resistance to flexion-compression is reduced, and pseudoalthrosis is likely to occur.

4.3.1.3
Group A3: Burst Fractures

Common Characteristics. The vertebral body is partially or completely comminuted with centrifugal extrusion of fragments. Fragments of the posterior wall are retropulsed into the spinal canal and are the cause of neural injury. The posterior ligamentous complex is intact. The injury to the arch, if present, is always a vertical split through the lamina or spinous process. Its contribution to instability is negligible. However, cauda fibers extruding through a tear outside the aura may become entrapped in the lamina fracture [13]. Superior, inferior, and lateral variants occur in burst fractures with partial comminution (A3.1, A3.2). In lateral variants with marked angulation in the frontal plane, a distractive lesion may be present on the convex side (compare Denis 1983; Fig. 4.11E). The frequency of neural injury is high (Table 4.5) and increases significantly from subgroup to subgroup.

A 3.1: Incomplete Burst Fracture (Fig. 4.7). The upper or lower half of the vertebral body has burst, while the other half remains intact. The stability of these injuries is reduced in flexion-compression. In particular, fragments of the posterior wall of the vertebral body may be further retropulsed into the spinal canal when the injury is exposed to flexion/compression [46].

A 3.2: Burst-Split Fracture (Fig. 4.8). In this injury, mentioned by Denis [10] and described extensively by Lindahl et al. [26], one-half of the vertebra (most often the upper half) has burst, whereas the other is split sagittally. The lamina or spinous processes are split vertically. Burst-split fractures are more unstable in flexion-compression and are more frequently accompanied by neurological injury than incomplete burst fractures.

A 3.3: Complete Burst Fracture. The entire vertebral body has burst. Complete burst fractures are unsta-

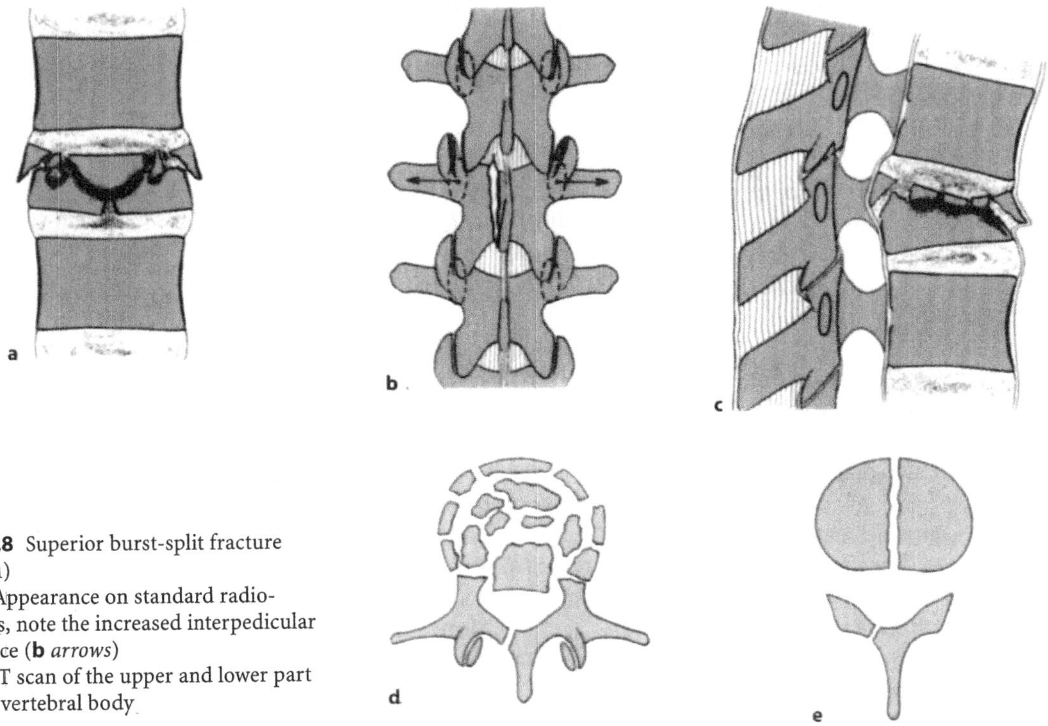

Fig. 4.8 Superior burst-split fracture (A3.2.1)
a–c Appearance on standard radiographs, note the increased interpedicular distance (**b** *arrows*)
d, e CT scan of the upper and lower part of the vertebral body

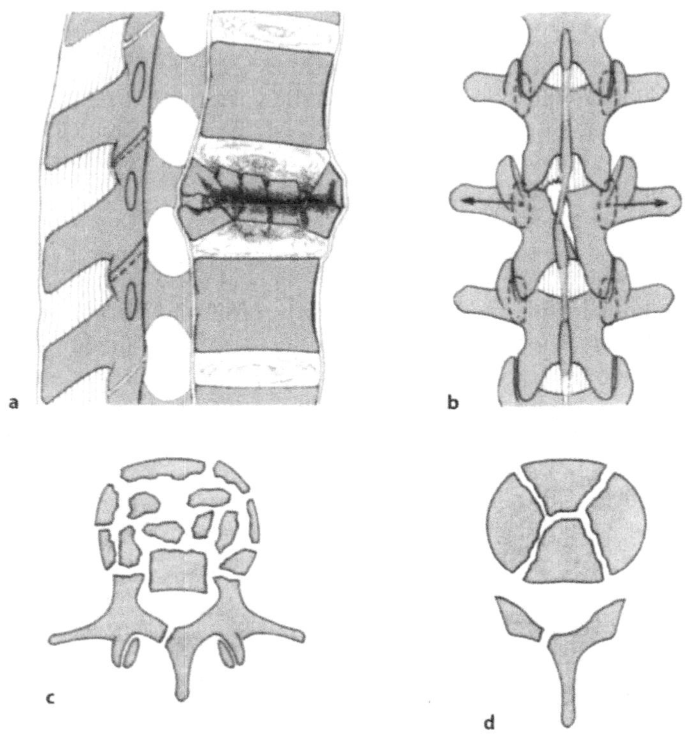

Fig. 4.9 Complete axial burst fracture (A3.3.3)
a, b Appearance on standard radiographs, note the increased interpedicular distance (*arrows*)
c, d CT scan of the upper and lower part of the vertebral body

ble in flexion-compression. Flexion and compression may result in an additional loss of vertebral body height. The spinal canal is often extremely narrowed by posterior wall fragments, and the frequency of neural injuries is accordingly high.

– *A 3.3.1: Pincer Burst Fracture.* In contrast to the simple pincer fracture (A2.3), the posterior wall of the vertebral body is fractured with fragments retropulsed into the spinal canal. The vertebral arch usually remains intact.

– *A3.3.2: Complete Flexion Burst Fracture.* The comminuted vertebral body is wedge shaped, resulting in a kyphotic angulation of the spine. The lamina or spinous processes are split vertically.

– *A 3.3.3: Complete Axial Burst Fracture (Fig. 4.9).* The height of the comminuted vertebral body is more or less evenly reduced. The lamina or spinous processes are split vertically.

4.3.1.4
Common Local Clinical Findings and Radiological Signs of Type A Injuries

Stable type A injuries may cause only moderate pain, so that patients are still able to walk. Unstable injuries are accompanied by significant pain and reduction of the patients' mobility. Marked wedging of the vertebral body produces a clinically visible gibbus. Posterior swelling and subcutaneous hematoma are not found since the injury to the posterior column, if at all present, does not involve the surrounding soft tissues. There is only tenderness at the level of the fracture.

The specific radiological appearances of the various type A injuries are shown in Figs. 4.2–4.9. Common radiological findings include: loss of vertebral body height, most often anteriorly, resulting in a kyphotic deformity; shortening of the posterior wall of the vertebral body, when fractured; a vertical split in the lamina accompanied by an increase of the horizontal distance between the pedicles (Figs. 4.8, 4.9); a vertical distance between the spinous processes is only somewhat increased in pronounced wedge-shaped fractures with an intact posterior wall. A significantly increased interspinous distance may well indicate the presence of a posterior distraction injury.

Fragments of the posterior wall are furthermore only displaced posteriorly into the spinal canal but not cranially and without significant rotation around the transverse axis (Figs. 4.7–4.9). On a CT scan, these fragments have a dense and smooth posterior border and appear blurred anteriorly. Translational dislocation in the horizontal plane does not occur in type A injuries.

4.3.2
Type B: Anterior and Posterior Element Injuries with Distraction

Common Characteristics. The main criterion is a transverse disruption of one or both spinal columns. Flexion-distraction initiates posterior disruption and elongation (groups B1 and B2), and hyperextension with or without anteroposterior shear causes anterior disruption and elongation (group B3).

In B1 and B2 injuries, the anterior lesion may be through the disk or a type A fracture of the vertebral body. Thus, type A fractures reoccur in these two groups, and the adjunction of their description is necessary for a complete definition of the injury. More severe B1 and B2 lesions may involve the erector spinae muscles or both these muscles and their fascia. Thus, the posterior disruption may extend into the subcutaneous tissue.

Translational dislocation in the sagittal direction may be present, and if not seen on radiographs, the potential for sagittal translocation should nonetheless be suspected. The degree of instability ranges from partial to complete, and the frequency of neurological impairment is altogether significantly higher than in type A injuries (Table 4.5).

4.3.2.1
Group B1: Posterior Disruption Predominantly Ligamentous

Common Characteristics (Fig. 4.16). The leading feature is the disruption of the posterior ligamentous complex with bilateral subluxation, dislocation, or facet fracture. The posterior injury may be associated with either a transverse disruption of the disk or a type A fracture of the vertebral body. Pure flexion-subluxations are only unstable in flexion, whereas pure dislocations are unstable in flexion and shear. B1 lesions associated with an unstable type A compression fracture of the vertebral body are additionally unstable in axial loading. Neurological deficit is frequent and caused by translational displacement and/or vertebral body fragments retropulsed into the spinal canal.

B 1.1: Posterior Disruption Predominantly Ligamentous Associated with Transverse Disruption of the Disk.

– *B 1.1.1: Flexion-Subluxation (Fig. 4.10A).* In this purely discoligamentous lesion, a small fragment not affecting the stability may be avulsed by the annulus fibrosus from the posterior or anterior rim of the end plate. Neurological deficit is uncommon.

– *B 1.1.2: Anterior Dislocation (Fig. 4.10B).* This purely discoligamentous lesion with a complete dislocation of the facet joints is associated with anterior translational displacement and narrowing of the spinal canal. The injury is rarely seen in the thoracolumbar spine [8, 47].

– *B 1.1.3: Flexion Subluxation or Anterior Dislocation with Fracture of the Articular Processes (Fig. 4.10C).* Either of the previously mentioned B1.1 lesions can be associated with bilateral facet fracture, resulting in a higher degree of instability, especially in anterior sagittal shear.

B 1.2: Posterior Disruption Predominantly Ligamentous Associated with Type A Fracture of the Vertebral Body. This combination might occur if the transverse axis of the flexion moment lies close to the posterior wall of the vertebral body. A severe flexion moment may then cause a transverse disruption of the posterior column and simultaneously a compression injury to the vertebral body which corresponds to an type A fracture.

– *B 1.2.1: Flexion-Subluxation Associated with Type A Fracture (Fig. 4.11).* The injury is unstable in flexion and axial compression. The latter corresponds to the impaired compression resistance of the vertebral body. Normally, the subluxation occurs in the upper facet joints (Fig. 4.11) of the fractured vertebra. Some cases of burst fractures have been reported in which the inferior facet joints were subluxed [25]. Neural injury may be due to kyphotic angulation or to fragments retropulsed into the spinal canal.

– *B 1.2.2: Anterior Dislocation Associated with a Type A Fracture (Fig. 4.12A).* The degree of instability as well as the risk of neural injury are higher than in the previously described injuries.

– *B 1.2.3: Flexion-Subluxation or Anterior Dislocation with Bilateral Facet Fracture Associated with Type A Fracture (Fig. 4.12B).* In the thoracic spine, this posterior injury is often combined with a complete burst fracture. The fracture of the articular process may extend into the pedicle. Some anterior translation is commonly present. The injury is very unstable, especially in anterior shear, and is frequently associated with complete paraplegia.

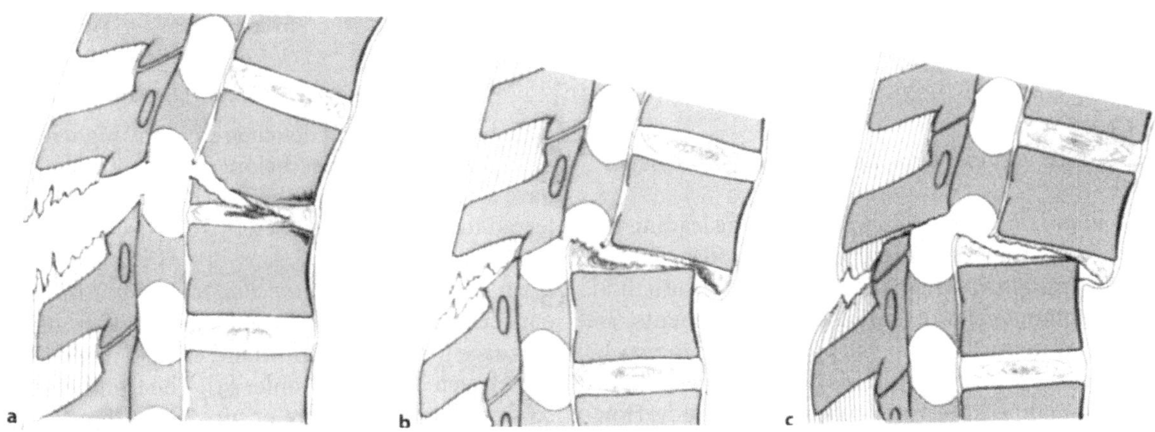

Fig. 4.10 Examples of posterior disruption (predominantly ligamentous) associated with an anterior lesion through the disk (B1.1)

a Flexion-subluxation (B1.1.1)
b Anterior dislocation (B1.1.2)
c Anterior dislocation with fracture of the articular processes (B1.1.3)

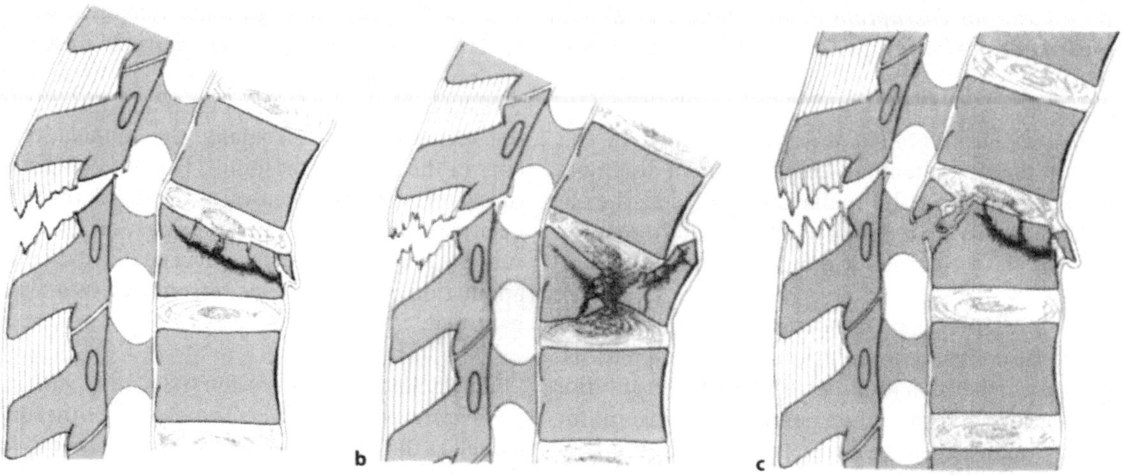

a b c

Fig. 4.11 Examples of posterior disruption predominantly ligamentous with subluxation of the facet joints associated with a type A fracture of the vertebral body (B1.2.1)
A Flexion-subluxation associated with a superior wedge fracture (Bl.2.1+A1.2.1)
B Flexion-subluxation associated with a pincer fracture (B1.2.1+A2.3)
C Flexion-subluxation associated with an incomplete superior burst fracture (B1.2.1+A3.1.1)

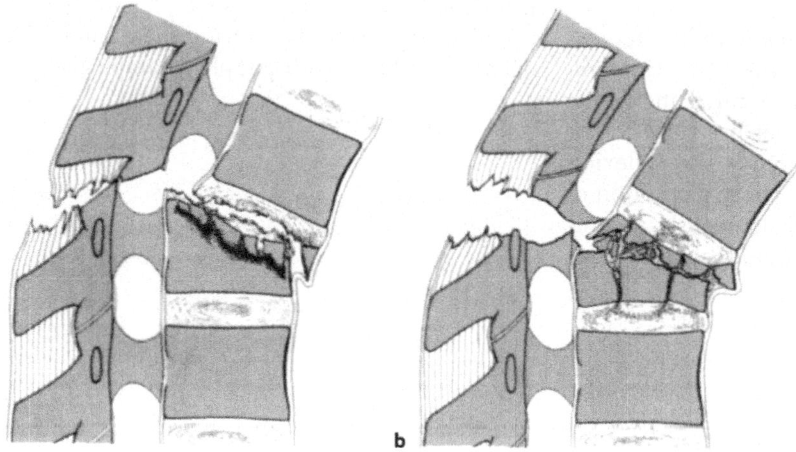

a b

Fig. 4.12 Examples of posterior disruption predominantly ligamentous associated with a type A fracture of the vertebral body
a Anterior dislocation associated with a superior wedge fracture (B 1.2.2+A1.2.1)
b Anterior subluxation with fracture of articular processes associated with a complete burst fracture (B 1.2.3+A3.3)

4.3.2.2
Group B2: Posterior Disruption Predominantly Osseous

Common Characteristics (Fig. 4.16). The leading criterion is a transverse disruption of the posterior column through the laminae and pedicles or the isthmi. Interspinous and/or supraspinous ligaments are torn. As in the B1 group, the posterior lesion may be associated with either a transverse disruption of the disk or a type A fracture of the vertebral body. However, there is no vertebral body lesion within type A that would correspond to the transverse bicolumn fracture. Except for Forsythe transverse bicolumn fracture, the degree of instability as well as the incidence of neurological deficit are slightly higher than in B1 injuries. Injuries belonging to this category have already been described by Bohler [3], who referred to a scheme designed by Heuritsch in 1933.

B 2.1: Transverse Bicolumn Fracture (Fig. 4.13). This particular lesion was first published in the English language literature by Howland et al. [23] and illustrated even earlier by Bohler [3]. The transverse bicolumn fracture usually occurs in the upper segments of the lumbar spine and is unstable in flexion. As it is a purely osseous lesion, it has excellent healing potential. Neurological deficit is uncommon.

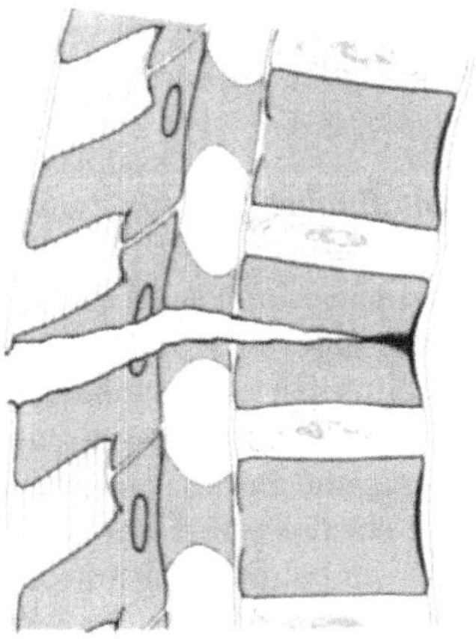

Fig. 4.13 Transverse bicolumn fracture (B2.1).

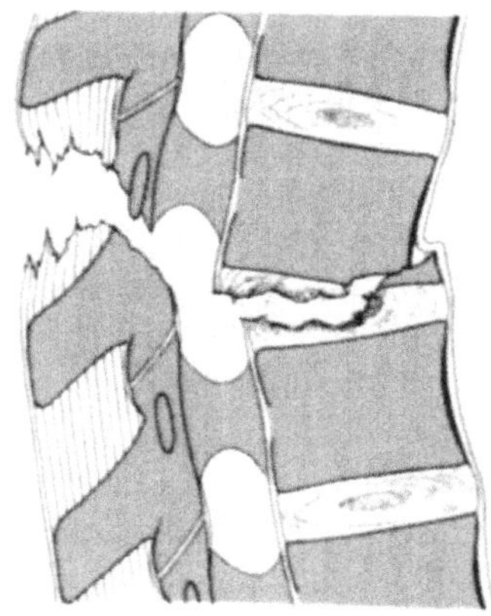

Fig. 4.14 Posterior disruption predominantly osseous associated with an anterior lesion through the disk: flexion-spondylolysis (B2.2.2)

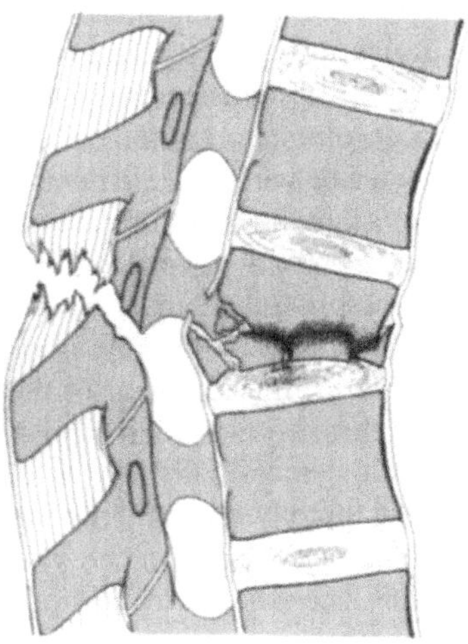

Fig. 4.15 Posterior disruption predominantly osseous associated with a type A fracture of the vertebral body: flexion-spondylolysis associated with an inferior incomplete burst fracture (B2.3.2+A3.1.3)

B 2.2: Posterior Disruption Predominantly Osseous with Transverse Disruption of the Disk

- *B2.2.1: Disruption Through the Pedicle and Disk (Fig. 4.16).* This rare variant is characterized by a horizontal fracture through the arch that exits inferiorly through the base of the pedicle.

- *B2.2.2: Disruption Through the Pars Interarticularis and Disk (Flexion-Spondylolysis) (Fig. 4.14).* A flexion-spondylolysis with minimal displacement is less likely to result in neurological deficit. However, displaced fractures with pronounced flexion-rotation of the vertebral body around the transverse axis are frequently combined with neural injury. This is due to narrowing of the spinal canal as the posterior inferior corner of the vertebral body approaches the lamina.

B 2.3: Posterior Disruption Predominantly Osseous Associated with Type A Fracture of the Vertebral Body.

- *B 2.3.1: Fracture Through the Pedicle Associated with a Type A Fracture.* The posterior injury is the same as described for B2.2.1.

- *B 2.3.2: Fracture Through the Isthmus Associated with a Type A Fracture (Fig. 4.15).* The posterior injury is the same as described for B2.2.2. The anterior column lesion is often an inferior variant of a type A fracture.

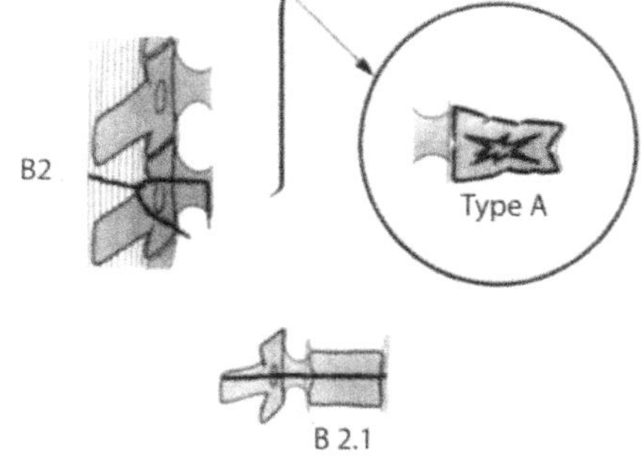

Fig. 4.16 In flexion-distraction injuries (B1–B2), the injury of the posterior column may be associated with either a rupture of the disk or a type A fracture of the vertebral body. Exception: the transverse hicolumn fracture

4.3.2.3
Common Local Clinical Findings and Radiological Signs of B1 and B2 Injuries

Marked tenderness, swelling, and subcutaneous hematoma at the site of the posterior injury as well as a palpable gap between the spinous processes are highly indicative of a distractive posterior lesion. Kyphotic deformity may be present. A step in the line of the spinous processes indicates anterior translational displacement.

A variety of radiographic signs are typical of B1 and B2 injuries (cf. Figs. 4.10–4.15): kyphotic deformity with significantly increased vertical distance between the two spinous processes at the level of the injury; anterior translational displacement; bilateral subluxation, dislocation, or bilateral fracture of the facet joints; horizontal or bilateral fracture of other posterior vertebral elements; avulsion of the posterior edge of the vertebral body; anterior shear-chip fracture of an end plate; and avulsion fracture of the supraspinous ligament from the spinous process.

In B1 and B2 injuries associated with burst-type fractures, the fragment of the posterior wall of the vertebral body is often displaced not only posteriorly but also cranially (Fig. 4.11C). It is sometimes rotated up to 90° around the transverse axis so that its surface consisting of the posterior part of the end plate faces the vertebral body. Unlike type A burst fractures, the anterior border of the fragment will then appear dense and smooth on a CT scan, while its posterior contour is blurred. This phenomenon may be called the 'inverse cortical sign.'

4.3.2.4
Group B3 Anterior Disruption Through the Disk

In the rare hyperextension-shear injuries, the transverse disruption originates anteriorly and may be confined to the anterior column or may extend posteriorly. Severe anteroposterior shear causes disruption of both columns. Denis and Burkus [14] saw a variety of hyperextension shear injuries due to direct trauma to the spine from behind. The anterior lesion was always through the disk. In the majority of cases, the posterior injury consisted of fractures of articular processes, lamina, or pars interarticularis. Eleven of 12 injuries were located in the thoracic spine and the thoracolumbar junction, and 11 patients suffered complete paraplegia. Sagittal translational displacement is not uncommon in these injuries. Anterior displacement can occur in B3.1 and B3.2 injuries, whereas posterior displacement is typical for the B3.3 subgroup.

B 3.1: Hyperextension-Subluxation (Fig. 4.17a). A spontaneously reduced, pure discoligamentous injury is difficult to diagnose. The presence of such an injury may be indicated by widening of the disk space and can be confirmed by magnetic resonance imaging scans [14]. Diskography may be helpful in the lumbar spine. Hyperextension-subluxations are

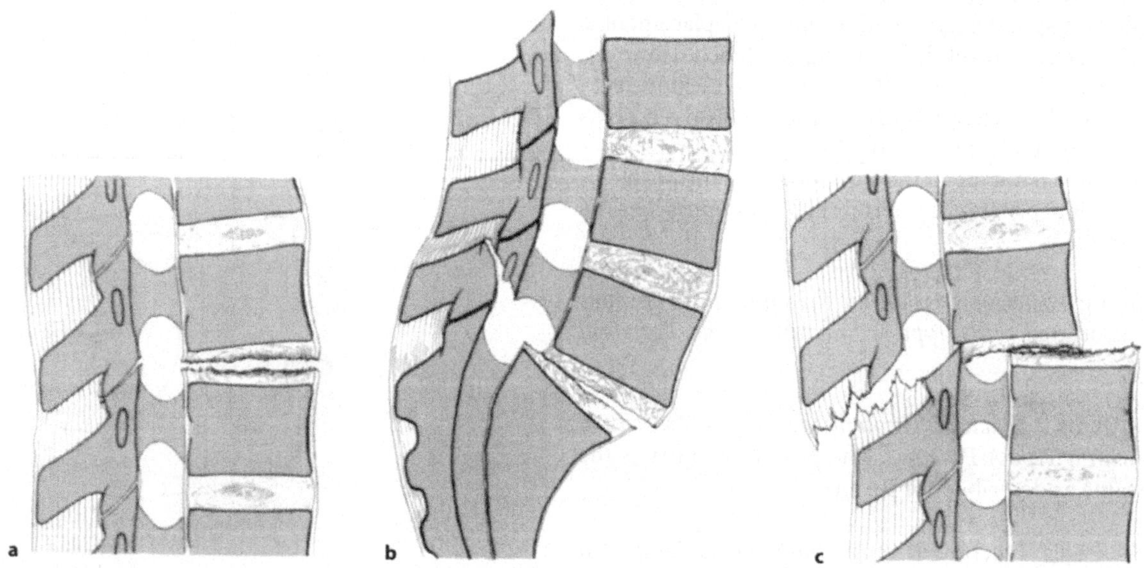

Fig. 4.17 Examples of anterior disruption through the disk (hyperextension-shear injuries)
a Hyperextension-subluxation without fracture of posterior vertebral elements (B3.1.1)
b Hyperextension-spondylolysis (B3.2) in the lower lumbar spine (cf. text)
c Posterior dislocation (B3.3)

sometimes associated with a fracture of the lamina or articular processes [14], or with a fracture of the basis of the pedicles [7].

B 3.2: Hyperextension-Spondylolysis (Fig. 4.17b). The few cases seen by us were located in the lowermost lumbar level. In contrast to flexion-spondylolysis, the sagittal diameter of the spinal canal was widened in these cases, as the vertebral body had shifted anteriorly, while the lamina remained in place. Consequently, there was no neurological deficit. The cases described by Denis and Burkus [14] occurred in the thoracic spine and were associated with severe neurological deficit.

B. 3.3: Posterior Dislocation (Fig. 4.17c). This is one of the severest injuries of the lumbar spine and is often associated with complete paraplegia. Lumbosacral posterior dislocations probably have a better prognosis [8].

4.3.2.5 Common Local Clinical Findings and Radiological Signs of B3 Injuries

Posterior tenderness, swelling, and subcutaneous hematoma are usually found in all injuries caused by a direct trauma to the back and other B3 lesions associated with significant injury to the posterior column and the surrounding soft tissues. The radiological signs and diagnostic possibilities have already been described earlier in this chapter, except for the avulsion and shear-chip fragments from end plates which can occur in all type B3 injuries [7].

4.3.3 Type C: Anterior and Posterior Element Injuries with Rotation

Out of the multitude of injury patterns, three groups of which each contains injuries with similar morphological patterns have been identified: (1) type A with superimposed rotation, (2) type B with superimposed rotation, and (3) rotation-shear injuries. Apart from a few exceptions, rotational injuries represent the severest injuries of the thoracic and lumbar spine and are associated with the highest rate of neurological deficit (Table 4.5). Neural injury is caused by fragments dislocated into the spinal canal and/or by the encroachment of the spinal canal resulting from translational displacement.

Common characteristics include two-column injury; rotational displacement; potential for translational displacement in all directions of the horizontal plane; disruption of all longitudinal ligaments and of disks; fractures of articular processes, usually unilateral; fracture of transverse processes; rib dislocations and/or fractures close to the spine; lateral avulsion fracture of the end plate; irregular fractures of the neural arch; and asymmetrical fractures of the vertebral body. These findings, typical sequelae of axial torque, are associated with the fundamental pattern of type A and B lesions, which can still be discerned. Since type A and B lesions have already been discussed in detail, the description of type C injuries can be confined to common characteristics and the special features of some injuries.

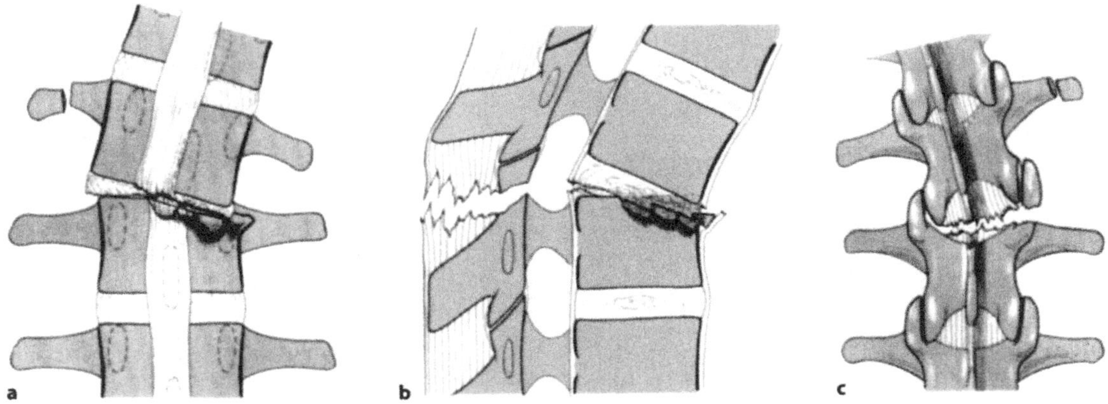

Fig. 4.18 Example of a type A fracture with rotation: rotational wedge fracture (C1.1)

4.3.3.1
Group C1: Type A with Rotation

This group contains rotational wedge, split, and burst fractures (Figs. 4.18–4.20). In type A lesions with rotation, one lateral wall of the vertebral body often remains intact. Therefore, a normal contour of a vertebral body (phantom vertebra) may radiographically appear in the lateral profile together with the fracture (Figs. 4.18, 4.20). As already mentioned, a sagittal split fracture (C1.2.1) may occur adjacent to a rotational burst fracture as a consequence of the axial torque. The vertebral body separation (C1.2.4) represents a contiguous, multilevel, coronal split lesion (Fig. 4.19). In this injury the spinal canal may be widened where it is involved in the lesion. The five patients treated by us as well as cases published to date [4, 19, 40, 42] suffered no neurological deficit.

4.3.3.2
Group C2: Type B with Rotation

The most commonly seen C2 lesions are different variants of flexion-subluxation with rotation (Fig. 4.21). Of the lateral distraction injuries pub-

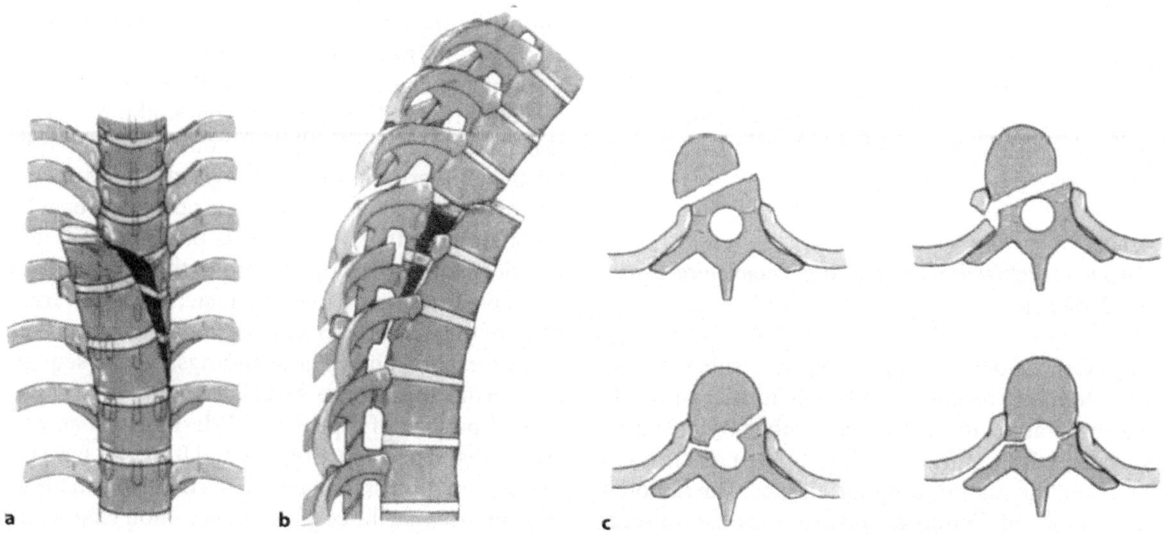

Fig. 4.19 Vertebral body separation (C1.2.4)
a, b Appearance on standard radiographs
c CT scans of the fractured vertebrae

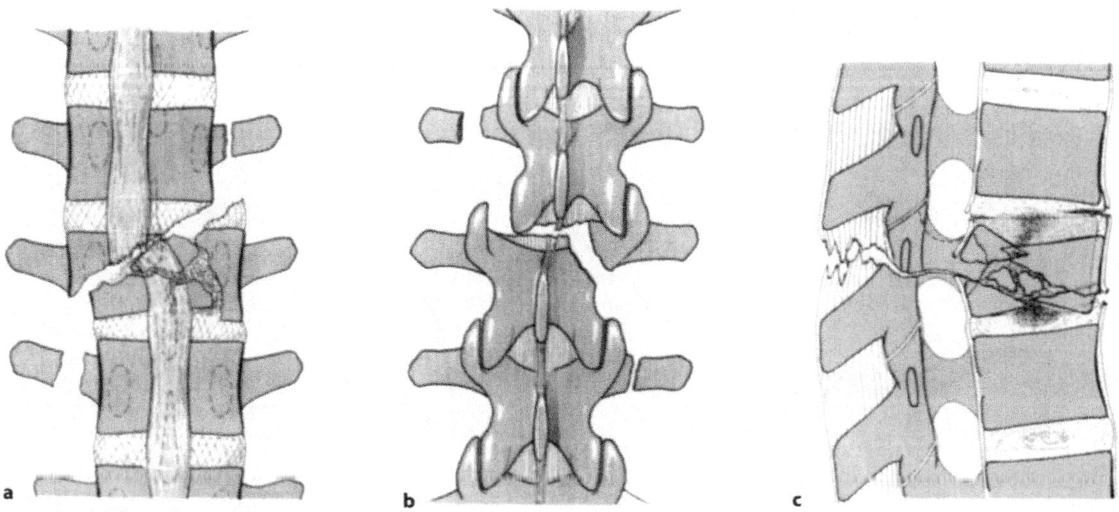

Fig. 4.20 Example of a type A fracture with rotation: complete burst fracture with rotation (C1.3.3)
a Vertebral body
b Posterior elements
c Lateral view

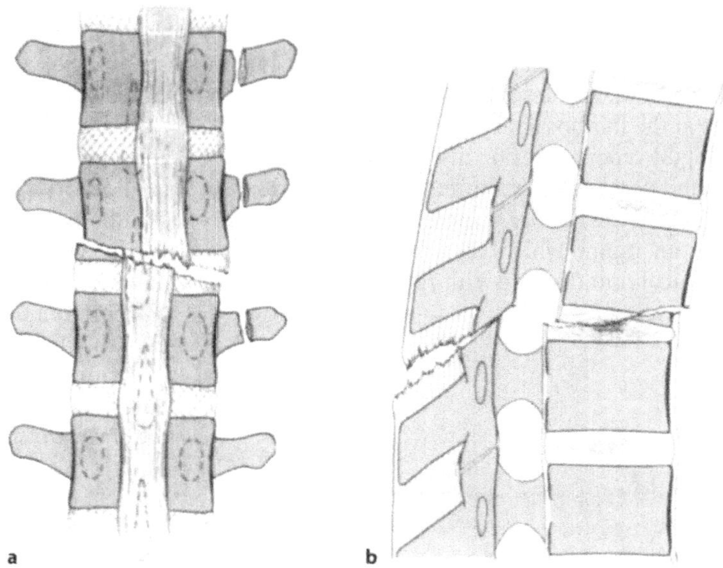

Fig. 4.21 Example of a type B injury with rotation: rotational flexion-subluxation (C2.1.1)
a Lateral view
b Posterior elements

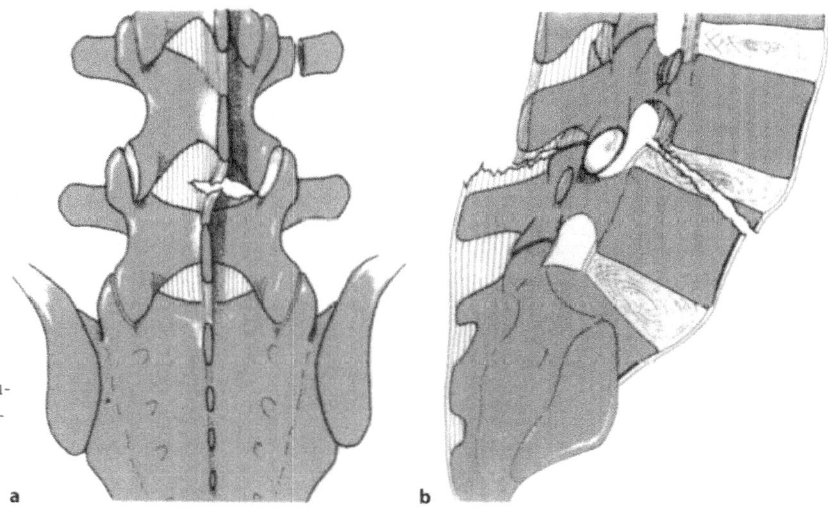

Fig. 4.22 Example of a type B injury with rotation: unilateral dislocation (C2.1.3)
a Lateral view
b Posterior elements

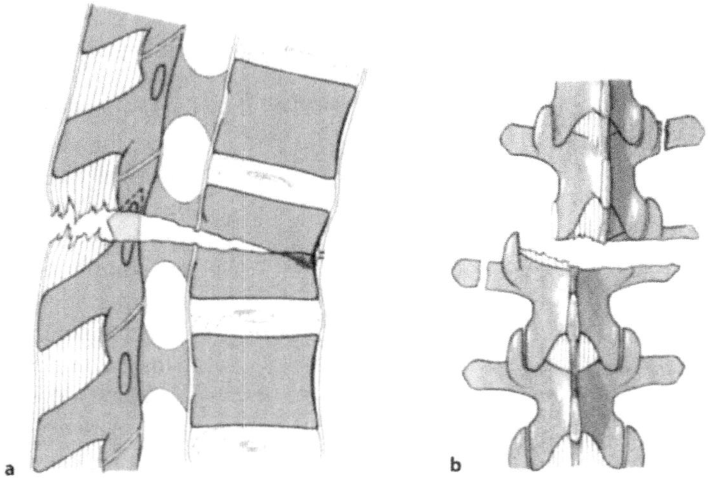

Fig. 4.23 Example of a type B injury with rotation: transverse bicolumn fracture with rotation (C2.2.1)
a Anterior elements
b Lateral view

lished by Denis and Burkus [12], we would ascribe at least one to type B with rotation. Unilateral dislocations are less frequent (Fig. 4.22). Boger et al. [2] and Conolly et al. [6] describe unilateral facet dislocations at the lumbosacral junction, and Roy-Camille et al. [38] report anterior dislocation with rotation and unilateral facet fracture. Amongst distraction fractures of the lumbar spine, Gumley et al. [20] describe an injury which corresponds to the transverse bicolumn fracture with rotation (Fig. 4.23).

4.3.3.3
Group C3: Rotational Shear Injuries

Holdsworth [22] stated that the slice fracture (Fig. 4.24) is "very common in the thoracolumbar and lumbar regions and is by far the most unstable of all injuries of the spine." With regard to frequency, this does not correspond with our experience, which is limited to three cases. Thirteen of our 16 C3 injuries were oblique fractures (Fig. 4.25). In our opinion, the oblique fracture is even more unstable than the slice fracture, as it completely lacks stability in compression. However, the slice fracture is obviously more dangerous to the spinal cord because of the shear in the horizontal plane.

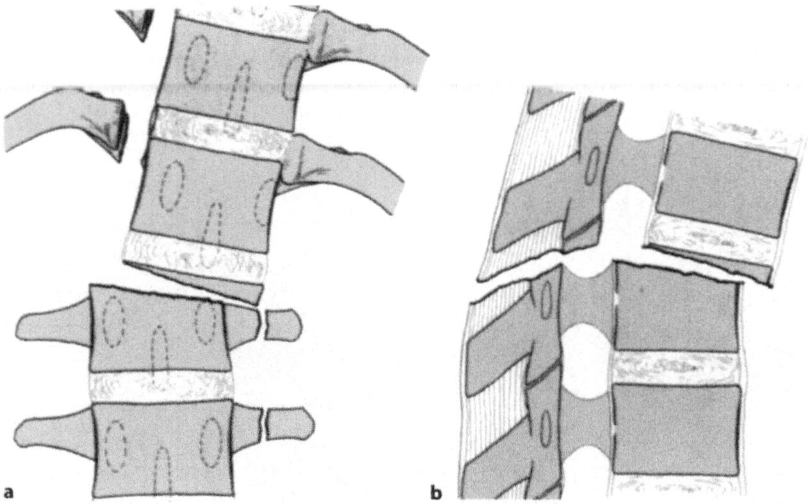

Fig. 4.24 Rotational shear injury: Holdsworth slice fracture (C3.1)
a Lateral view
b Anterior view

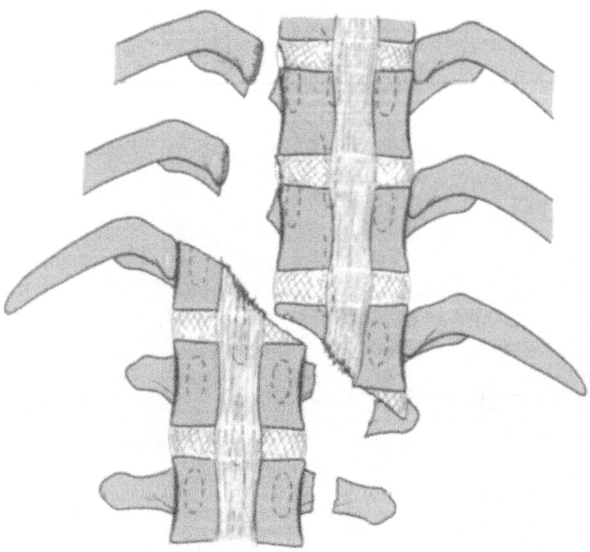

Fig. 4.25 Rotational shear injury: oblique fracture of the vertebra (C3.2)

4.3.3.4
Common Clinical Findings and Radiological Signs of Type C Injuries

The type of accident, e.g., a fall from a great height, injuries caused by a heavy object falling on the bent back, or when the patient was thrown some distance, may be enough to suggest that axial torque was involved in the mechanism of injury. Local findings are the same as those described for type B injuries. The radiological appearance of the various type C injuries is shown in Figs. 4.18–4.25, and the characteristic signs of rotation have been described above. Fractures of transverse processes are the principal indicator of rotational injuries of the lumbar spine. Therefore, even if they seem isolated, their presence should always trigger an intense search for a hidden type C injury.

4.4 Epidemiological Data

The 1445 cases investigated were also analyzed with regard to: (1) the level of the main injury, (2) the frequency of the types and groups, and (3) the incidence of the neurological deficit related to types and groups. A more detailed analysis of the epidemiological data is the subject of another study to be published.

4.4.1 Level of Main Injury

Figure 4.26 demonstrates the distribution of the level of the monosegmental lesions and the level of the main injury in multisegmental injuries. As expected, most injuries were located around the thoracolumbar junction. The upper and lower end of the thoracolumbar spine as well as the T10 level were the areas most infrequently injured.

Injuries to the spine often involve more than one segment, especially in polytraumatized patients [34]. Of the 468 consecutive cases which were analyzed in more detail, 23% had multisegmental injuries of the thoracolumbar spine.

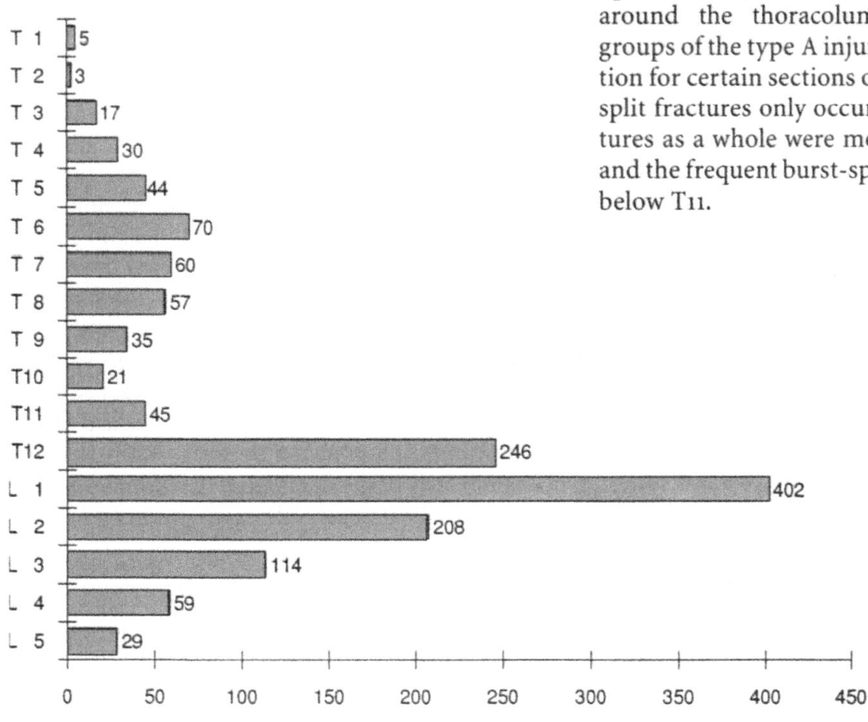

Fig. 4.26 The main level of injury in 1445 patients

Table 4.4 Number and percentage of injuries per type and group ($N = 1445$)

	Cases	Percentage of total [%]	Persentage of type [%]
Type A	*956*	*66.16*	
A1	502	34.74	52.51
A2	50	3.46	5.23
A3	404	27.96	42.26
Type B	*209*	*14.46*	
B1	126	8.72	60.29
B2	80	5.54	38.28
B3	3	0.21	1.44
Type C	*280*	*19.38*	
C1	156	10.80	55.71
C2	108	7.47	38.57
C1	16	1.11	5.71

4.4.2 Frequency and Distribution of Types and Groups

Type A fractures represented two-thirds of all injuries (Table 4.4). Type B and C lesions, although they encompass a great variety of injuries, altogether only accounted for one-third. Stable type A injuries alone exceeded more than one-third of the total.

Detailed analysis of the 468 cases mentioned above revealed that the frequency of type A injuries decreases from cranial to caudal, whereas type C injuries are more frequently located in the lumbar spine, and type B injuries are more often found around the thoracolumbar junction. Also, the groups of the type A injuries showed some predilection for certain sections of the thoracolumbar spine: split fractures only occurred below T10; burst fractures as a whole were more often found below T12; and the frequent burst-split fractures were only seen below T11.

Table 4.5 Incidence of neurological deficit in 1212 patients

Types and groups	Number of injuries	Neurological deficit [%]
Type A	*890*	*14*
A1	501	2
A2	45	4
A3	344	32
Type B	*145*	*32*
B1	61	30
B2	82	33
B3	2	50
Type C	*177*	*55*
C1	99	53
C2	62	60
C3	16	50
Total	*1212*	*22*

4.4.3 Incidence of Neurological Deficit

The neurological deficit, ranging from complete paraplegia to single root lesions, was evaluated in 1212 patients (Table 4.5). The overall incidence was 22% and increased significantly from type to type. Neurological deficit is very rare in A1 and A2 injuries. Neural injury of A1 fractures may be attributed to severe kyphotic angulation resulting from multisegmental wedge fractures in the thoracic spine [31]. However, it may also be possible that some wedge fractures of the thoracic spine were in fact hidden B1.2 injuries in which the posterior lesion was not discernible on standard radiographs. The striking increase of neural injury between the A2 and the A3 group may be attributed to the high proportion of severe burst fractures in the A3 group. This high proportion of severe burst fractures also accounts for the fact that the frequency of neural injury in the A3 group is similar to that in the B1 and B2 groups. Another reason for this similarity may be that anterior dislocation with its high risk of neural injury rarely occurs in the thoracolumbar spine. An explanation for the decrease of neurological deficits from the C2 to the C3 group can be found in the rather small number of the neurologically most dangerous Holdsworth slice fractures in group C3 of this series.

4.5 Discussion

A classification of spinal injuries should meet several requirements. It should be clearly and logically structured and should furthermore provide an easily understandable terminology, information regarding the severity of the injury, and guidance as to the choice of treatment. The classification should be comprehensive so that every injury can be precisely defined, itemized, and retrieved, as necessary. In addition, the structure of the classification should also allow it to be used in a simplified form without impairment of information most essential for clinical practice. Several criteria have been employed to classify spinal injuries, e.g., stability, mechanism of injury, and involvement of anatomical structures. Though each of the existing classifications has certain merits, none would seem to meet all the requirements.

The classification proposed is the result of more than 10 years of intense consideration of the subject matter [29] and a thorough review of 1445 consecutive thoracolumbar injuries at five institutional*. During this time we tested several existing classification systems and worked on our own approaches to a new system until finally agreeing on the version presented here.

The new classification is primarily based on the pathomorphology of the injury. Emphasis was placed on the extent of involvement of the anterior and posterior elements, with particular reference to soft-tissue injury, as well as ancillary bony lesions. Analysis of the injury pattern provides information on the pathomechanics of the injury, at least regarding the main mechanisms. For example, loss of vertebral height implies a compressive force, transverse disruption suggests distraction or shear, and rotational displacement in the vertical axis indicates torsion. Each of these mechanisms produces injuries with its own characteristic fundamental pattern.

Although compression may be purely axial or combined with flexion, distraction and torsion usually occur in combination with compression, flexion, extension, and/or shear. Deviations and combinations of forces and moments as well as their varying magnitude and rate modify the fundamental patterns. The natural variations in the anatomical and mechanical properties of the different sections of the thoracolumbar spine itself are responsible for the fact that some injury patterns are typical of certain sections. Age-related differences in the strength of the affected tissue determine that some forms of injury are typical of juvenile or osteoporotic spines.

* Department of Orthopaedic Surgery, Kantonsspital, St. Gallen; Department of Orthopaedic Surgery, Inselspital, Bern; Sunnybrook Health Service Centre, Toronto; Rehabitilations-krankenhaus, Karlsbad-Langensteinbach; Hôpital de la Conception, Marseille

Because the fundamental pattern of injury still remains recognizable in almost every case, the main mechanisms of injury can be used to establish principal categories, each of which is characterized by common morphological findings. In view of the great variability of the forces and moments, it would, however, hardly be feasible to use the mechanism of injury as an order principle throughout the classification.

To provide an easily recognizable grid for classifying the injuries, the 3-3-3 scheme of the AO fracture classification was applied as far as possible. The three principle categories, the types, are determined by the three most important mechanisms acting on the spine [46]: compression, distraction, and torsion. Predominantly morphological criteria are used for all further grouping.

Every injury can be defined alphanumerically or by a descriptive name, e.g., wedge impaction fracture, anterior dislocation, or rotational burst fracture. The specifications describe the injuries most precisely. In clinical practice, application of the classification can be restricted to subgroups or even groups without the loss of information which is most important for defining the principal nature of the injury and the choice of treatment.

As already mentioned, distraction as well as torsion usually occur in combination with other mechanisms. Since posterior distraction is often combined with anterior compression, type A fractures reoccur in type B as the anterior component of flexion-distraction lesions. Torsion is frequently associated with compression or distraction. Consequently, type A and B lesions appear in type C modified by the axial torque. Thus, several type B and C injuries are based on preceding types. This concept permits the inclusion of various combinations of injuries, facilitates their proper identification, and avoids the need to memorize every particular form of injury.

It is quite natural that injuries occur which constitute transient forms between types as well as between subdivisions of the classification. For example, a type A injury can become type B when the degree of flexion exceeds the point beyond which the posterior ligament complex definitely fails. Transient forms with partial rupture of the posterior ligaments occur in cases in which the degree of flexion has just become critical. The same applies for transient forms between type A or B and type C injuries. Here, the degree of axial torque determines whether a partially or fully developed rotational injury will result. Transient forms may either be allocated to the lesser or more severe category, depending on which characteristics predominate.

While dealing with the subject, all injuries described in the classification were seen by us. Regarding statistical data, there is good reason to assume that in the review of the 1445 cases, some type B injuries of the thoracic spine were missed and classified as type A injuries when only standard radiographs were available. Correct diagnosis of posterior distraction injuries is often difficult since some of them can look like plain type A lesions, especially in the thoracic spine. Therefore, it is of the utmost importance to search for clinical and radiological signs of posterior disruption to unmask the true nature of the injury. Radiographically, a posterior lesion is often only identifiable by lateral tomography or sagittal reconstruction of thin CT slices.

The severity of trauma has been considered in the organization of the classification whenever possible. Severity is defined by several factors such as impairment of stability, risk of necrological injury, and prognostic aspects. In this classification, the loss of stability constitutes the primary determining factor for ranking the injuries because it is the most important one for choosing the form of treatment.

This study confirms that the risk of neural injury is largely linked to the degree of instability (Table 4.5). The separation of discoligamentous injuries from osseous lesions was undertaken in consideration of prognostic aspects important for the treatment. Because discoligamentous injuries have a poor healing potential [28], surgical stabilization and fusion should be considered to avoid chronic instability.

The term 'instability' on its own is of little use if it is not related to parameters defining the load beyond which a physical structure fails. For understanding traumatic spinal instability, the definition of stability as formulated by Whitesides [46] may be helpful: "A stable spine should be one that can withstand axial forces anteriorly through the vertebral bodies, tension forces posteriorly, and rotational stresses..., thus being able to function to hold the body erect without progressive kyphosis and to protect the spinal canal contents from further injury." In this sense, any reduction of the compressive, tensile, or torsional strength impairing the spine from functioning in the upright position as outlined by Whitesides would, by inverse definition, be instability. Whitesides' definition also implies that forces and moments most important for the spine can be reduced to compressive forces, tensile forces, and axial torque. With the proviso that tensile forces can also act anteriorly, Whitesides' primary forces correspond to those responsible for the fundamental injury patterns of the types in our classification: Type A injuries are primarily caused by compression, type B injuries by tension, and type C injuries by axial torque.

Though any reduction of resistance against primary forces may be termed 'instability,' a more precise identification of the type and degree of instability is necessary for the treatment modalities. There are injuries which are clearly stable and those which are clearly unstable when subject to forces of any direction and magnitude. Between these two extremes, there are many injuries of varying instability with flowing transitions regarding the quality and magnitude of the instability. There are those with 'partial instability' and simultaneously 'residual stability.' For example, most type A injuries are unstable in compression but stable in distraction, shear, and torque. An anterior dislocation is unstable in flexion and anterior shear; in extension and compression, however, it is stable when reduced. Both residual stability and the type of instability must be considered when selecting the most rational form of treatment, i.e., restoring stability with minimum expenditure and invasiveness. Thus, understanding the individual aspects of instability helps determine the appropriate treatment.

Overlap of some categories regarding instability was accepted for the sake of morphological uniformity. Furthermore, because the precise degree of instability cannot be defined for every injury, it would hardly be feasible to classify spinal injuries on a strictly progressive scale of instability. Generally, however, instability increases from type to type and within each subdivision of the classification. The progression of instability and its consequences for the choice of treatment can be described as follows.

4.5.1 Type A

The stability in compression may be intact, impaired, or lost, depending on the extent of destruction of the vertebral body. The stability in flexion may be intact, or it may be reduced due to the impaired compressive resistance of the vertebral body. However, stability in flexion is never completely lost since, by definition, the posterior ligament complex must be intact in type A injuries. Really stable injuries only occur in type A. The degree of instability progresses gradually from the stable Al fractures to the very unstable A3.3 burst fractures. Translation in the horizontal plane does not occur in this type.

The intactness of the posterior ligament complex and the anterior longitudinal ligament [48] accounts for the unimpaired tensile strength of the spine, which is in turn important for treatment modalities. Application of longitudinal traction, e.g., by Harrington distraction rods or an internal fixator, does not result in overdistraction.

The spine is stable in extension as the strong anterior longitudinal ligament is preserved [48], and the posterior vertebral elements maintain their stabilizing function despite a possible split of the lamina. Because the posterior vertebral elements can act as a fulcrum, extension can be used for reduction of type A fractures in conservative treatment [3, 44]. Only complete burst fractures with markedly splayed laminae may constitute exceptions in this regard.

4.5.2 Type B

The leading criterion is the partial or complete loss of the tensile strength of the spine, often in addition to the loss of stability in axial compression. Sagittal translation can occur either anteriorly or posteriorly.

4.5.2.1 B1 and B2 Injuries

Due to the transverse posterior disruption, stability in flexion is always completely lost, sometimes together with the loss of stability in anterior shear. These instabilities are combined with a reduced stability in axial compression if the posterior injury is associated with a type A fracture. Stability in extension is generally preserved because the anterior longitudinal ligament is most often stripped off the vertebral body. Anterior subluxation or dislocation can occur, and, if not present, the potential presence of anterior sagittal translation should be taken into consideration.

Application of posterior distraction can result in kyphosis or even overdistraction. Stabilization of these injuries should therefore involve posterior compression and restoration of the compressive resistance of the anterior column, where necessary. This can be accomplished by either conservative or surgical treatment modalities. Conservative treatment with immobilization in hyperextension may be adequate for predominantly osseous injuries in which intact articular processes prevent anterior translational displacement. This treatment may also be applied to transverse bicolumn fractures since the friction in the rough and large bony surfaces would prevent secondary anterior displacement. However, mainly discoligamentous injuries necessitate surgical treatment, including fusion, because of their poor healing potential [28].

4.5.2.2
B3 Injuries

These injuries are unstable in extension and stable in axial compression, at least when reduced. Injuries with a preserved posterior ligament complex are also stable in flexion. On the other hand, injuries with additionally disrupted posterior structures, as with posterior dislocation and some of the shear fracture dislocations described by Denisand Burkus [14], completely lack tensile and shear resistance. True anterior translational displacement may be found in shear fracture dislocations [14], whereas in hyperextension spondylolyses only the vertebral body is displaced anteriorly. Posterior translational displacement is typical of posterior dislocations.

Since the disk is damaged in all B3 injuries, surgical treatment is indicated, including fusion. Anterior fusion supplemented by tension band fixation or followed by postoperative immobilization in slight flexion can be applied in injuries with preserved stability in flexion. Posterior dislocations and some shear fracture dislocations require combined anterior and posterior stabilization or the application of a fixator system.

4.5.3
Type C

These injuries are unstable in axial torque. In most cases, instability in axial torque is superimposed on the instabilities already present in types A or B. Instability in torque is caused by the patterns of the vertebral fracture itself as well as by avulsion of soft-tissue attachments (e.g., disk, ligaments, muscles) and fractures of bony structures (e.g., transverse processes, ribs) which control rotation. Except for some incomplete lesions, the majority of type C injuries seen in clinical practice represent the most unstable injuries with the highest incidence of neurological deficit (Table 4.5). The potential for horizontal translation in every direction is present in the vast majority of cases, regardless of the radiographic appearance. Since these lesions can spontaneously reduce, translation may not be seen on any given set of radiographs.

Because of the high degree of instability and the poor healing potential of mainly discoligamentous rotational injuries, treatment should be surgical. Whereas in type A and B injuries the internal fixation must resist shortening, flexion, or extension, and sometimes sagittal shear, the system used for fixation of rotational injuries must additionally withstand axial torque and any shearing in the horizontal plane.

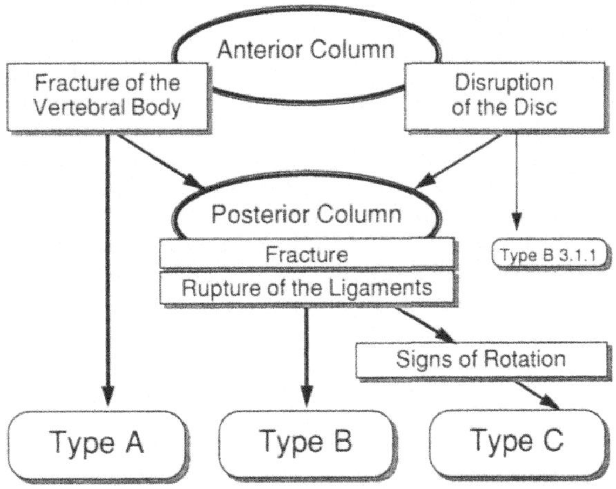

Fig. 4.27 Algorithm for determination of the injury types

4.6
Conclusions

Experience has shown that to a great extent this classification meets the previously outlined requirements. The injuries are logically grouped into different categories according to main mechanisms of injury and pathomorphological uniformity, and with prognostic aspects in mind. Its organization presents a progressive scale of morphological damage by which the degree of instability is determined. Thus, the severity of the injury in terms of instability is expressed by its ranking within this classification system. The degree of instability and prognostic aspects indicate the treatment to be applied.

The classification is comprehensive as almost any injury can be itemized according to easily recognizable and consistent radiographic and clinical findings. It can, however, also be used in an abbreviated form without impairment of the information most important for clinical practice. Recognition of the fundamental nature of an injury is facilitated by using a simple algorithm (Fig. 4.27).

Furthermore, the system presented also permits the classification of injuries occurring in the lower cervical spine (C3–7). Our current experience with the classification of these injuries has so far confirmed that they can be logically integrated into the new system without difficulty.

Any classification serves several purposes. Besides providing a common terminology, facilitating the choice of treatment is considered to be the main goal for clinical practice. We believe that this classification provides a sound basis for determining a rational approach to the management of the injuries, and that it will prove its value for documentation of the injuries and for future research.

References

1. Arciero R, Leung K, Pierce J (1989) Spontaneous unstable burst fracture of the thoracolumbar spine in osteoporosis. Spine 14: 114–117
2. Boger DC, Chandler RW, Pearce JG, Balciunas A (1983) Unilateral facet dislocation at the lumbosacral junction. J Bone Joint Surg [Am] 65: 1174–1178
3. Bohler L (1951) Die Technik der Knochenbruchbehandlung, 12–13 edn, vol 1. Maudrich, Vienna, pp 318–480
4. Bohler J (1983) Bilanz der konservativen und operativen Knochenbruchbehandlung – Becken und Wirbelsäule. Chirurg 54: 241–247
5. Chance CQ (1948) Note on a type of flexion fracture of the spine. Br J Radiol 21: 452–453
6. Conolly PI, Esses StI, Heggeness MH, Cook StS (1992) Unilateral facet dislocation of the lumbosacral junction. Spine 17: 1244–1248
7. De Oliviera J (1978) A new type of fracture-dislocation of the thoracolumbar spine. J Bone Joint Surg [Am] 60: 481–488
8. Delplace J, Tricoit M, Sillion D, Vialla IF (1983) Luxation postérieure de L5 sur le sacrum. A propos d'un cast Rev Chir Orthop 69: 141–145
9. Denis F (1982) Updated classification of thoracolumbar fractures. Orthop Trans 6: 8–9
10. Denis F (1983) The three column spine and its significance in the classification of acute thoracolumbar spinal injuries. Spine 8: 817–831
11. Denis F (1984) Spinal instability as defined by the three-column spine concept in acute spinal trauma. Clin Orthop 189: 65–76
12. Denis F, Burkus JK (1991) Lateral distraction injuries to the thoracic and lumbar spine. A report of three cases. J Bone Joint Surg [Am] 73: 1049–1053
13. Denis F, Burkus JK (1991) Diagnosis and treatment of cauda equina entrapment in the vertical lamina fracture of lumbar burst fractures. Spine [Suppl] 16: 433–439
14. Denis F, Burkus JK (1992) Shear fracture dislocation of the thoracic and lumbar spine associated with forceful hyperextension (lumberjack paraplegia). Spine 17: 156–161
15. Ferguson RL, Allen BL Jr (1984) A mechanistic classification of thoracolumbar spine fractures. Clin Orthop 189: 77–88
16. Fuentes JM, Bloncourt J, Bourbotte G, Castan P, Vlahovitch B (1984) La fracture du chance. Neurochirurgie 30: 113–118
17. Gertzbein SD, Court-Brown CM (1988) Flexion/distraction injuries of the lumbar spine. Mechanisms of injury and classification. Clin Orthop 227: 52–60
18. Gertzbein SD, Court-Brown CM (1989) The rationale for management of flexion/distraction injuries of the thoracolumbar spine, based on a new classification. J Spinal Disord 2: 176–183
19. Gertzbein SD, Offierski C (1979) Complete fracture-dislocation of the thoracic spine without spinal cord injury. A case report. J Bone Joint Surg [Am] 61: 449–451
20. Gumley G, Taylor TKF, Ryan MD (1982) Distraction fractures of the lumbar spine. J Bone Joint Surg [Br] 64: 520–525
21. Holdsworth FW (1963) Fractures, dislocations, and fracture dislocations of the spine. J Bone Joint Surg [Br] 45: 6–20
22. Holdsworth FW (1970) Review article: fractures, dislocations, and fracture-dislocations of the spine. J Bone Joint Surg [Am] 52: 1534–1551
23. Howland WJ, Curry JL, Buffington CD (1965) Fulcrum injuries of the lumbar spine. JAMA 193: 240–241
24. Jeanneret B, Ward J-C, Magerl F (1993) Pincer fractures: a therapeutic quandary. Rev Chir Orthop 79 (Spécial): Abstract 38
25. Jeanneret B, Ho PK, Magerl F (1993) "Burst-shear" flexion/distraction injuries of the lumbar spine. J Spinal Disord 6: 473–481
26. Lindahl S, Willen J, Norwall A, Irstam L (1983) The crush-cleavage fracture. A "new" thoracolumbar unstable fracture. Spine 8: 559–569
27. Lob A (1954) Die Wirbelsäulen-Verletzungen und ihre Ausheilung. Thieme, Stuttgart
28. Louis R (1977) Les théories de l'instabilite. Rev Chir Orthop 63: 423–425

29a Magerl F, Harms J, Gertzbein SD, Aebi M, Nazarian S (1990) A new classification of spinal fractures. Presented at the Société Internationale de Chirurgie Orthopédique et de Traumatologie (SICOT) Meeting, Montreal, September 9, 1990

29b Magerl F, Aebi M, Gertzbein SD, Harms J, Nazarian S (1994) A comprehensive classification of thoracic and lumbar injuries. Eur Spine J

30. Maruo S, Tatekawa F, Nakano K (1987) Paraplegie infolge von Wirbelkompressionsfrakturen bei seniler Osteoporose. Z Orthop 125: 320–323
31. McAfee PC, Yuan HA, Fredrickson BE, Lubicky JP (1983) The value of computed tomography in thoracolumbar fractures. An analysis of one hundred consecutive cases and a new classification. J Bone Joint Surg [Am] 65: 461–479
32. Müller ME, Nazarian S, Koch P (1987) Classification AO des fractures. I Les os longs. Springer-Verlag, Berlin Heidelberg New York
33. Nicoll EA (1949) Fractures of the dorso-lumbar spine. J Bone Joint Surg [Br] 31: 376–394
34. Powell J, Waddell J, Tucker W, Transfeldt E (1989) Multiple-level noncontiguous spinal fractures. J Trauma 29: 1146–1150
35. Rennie W, Mitchell N (1973) Flexion distraction injuries of the thoracolumbar spine. J Bone Joint Surg [Am] 55: 386–390
36. Roy-Camille R, Saillant G (1984) Les traumatismes du rachis sans complication neurologique. Int Orthop 8: 155–162
37. Roy-Camille R, Saillant G, Berteaux D, Marie-Anne S (1979) Early management of spinal injuries. In: McKibbin B (ed) Recent advances in orthopaedics 3. Churchill Livingstone, Edinburgh, pp 57–87
38. Roy-Camille R, Gagnon P, Catonne Y, Benazet JB (1980) La luxation antero-laterale du rachis lombo-sacre. Rev Chir Orthop 66: 105–109
39. Salomon C, Chopin D, Benoist M (1988) Spinal cord compression: an exceptional complication of spinal osteoporosis. Spine 13: 222–224
40. Sasson A, Mozes G (1987) Complete fracture-dislocation of the thoracic spine without neurologic deficit. A case report. Spine 12: 67–70
41. Shikata J, Yamamuro T, Iida H, Shimizu K, Yoshikawa J (1990) Surgical treatment for paraplegia resulting from vertebral fractures in senile osteoporosis. Spine 15: 485–489
42. Simpson AHRW, Williamson DM, Golding SJ, Houghton GR (1990) Thoracic spine translocation without cord injury. J Bone Joint Surg [Br] 72: 80–83
43. Smith WS, Kauter H (1969) Patterns and mechanics of lumbar injuries associated with lap seat belts. J Bone Joint Surg [Am] 51: 239–254

44. Trojan E (1972) Langfristige Ergebnisse von 200 Wirbelbrüchen der Brust- und Lendenwirbelsäule ohne Lähmung. Z Unfallmed Berufskr 65: 122–134
45. White AA III, Panjabi MM (1978) Clinical biomechanics of the spine. Lippincott, Philadelphia
46. Whitesides TE Jr (1977) Traumatic kyphosis of the thoracolumbar spine. Clin Orthop 128: 78–92
47. Willems MHA, Braakman R, Van Linge B (1984) Bilateral locked facets in the thoracic spine. Acta Orthop Scand 55: 300–303
48. Willen J, Lindahl S, Irstam L, Aldman B. Norwall A (1984) The thoracolumbar crush fracture. An experimental study on instant axial dynamic loading: the resulting fracture type and its instability. Spine 9: 624–630

CHAPTER 5

Stabilization Techniques: Upper Cervical Spine

Atlanto-axial fusions may be indicated in certain cases of acute or chronic atlanto-axial instability. There are a number of approaches and surgical techniques to stabilize the C1–2 segment. Anterior transoral techniques carry well-known risks, particularly infection. Both the lateral and the combined anterior/posterior techniques require two surgical approaches. For most lesions in the upper cervical spine, we prefer the posterior surgical approach.

5.1 Posterior Wiring Techniques

5.1.1 Standard Technique (After Gallie) (Fig. 5.1)

Principle
This technique provides a posterior stable construct for C1–2 instability particularly resistant to flexion forces.

Indications
- Fractures of the odontoid (dens) with anterior displacement.
- Rupture of the transverse ligament of C1.

Advantages
- Relatively easy technique.
- The graft firmly fixed between the two arches of C1 and C2.
- Aids in reduction of the anterior subluxation.

Disadvantages
- Sublaminar wiring technique.
- Cannot be used with associated fractures of the C1 arch.
- Is not suitable for posterior displacement of the atlas.

Surgical Technique
The patient is placed prone with Gardner-Wells traction or with a Mayfield clamp installed. Lateral image intensification is used to check position and reduction. A midline incision extends from the occiput to C4. The soft tissues are cleared from the occiput, C1 and C2. Lateral dissection beyond a maximum of 2 cm from the midline, particularly at C1, is avoided to prevent injury to the vertebral artery and venous plexus. The soft tissues are cleared circumferentially around the C1 posterior arch in the midline to allow easy passage of the wire.

A 1.2-mm wire is fashioned into a loop with a hook configuration. The wire is passed from the inferior aspect of C1 cranially and looped over the superior surface of C1 (Fig. 5.1a). The loop is carefully pulled backwards and distally sufficiently far to loop over the spinous process of C2 (Fig. 5.1b). Unless the vertebrae are sufficiently reduced prior to insertion of the wire, there is a risk of damage to the spinal cord during this process. The arch of C1 and the lamina of C2 are decorticated by means of a high-speed burr.

A cortico-cancellous rectangular bone graft measuring 34 cm is removed from the posterior iliac crest. The graft is fashioned into an H configuration to fit snugly around the spinous process and over the lamina of C2. It is also notched laterally (Fig. 5.1c).

The cancellous surface of the graft is shaped to conform with the slope of the arch of C1 and the lamina of C2 in order to provide maximal contact. The two free ends of the wire, which are laterally placed, are then brought across to the midline after the graft has been applied to the posterior surfaces of C1 and C2 (Fig. 5.1d). The notches provide better fixation of the bone graft when tightening the wires. During the process of tightening, the remaining reduction is achieved. Fragments of cancellous bone can then be packed around the bone graft between C1 and C2 (Fig. 5.1e).

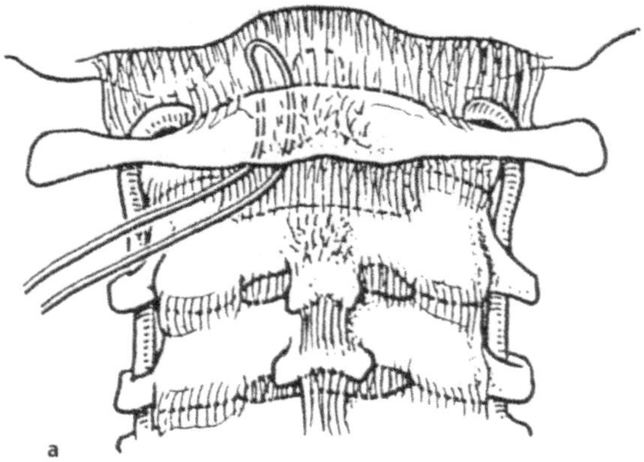

a

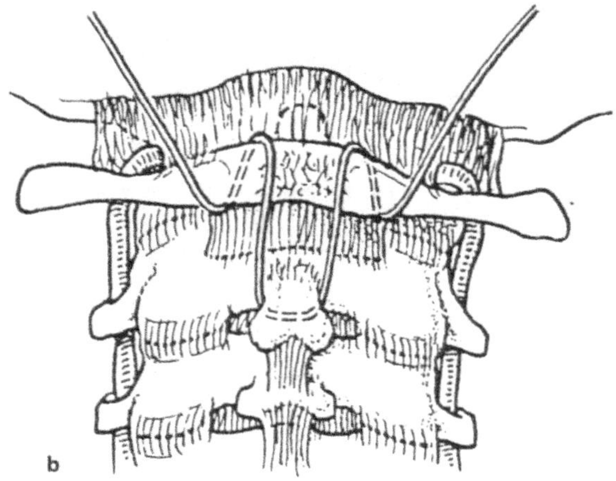

b

Fig. 5.1 Standard technique of C1–2 stabilization (Gallie).
a The 1.2-mm wire is fashioned into a loop with a hook configuration and then passed from the inferior aspect of C1 anteriorly and cranially and looped over the superior surface of C1
b The loop is carefully pulled backwards and distally sufficiently far to loop over the spinous process of C2
c A cortico-cancellous rectangular bone graft measuring 34 cm is fashioned into an H configuration to fit around the spinous process and over the lamina of C2
d The two free ends of the wire, which are laterally placed, are then brought across to the midline after the graft has been applied to the posterior surfaces of C1 and C2
e Fragments of cancellous bone can be packed around the bone graft between C1 and C2

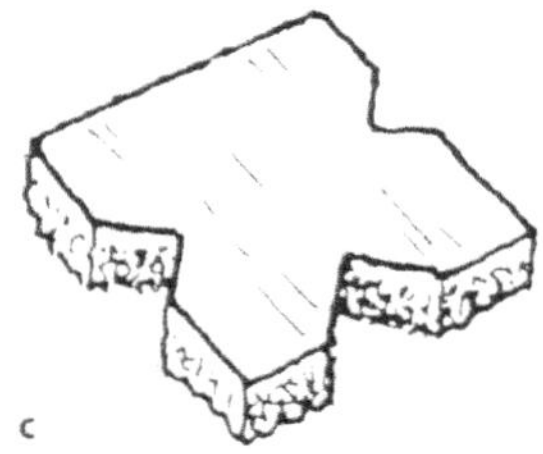

c

Postoperative Care
A firm collar preventing extension of the neck for a period of 6–10 weeks is recommended. It may be removed for daily care and, after 6 weeks, while resting.

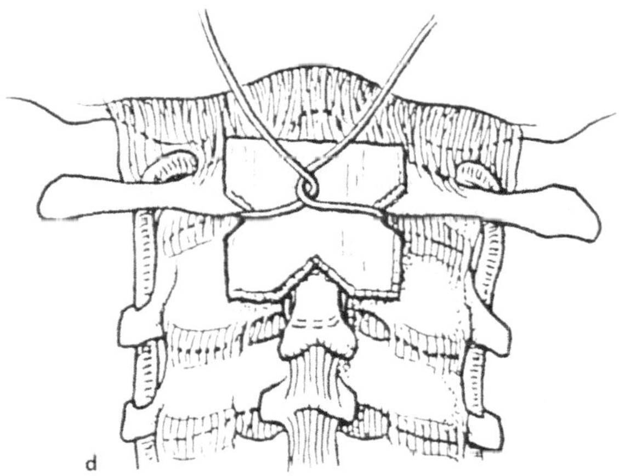

d

5.1.2 Wedge Compression Technique (After Brooks and Jenkins) (Fig. 5.2)

Principle
The construct is similar to that used in the standard technique but provides more rotational and tensile strength.

Indications
- Similar to those for the Gallie fusion, with the addition of posterior displacement of C1.

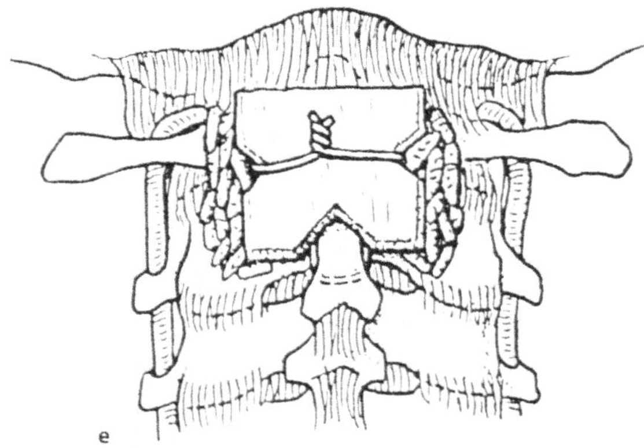

e

Advantage
- Biomechanically superior to the standard technique.

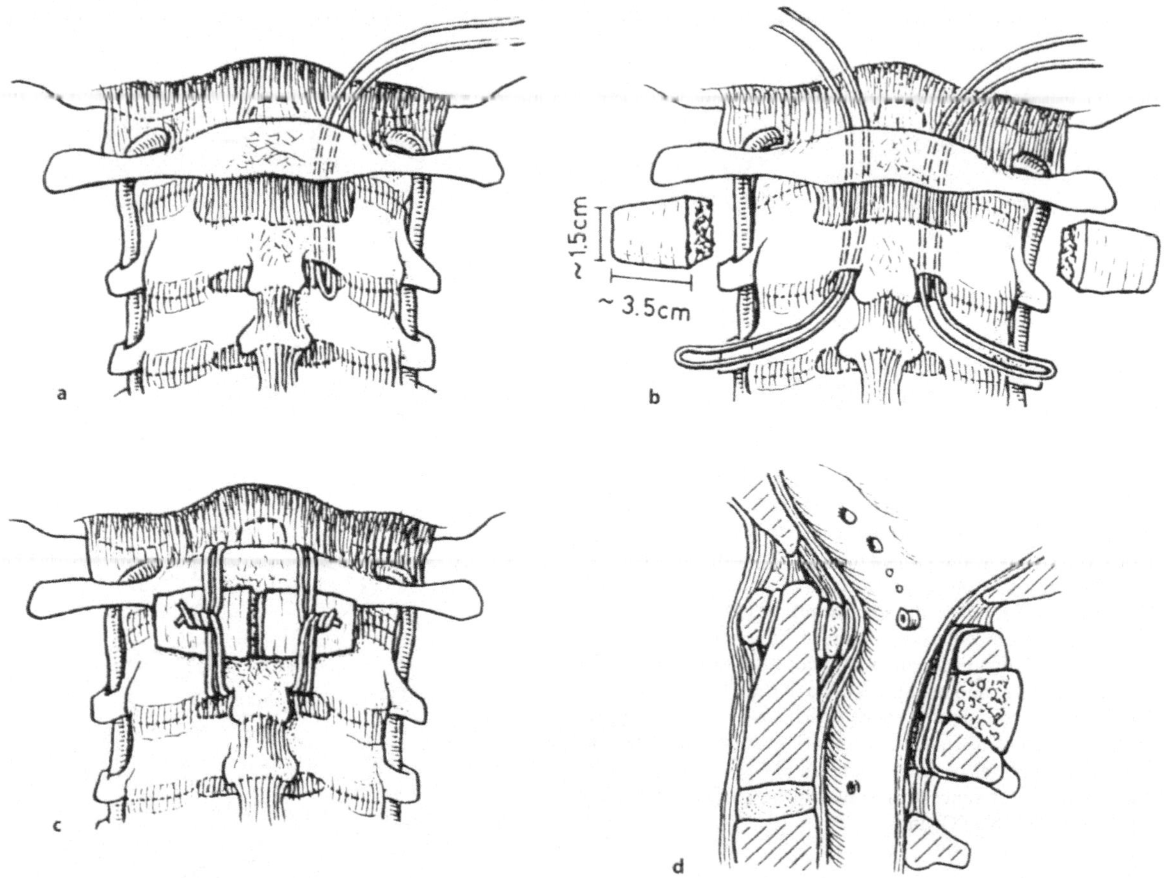

Fig. 5.2 C1–2 stabilization according to Brooks and Jenkins
a A wire loop is passed from the superior aspect of C1 around the arch of C1 and further distally beneath the lamina of C2
b A second wire is inserted on the opposite side. Two cortico-cancellous bone grafts measuring approximately 1.5 × 3.5 cm are fashioned into a wedge with the cortical portion posterior
c After the two wedges of bone have been placed between the two vertebral arches and after the undersurface of C1 and the superior surface of C2 have been decorticated, the double wires are then twisted to press the bone graft against the vertebral arches
d Lateral view

Disadvantages
- Requires the passage of sublaminar wires at two levels.
- Cannot be used for associated fractures of the C1 arch.

Surgical Technique
The approach is similar to that for the standard technique. In addition, the soft tissues anterior to the arch of C2 must be cleared, leaving the atlanto-axial membrane intact. A wire loop is then passed from the superior aspect of C1 around the arch of C1 and further distally beneath the lamina of C2 (Fig. 5.2a). A second wire is inserted on the opposite side (Fig. 5.2b). Two cortico-cancellous bone grafts, measuring approximately 1.5 × 3.5 cm, are taken from the posterior iliac crest. They are fashioned into a wedge with the cortical portion posterior. The wedges of bone are placed between the two vertebral arches after the undersurface of C1 and the superior surface of C2 have been decorticated by a high-speed burr (Fig. 5.2c). The double wires are then twisted to press the bone graft against the vertebral arches (Fig. 5.2d). One double wire provides the necessary stability, whereas four separate wires would just double the risk of neural injury.

Postoperative Care
Postoperative care is the same as in the standard technique.

5.2 Transarticular Screw Fixation

Indications

Acute and chronic atlanto-axial instability.

Advantages

- Biomechanically superior to wiring technique.
- Maintenance of reduction possible.
- Integrity of posterior arch of C1 is not necessary.

Disadvantage

- Technically demanding.

Instruments (Fig. 5.3)

- Drill guide.
- Cannulated 2.5-mm drill.
- Different screw sizes: 3.5-mm screw, 3.5-mm cannulated odontoid screw.
- Oscillating drill.
- Countersink (special).
- Special sleeve for K-wires.
- Measuring device for the protruding K-wires.
- Small hook or Penfield.

Surgical Technique

The patient lies in the prone position and the reduction of C1–2 is checked using lateral image intensifier control. The reduction is facilitated by either traction with Gardner-Wells tongs/Halo or a Mayfield clamp, the latter controlling translation more easily. The neck is flexed as much as possible to facilitate insertion of the screws, and the image intensifier is used to exclude redislocation.

A midline incision is performed from the occiput to the tip of the spinous process of C5. The arch of C1, the spinous processes, lamina and inferior articular processes of C2 and the lamina and articular masses of C3 are exposed subperiosteally. Persistent anterior dislocation of C1 or C2 may be reduced by pushing on the spinous process of C2 and/or by pulling gently on the posterior arch of C1, either with a towel clamp or with a sublaminar wire. Persistent posterior dislocation requires opposite forces.

A small dissector is used to expose the cranial surface of the lamina and isthmus of C2 by careful subperiosteal dissection up to the posterior capsule of the atlanto-axial joint (Fig. 5.4a).

Medial to the isthmus the atlanto-axial membrane is visible. The laterally situated vertebral artery is not exposed.

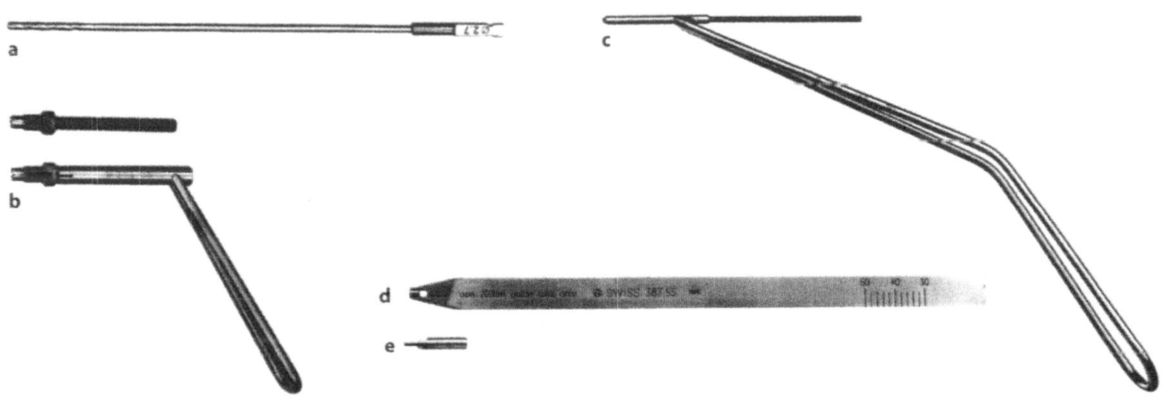

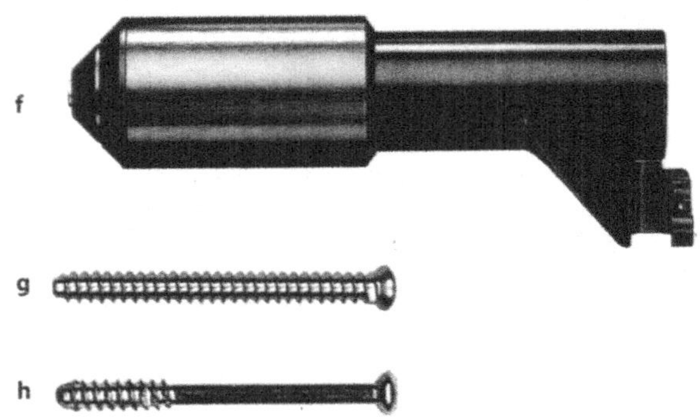

Fig 5.3
a Drill bit 2.5, cannulated
b Drill guide with stop
c Drill sleeve 1.25 mm flexible proximal tube
d Direct measuring device
e Countersink
f Oscillating drill attachment
g 3.5 mm cannulated screw, fully threaded
h 3.5 mm cannulated screw, short thread

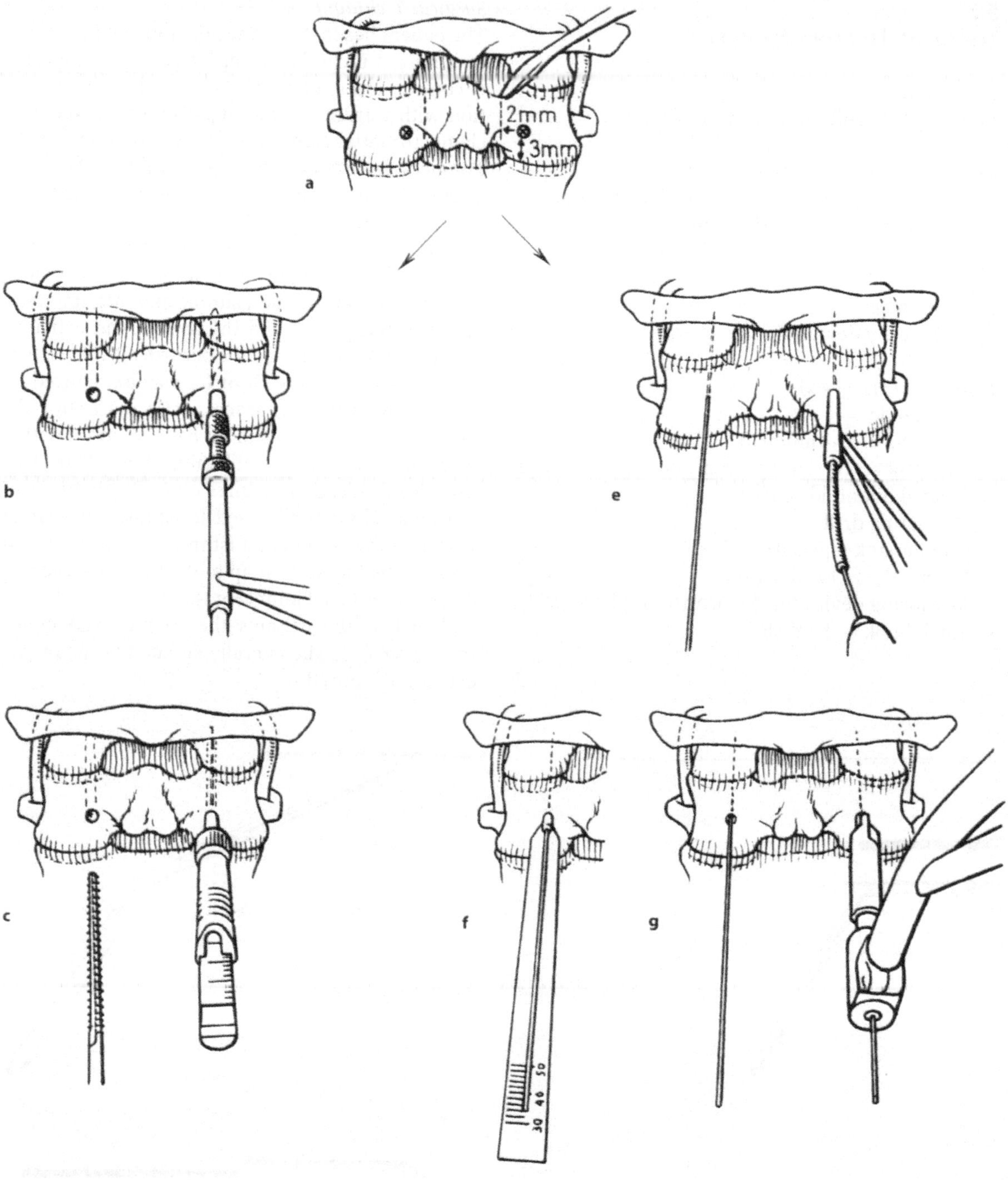

Fig. 5.4 Transarticular screw fixation of C1–2

a The small dissector is used to expose the cranial surface of the lamina and isthmus of C2 by careful subperiosteal dissection up to the posterior capsule of the atlanto-axial joint. The entry point is shown

b The entry point of the drill is at the lower edge of the caudal articular process of C2. The drill goes through the isthmus near to its posterior and medial surface. It then enters the lateral mass of the atlas

c Measuring of the screw length and tapping of the screw hole with the 3.5-mm cortical tap

d Insertion of 3.5-mm cortical screw with screwdriver

e Insertion of 1.5-mm K-wire with special drill sleeve (see Fig. 5.3c)

f Measuring the length of screw using the special measuring device

g Opening of near cortex with the countersink

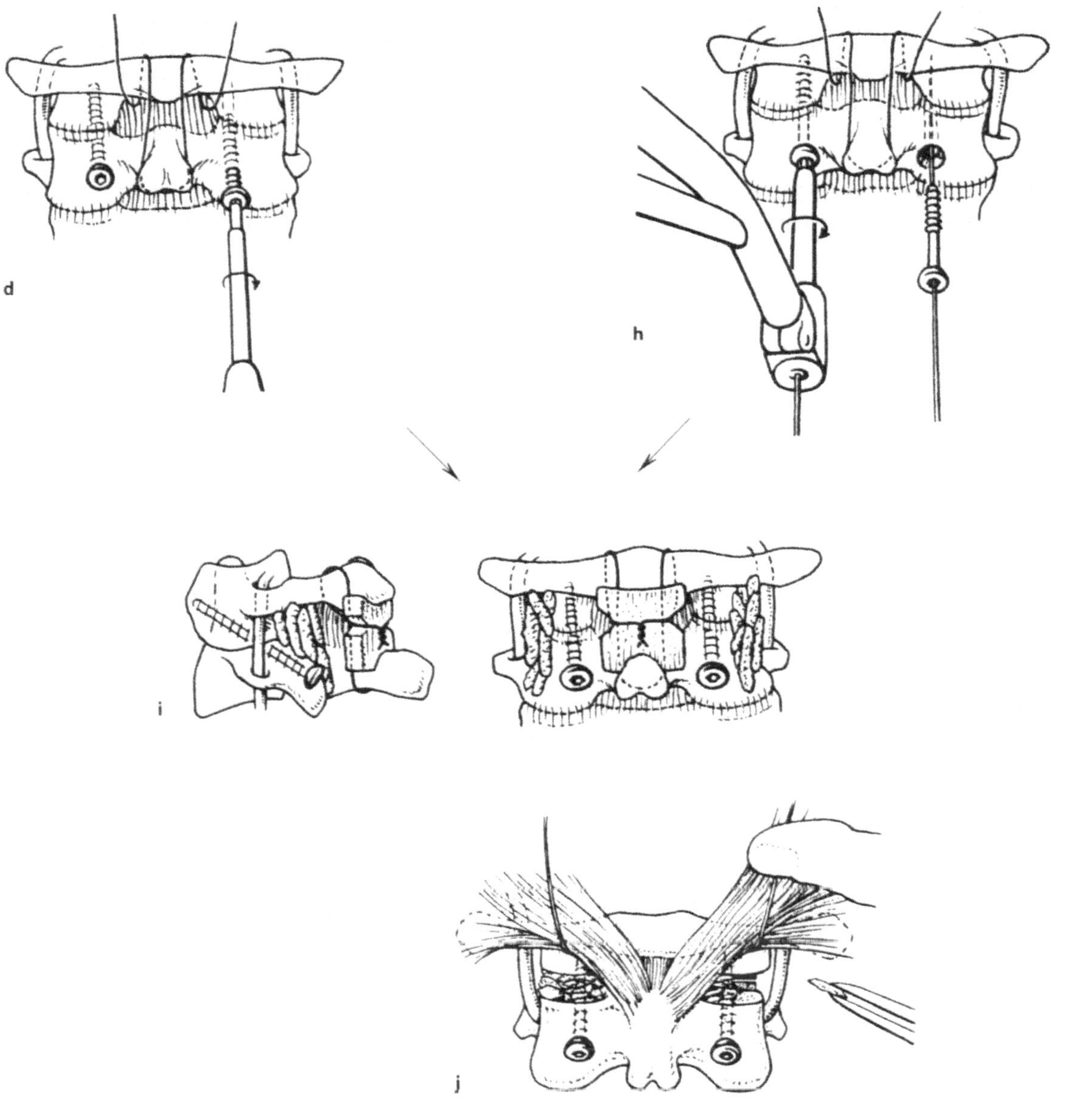

(Fig. 5.4)
h Insertion of the cannulated self-cutting odontoid type screw with the special angulated screwdriver
i Following bilateral screw fixation, a posterior C1–2 fusion is performed and the graft is supplemented with a posterior wiring technique
j Direct fusion of the atlanto-axial joints with insufficient stability of the posterior arch of C1 or absence of it: exposure of the atlanto-axial joint, removal of the cartilage of the posterior half of the facet joint, and packing of the resulting defect with cancellous bone

5.2.1 Standard Technique

Using lateral image intensifier control, a long 2.5-mm drill is inserted in a strictly sagittal direction (Fig. 5.4b). The oscillating drill prevents soft tissue being wrapped around the drill. The entry point of the drill is at the lower edge of the caudal articular processes of C2 (Fig. 5.4a). The drill goes through the isthmus near to its posterior and medial surface. It then enters the lateral mass of the atlas close to its posterior-inferior edge. Anteriorly, the drill perforates the cortex of the lateral mass of C1. The screw length is measured and the direction of the screw canal is checked using the image intensifier (Fig. 5.4c). The screws are inserted after tapping with a 3.5-mm cortical tap across the C1–C2 joint – the anterior cortex of C1 must not be tapped (Fig. 5.4d). Proper caudo-cranial drilling may sometimes be difficult because the neck muscles and the upper torso prevent the correct placement of the drill. Gently pulling the spinous process of C2 cranially with a towel clamp facilitates drilling. It is sometimes necessary to drill through a distal percutaneous stab wound in order to place the drill in the correct angle.

Drilling in a horizontal direction must be avoided because:

- At the level of C2 the vertebral artery runs upward anteriorly to the C1–C2 joint and could be damaged.
- The screw could exit C2 anteriorly and not enter the atlas.

5.2.2 Cannulated Screw Technique

Using lateral image intensifier control, 1.2-mm K-wire is inserted with a surgical drill guide in a strictly sagittal direction on each hole (Fig. 5.4e). The entry point/or the K-wire is at the lower edge of the caudal articular process of C2 (Fig. 5.4a). The length of the screw is established with a special ruler by measuring the protruding part of the guide wire (Fig. 5.4f). Before inserting the cannulated screw over the K-wire, the entrance for the screw is prepared by a cannulated special 3.5-mm countersink drill (Fig. 5.4g) in order to facilitate the starting bite of the screw. The appropriate self-cutting, cannulated 5-mm cancellous screw (same screw as for odontoid fixation, usually around 45 mm long) is inserted over the guide wires (Fig. 5.4h). The progress of the screw *must* be observed with an image intensifier to ensure that the Kirschner wire does not migrate proximally beyond the C1 arch.

In severe degenerative disease the sclerotic subcortical bone of the C2 joint may prevent insertion of the self-tapping screw. In this case a 2.7-mm cannulated drill is used to cross the joint and a cannulated fully threaded 3.5-mm screw can be inserted, after regular tapping of the drill hole.

Following bilateral screw fixation, a posterior C1–C2 fusion is performed. It is preferable to supplement the graft with a posterior wiring technique, as this increases the stability of the fixation and the fusion rate (Fig. 5.4i).

When there is a defect or fracture of the posterior arch of C1, a fusion of the atlanto-axial joint must be performed. For visualization of the atlanto-axial joint, Kirschner wires are drilled into the posterior aspect of the lateral mass of the atlas. For this purpose, the greater occipital nerve is retracted cranially, the soft tissues containing the greater occipital nerve, and its accompanying venous plexus can be retracted. The atlanto-axial joints are exposed by opening the posterior capsule, thus allowing visualization of the C1–C2 joint (Fig. 5.4k). The articular cartilage of the posterior half of the facet joint is removed with either a small chisel or a sharp curette, after which the joints are packed with cancellous bone and the screws are inserted.

Postoperative Care
Patients are immobilized in a firm collar for a period of 6–8 weeks but are allowed to remove the collar for daily care. After 6–8 weeks, the collar can be discarded when resting. If additional posterior wiring has been used, a soft collar can be worn instead of a firm collar.

5.3 Anterior Screw Fixation of Odontoid (Dens) Fractures (Figs. 5.5–5.9)

Implants and Instruments
The implants and instruments required are shown in Fig. 5.5 (see also Fig. 5.3).

Principle
The technique provides a direct screw fixation of a type II odontoid fracture, using the axial compression lag screw principle and avoiding a fusion of C1/C2 (Fig. 5.6a).

Indications
- The ideal indication is the transverse fracture of the neck of the odontoid process (type II and certain type III fractures).
- Nonunion of odontoid fracture.

Advantages
- This procedure preserves the C1–C2 motion segment.
- Simple postoperative care and immobilization.
- Anterior approach less traumatic than posterior surgery.

Disadvantages
- Should not be used in the oblique flexion fracture of the neck of the odontoid (Fig. 5.6b).
- Technically difficult or impossible in short-necked patients, in patients with limited motion of the cervical spine and in patients with pronounced kyphosis of the upper thoracic spine.

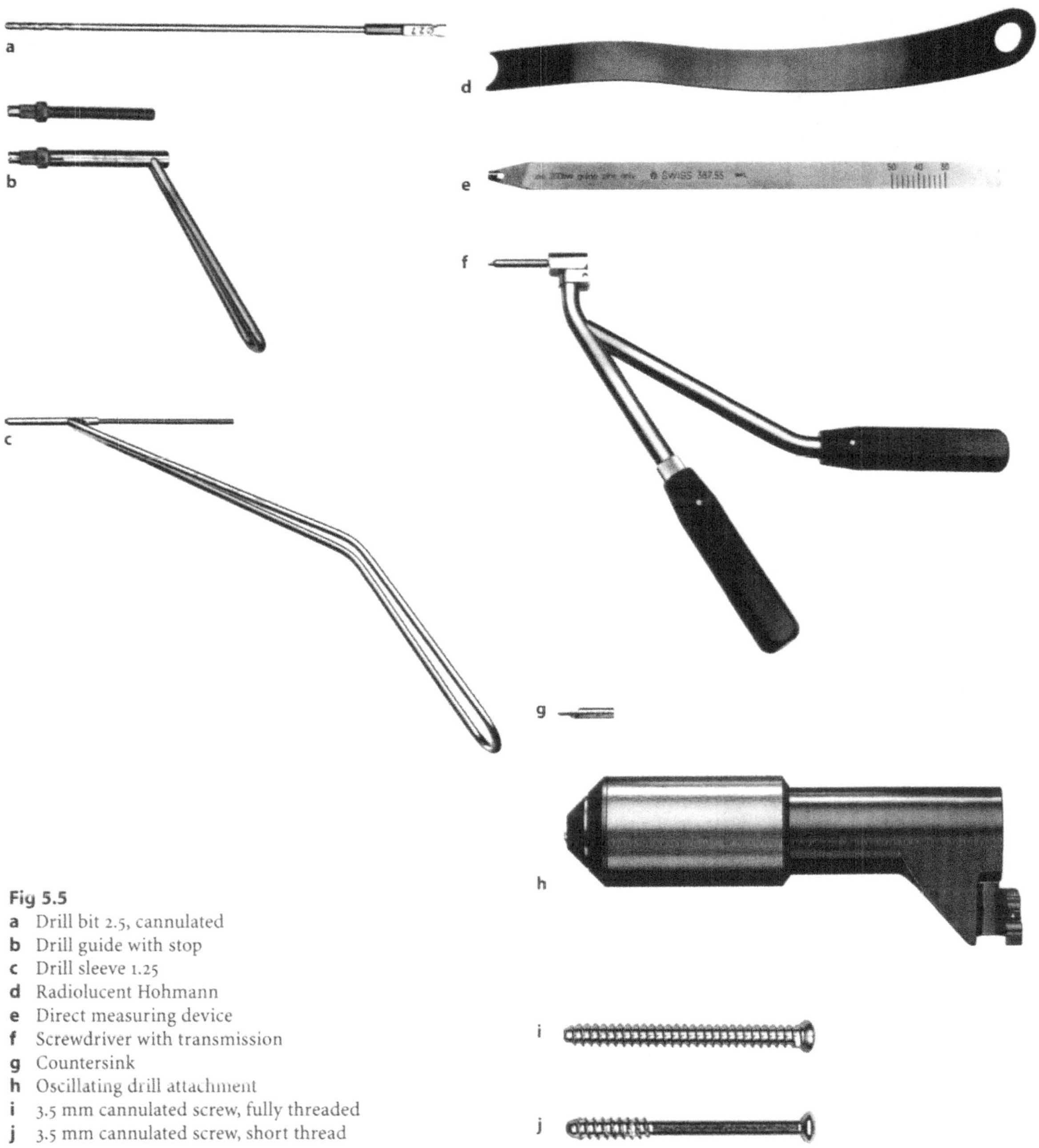

Fig 5.5
a Drill bit 2.5, cannulated
b Drill guide with stop
c Drill sleeve 1.25
d Radiolucent Hohmann
e Direct measuring device
f Screwdriver with transmission
g Countersink
h Oscillating drill attachment
i 3.5 mm cannulated screw, fully threaded
j 3.5 mm cannulated screw, short thread

- Requires high-resolution two-plane imaging (Fig. 5.7).
- Spinal stenosis is a contraindication because of the danger of cord injury associated with hyperextension of the neck.

Surgical Technique
The patient is in a supine position. Two image intensifiers are necessary to identify the odontoid process in the anteroposterior and lateral projections (Fig. 5.7). Without this help, this technique cannot be carried out. The head is placed in the extended position to reduce the fracture and to facilitate the insertion of the screws. An anteromedian approach is used. The placement of the incision is determined by placing a long Kirschner wire along the side of the neck in the intended direction of the screw and viewing on the image intensifier. The transverse incision can then be made in the neck where the K-wire is likely to exit the skin.

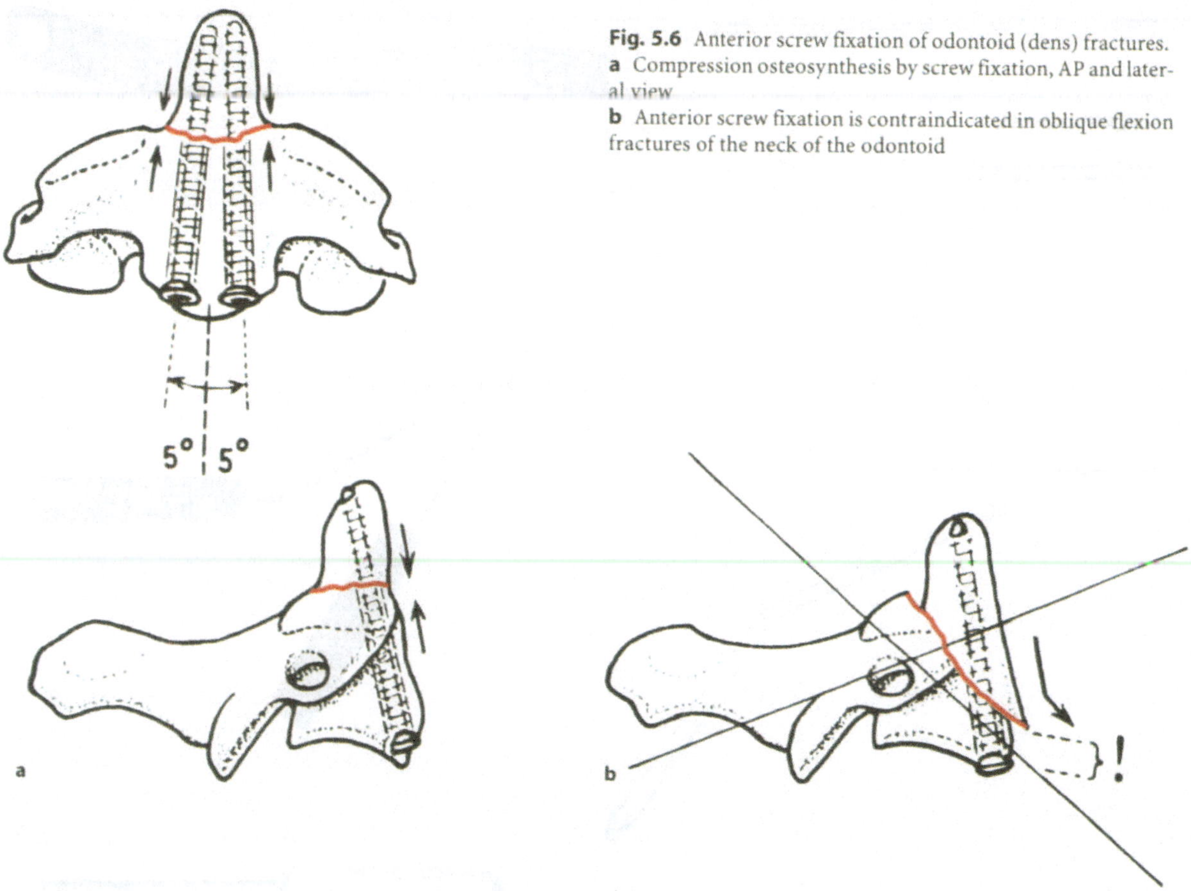

Fig. 5.6 Anterior screw fixation of odontoid (dens) fractures.
a Compression osteosynthesis by screw fixation, AP and lateral view
b Anterior screw fixation is contraindicated in oblique flexion fractures of the neck of the odontoid

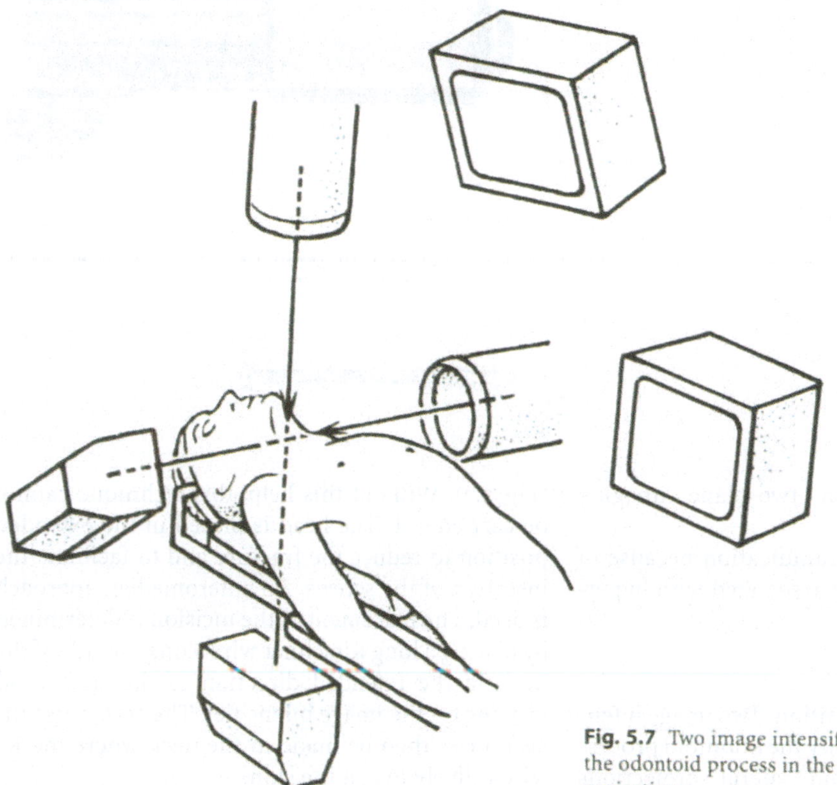

Fig. 5.7 Two image intensifiers are necessary to identify the odontoid process in the anteroposterior and lateral projections

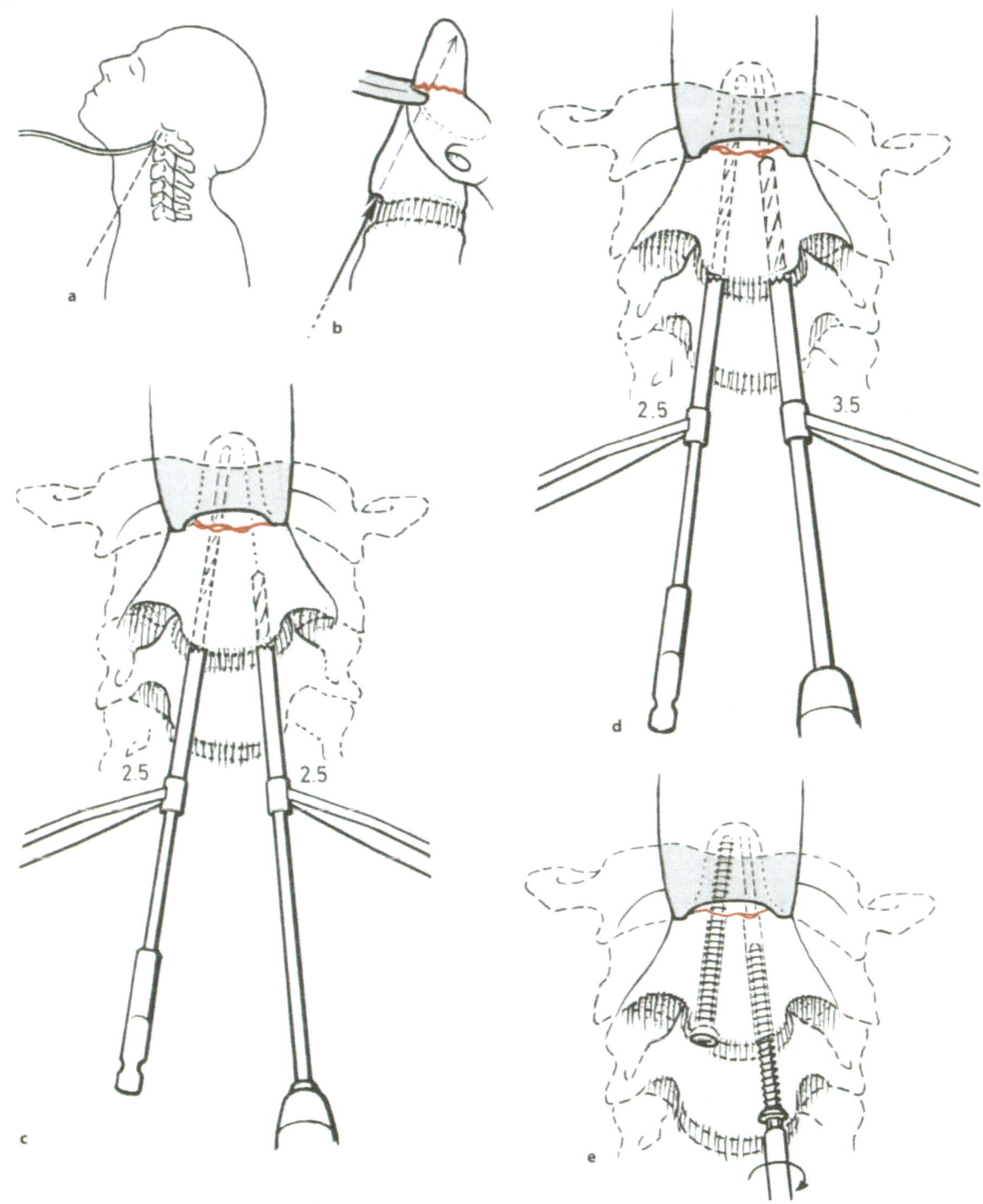

Fig. 5.8 Exposure of the segment C2–3

a Two Hohmann retractors are inserted, one on either side of the odontoid, to expose the body of the axis, or a special large radiolucent carbon fiber Hohmann can be used (as shown in the figure)

b A long 2.5-mm drill is inserted into the antero-inferior edge of the C2 body. In the sagittal plane, the drill should be angled slightly posteriorly in order to exit at the posterior half of the tip of the odontoid

c In the frontal plane the drill should be angled a few degrees towards the midline. A second drill is inserted in the same manner

d One drill is removed and the entire hole in the distal fragment is overdrilled using a 3.5 mm drill

e Insertion of a 3.5 mm cortical screw with a screwdriver

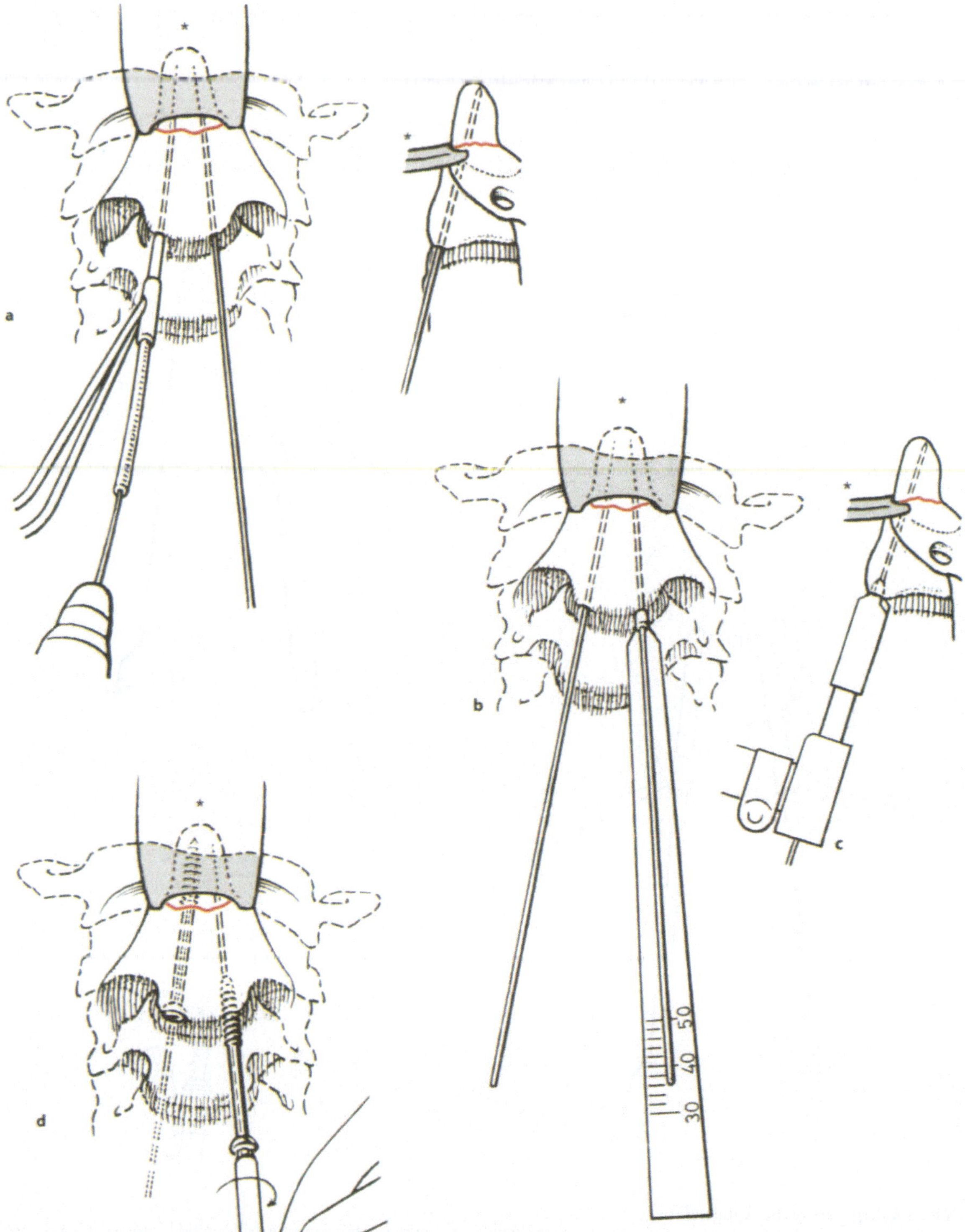

Fig. 5.9
a Insertion of a 1.2-mm K-wire with a special drill sleeve (see Fig. 5.3c)
b Measuring the length of screw using a specialized designed ruler
c Opening of near cortex with the cannulated countersink
d Insertion of the cannulated self-cutting odontoid-type screw with the special angled screwdriver
* Radiolucent Hohmann (see Fig. 5.5d)

The vertebral column is exposed anteriorly by blunt dissection and then exposed cranially until the inferior edge of the body of the second cervical vertebra is identified. Two Hohmann retractors or a specially curved radiotranslucent retractor are then inserted on either side of the odontoid (dens) to expose the body of the axis (Fig. 5.8a-c).

5.3.1 Standard Lag Screw Technique (Fig. 5.8a-e)

A long 2.5-mm drill is inserted into the anterior inferior edge of the C2 body. In the sagittal plane, the drill should be angled slightly posteriorly in order to exit at the posterior half of the tip of the odontoid (Fig. 5.8a, b, see also Fig. 5.9a, c). Furthermore, in the frontal plane, the drill should be angled a few degrees towards the midline (Fig. 5.8c). A second drill is inserted in the same manner (Fig. 5.8c). One drill is removed and the entire hole in the distal fragment is overdrilled by a 3.5-mm drill (Fig. 5.8d). The depth of the hole to the tip of the odontoid is measured, tapped and the appropriate-length 3.5-mm cortex screw inserted (Fig. 5.8e). The same technique is used for the second screw.

It is absolutely essential that tissue protectors are used when drilling and tapping, to avoid damaging vital structures. *The oscillating attachment should be used to avoid soft tissue damage.*

In patients of small stature, 2.7-mm screws are used with their appropriate drills and tap.

5.3.2 Cannulated Screw Technique (Fig. 5.9)

To facilitate the placement of screws and decrease the risk of neurovascular damage, a cannulated screw technique has been developed, which is based on the odontoid cannulated screw set. Using lateral image intensifier control, a 20-cm-long 1.2-mm-diameter K-wire is inserted in a strictly sagittal direction on both sides. The K-wire should be angled slightly posteriorly in order to exit the posterior half of the tip of the odontoid. Furthermore, in the frontal plane, the K-wire should be angled a few degrees towards the midline (Fig. 5.9a). The length of K-wire in the bone is measured with the special ruler (Fig. 5.9b), indicating the length of screw required. In order to allow the self-cutting screw to start in the near cortex, it is perforated with the special cannulated countersink (Fig. 5.9c). The appropriate-length odontoid screw is inserted using the special cannulated screwdriver (Fig. 5.9d).

N.B. During insertion of the cannulated odontoid screw, it is essential to observe this on the lateral image-intensifier to ensure the K-wire does not advance anteriorly.

Postoperative Care

Patients are immobilized in a firm collar for a period of 10 – 12 weeks but are allowed to remove the collar for daily care. After 6 weeks, the collar can be discarded when resting. If additional posterior wiring has been used, a firm collar need only be worn for 3 weeks.

CHAPTER 6

Stabilization Techniques: Lower Cervical Spine

6.1 Posterior Techniques

6.1.1 Wiring Technique

There are many wiring techniques for posterior fixation of the lower cervical spine. The most simple and least dangerous is interspinous wiring (Fig. 6.1).

Principle
This technique applies the tension band principle.

Indications
- Injuries of the posterior complex involving predominantly soft tissue with insignificant damage to the vertebral body.
- Enhancement of other posterior fusion techniques.

Advantages
- Relatively easy.
- Safe.
- Large surface area for fusion.
- Short segment stabilization.

Disadvantages
- Wire breakage.
- Wire cut-out.
- Cannot be used in fractures of the vertebral arch including the spinous processes.
- Poor biomechanical fixation – especially in rotation.
- Failure to maintain lordosis.

Surgical Technique
A midline posterior approach is used. It is essential to identify radiographically the levels to be fused. A hole is drilled on each side of the base of the spinous process of the upper vertebra of the injured segment (Fig. 6.1a). The entry point corresponds to the junction of the base of the spinous process and the lamina. A towel clip is placed in the holes, and with a gently rocking movement the holes are connected (Fig. 6.1b). A 1.2-mm wire is passed through the hole and then around the base of the inferior spinous processes, leaving the interspinous soft tissue intact (Fig. 6.1c). The two ends of the wires are tightened. Lastly, the wire ends are curved around the inferior spinous process and twisted tight (Fig. 6.1d). The laminae are decorticated with a high-speed burr, and the cancellous bone graft is applied (Fig. 6.1e).

Postoperative Care
Postoperative care is similar to that for the posterior wiring techniques for the atlas and axis described above.

6.1.2 Plate Technique

6.1.2.1 Screw Placement

6.1.2.1.1 Mid and Lower Cervical Spine (Fig. 6.2)

Viewed from dorsally a valley exists at the junction of the lamina and lateral mass. Directly anteriorly lies the vertebral artery and the most posterior aspect of the exiting nerve root. Screws placed into the lateral mass must start lateral to the valley and can be directed outward to avoid neurovascular damage. Screw placement from C3–C7 is in the lateral mass and not transpedicular.

Following exposure, the boundaries of the lateral mass are identified. The medial border is the valley at the junction of the lamina and lateral mass. The lateral boundary is the far edge of the lateral mass. The superior and inferior borders are the respective cranial and caudal facet joints.

According to Magerl, the starting point for screw insertion is 2 mm medial to the center of the lateral mass (Fig. 6.2a). The screw orientation is about $20°-25°$ outwards (Fig. 6.2b) and $30°-40°$ cranially. The cranial angulation attempts to parallel the facet joints (Fig. 6.2c). An alternative technique has been described by Roy-Camille (1980), where screws are placed perpendicular to the posterior cortex in the sagittal direction (Fig. 6.2e, f). The entry point is the junction of the upper and middle third of the lateral

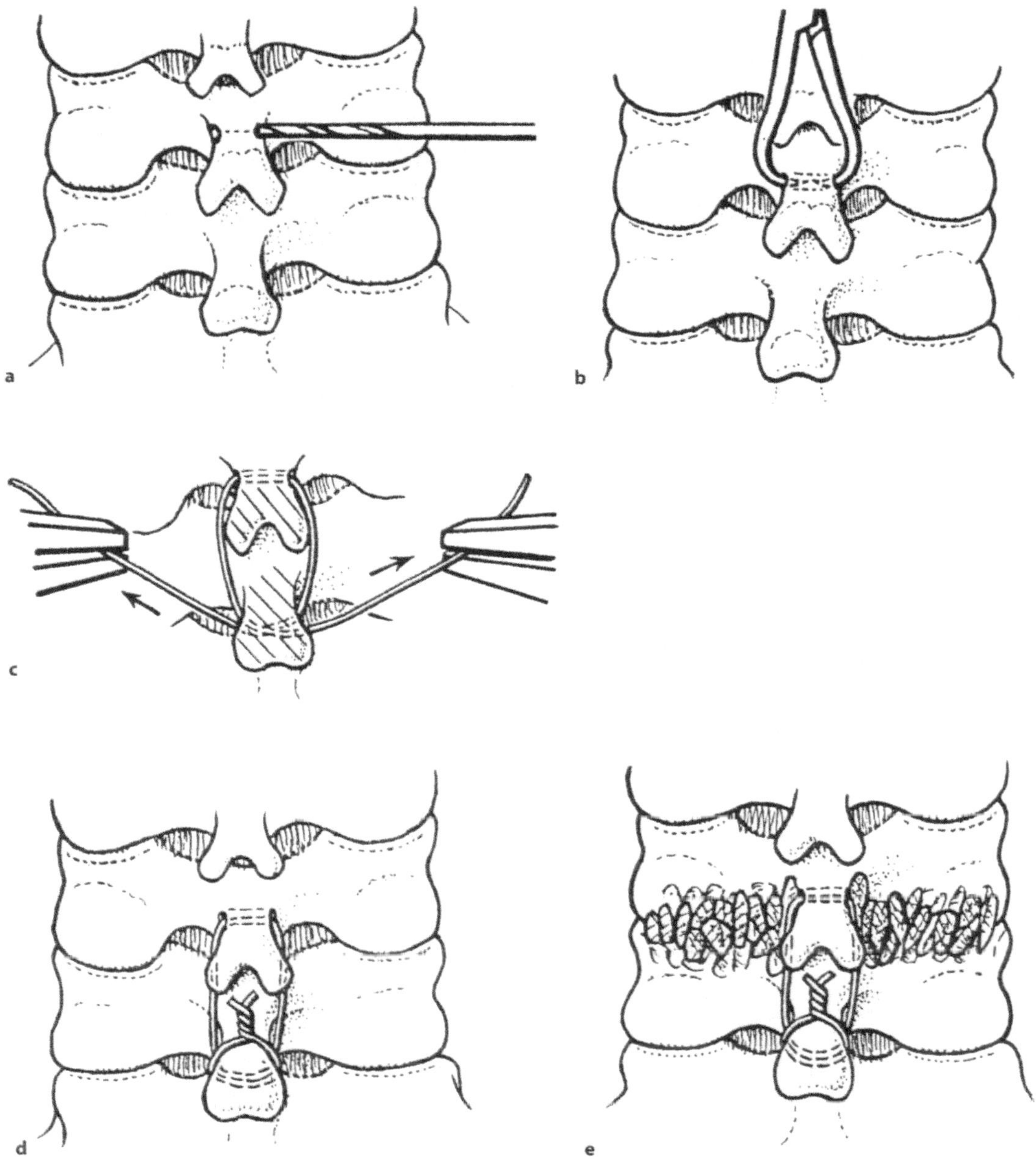

Fig. 6.1 Interspinous wiring of the lower cervical spine
a A hole is made on each side of the base of the spinous process of the upper vertebra of the injured segment, using a drill
b The two tips of a towel clamp are placed in the holes, and with a gentle rocking movement the holes are connected
c A 1.2-mm wire is passed through the hole and then around the base of the inferior spinous process, leaving the interspinous soft tissues intact
d The two ends of the wire are tightened, curved around the inferior spinous process and twisted tight
e The lamina are decorticated and cancellous bone graft is applied

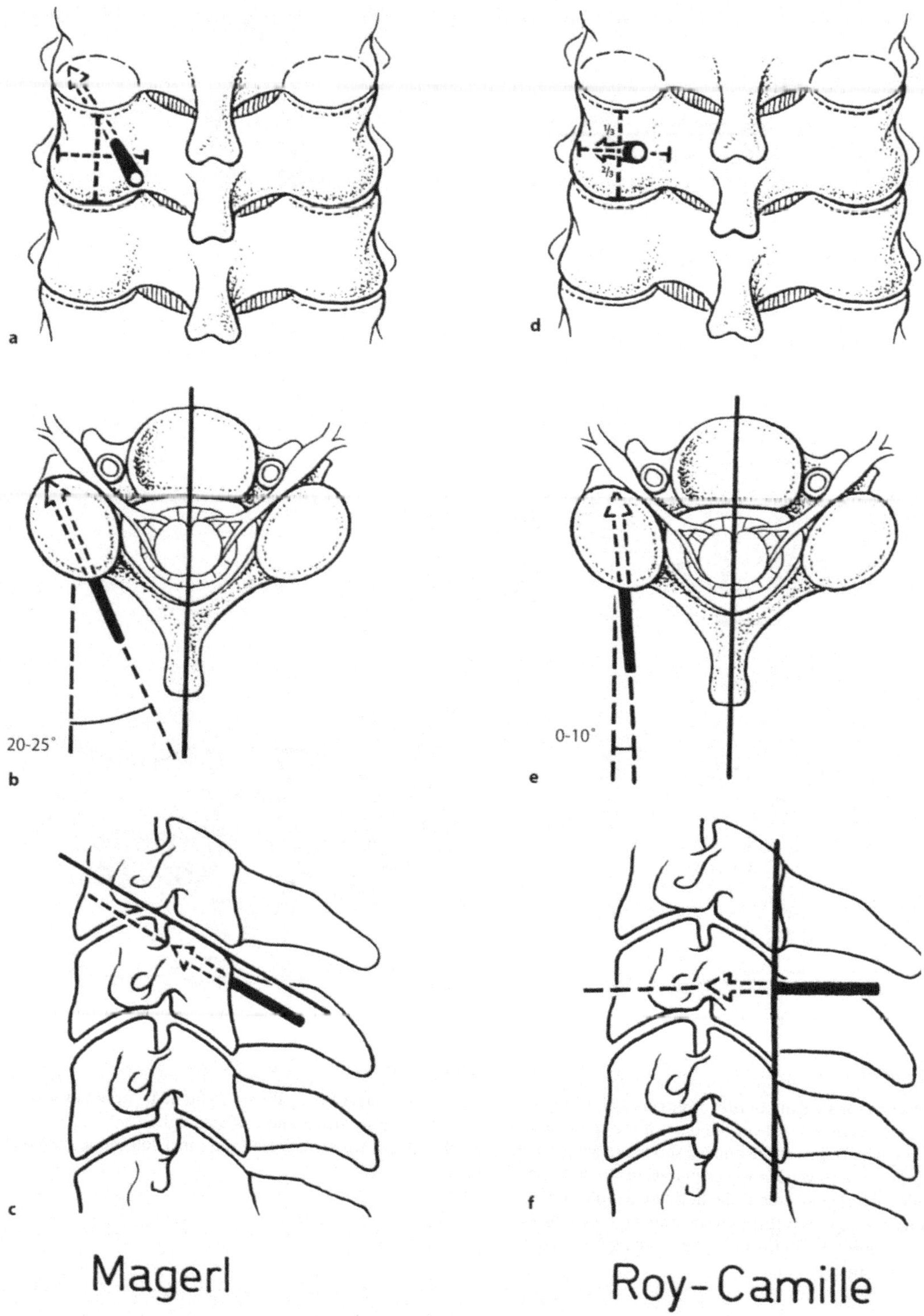

Fig. 6.2 Screw technique
a The entry point for the screws lies 2 mm medially and cranially to the center of the articular mass
b Each screw diverges by 20°–25° anterolaterally and runs parallel to the surface of the intervertebral joints. Note the relationship to the neuromuscular structures
c The inclination of the surface can be determined by inserting a fine dissector into the joint
d–f The alternative technique according to Roy-Camille

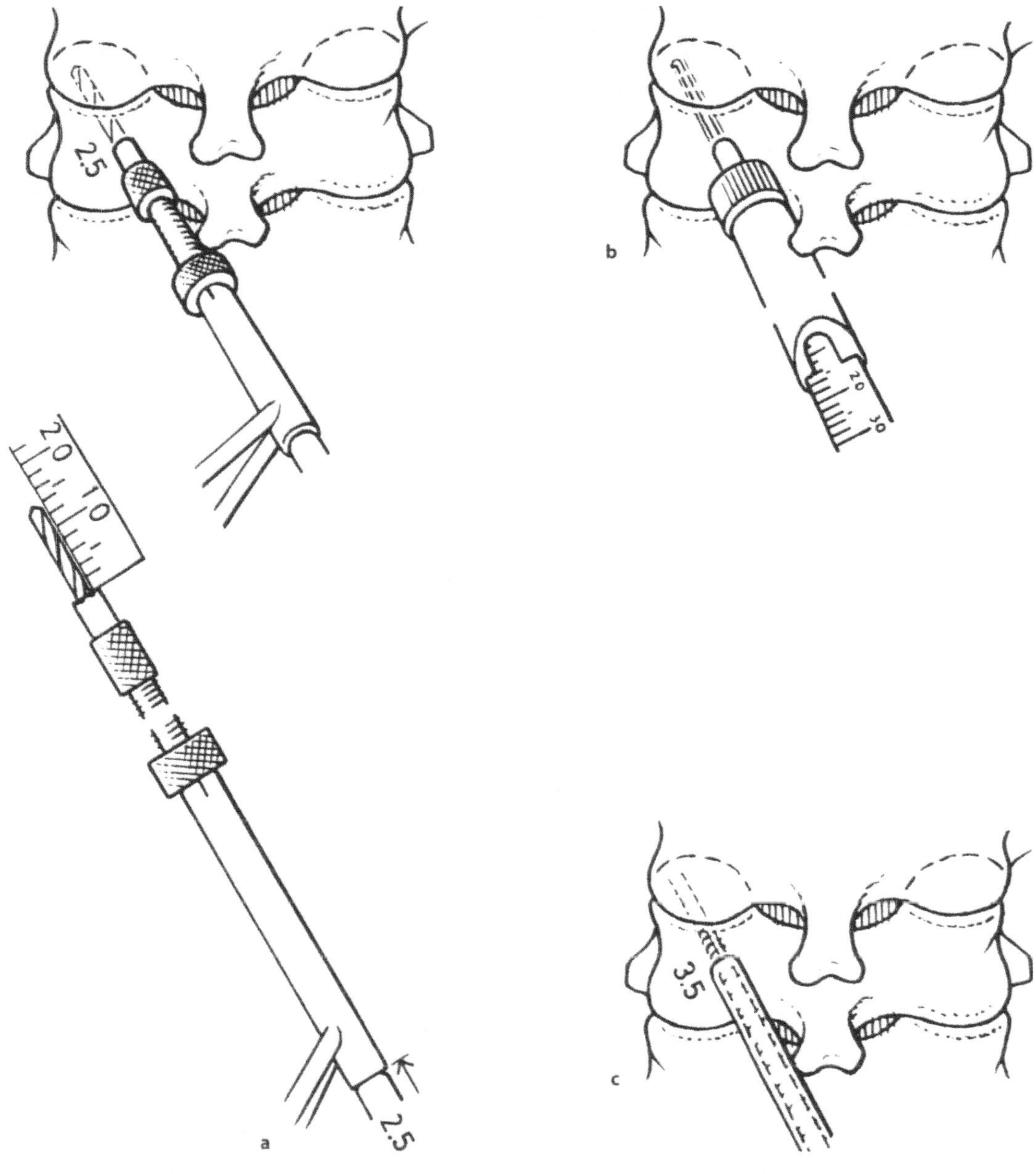

Fig. 6.3 Drilling of the lateral mass
a A 2.5-mm drill with an adjustable drill guide is used. The drill guide is primarily set at 14 mm. The adjustable drill guide is increased by 2-mm increments until the drill then penetrates the far cortex
b The hole is checked for penetration with the depth gauge
c The proximal cortex only is tapped with the 3.5-mm cancellous tap

mass in the midline (Fig. 6.2d). However, we do not recommend it as a standard technique because screw length is shorter and the purchase in bone is less satisfactory. We feel there is more likelihood of damage to neurovascular structures.

Once the starting point has been identified, a 2.5-mm drill is used. An adjustable 2.5-mm drill guide is set to allow an initial maximal penetration of 14 mm (Fig. 6.3a). The length of the adjustable drill guide is increased by 2-mm increments until the drill penetrates the far cortex. The hole is checked for penetration with a depth gauge (Fig. 6.3b) and the depth is measured. The *proximal cortex only* is tapped with a 3.5-mm cancellous tap (Fig. 6.3c).

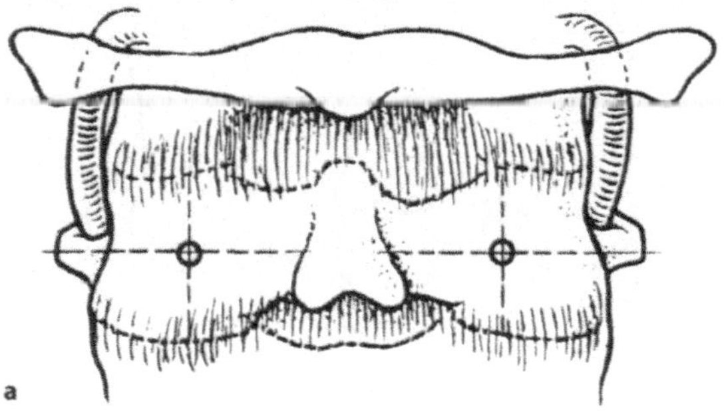

a

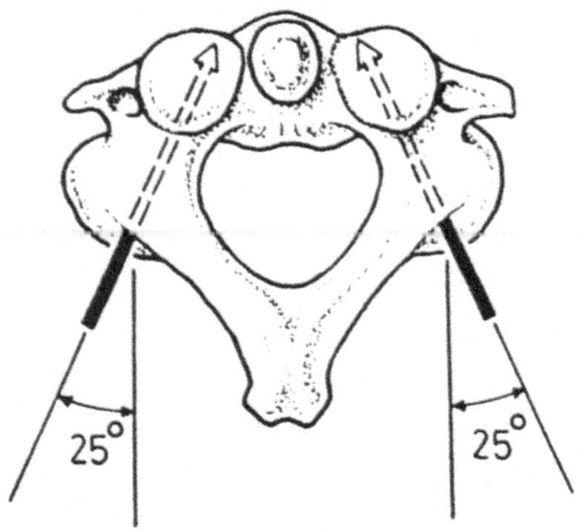

b

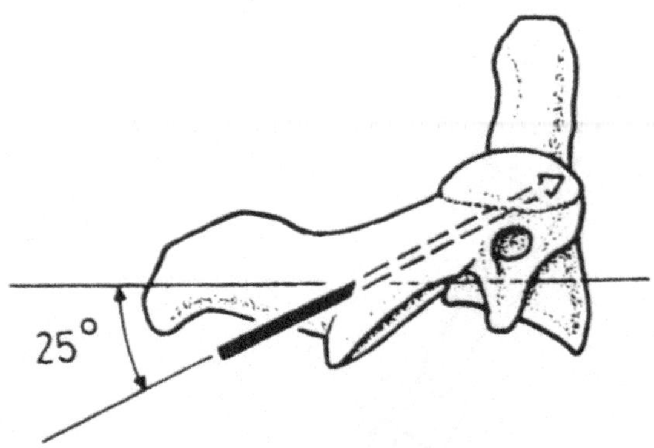

c

Fig. 6.4 Screws inserted into the lateral mass of C2
a Entry point for the drill halfway between the upper and lower articular surfaces of C2 at a vertical line bisecting the articular mass
b The screw is oriented 25° upwards
c The screw is oriented 15°–25° medially

6.1.2.1.2
Upper Cervical Spine (Fig. 6.4)

Screws inserted into C2 must be directed medially and passed through the isthmus of C2 to avoid injury to the vertebral artery. The directions are determined by subperiosteal dissection of the soft tissues from the superior aspect of the isthmus. The dissector is placed medial to the isthmus to identify the medial border in order to prevent penetration of the drill to the spinal canal. The drill is inserted halfway between the upper and lower articular surfaces of C2 at a vertical line bisecting the articular mass (Fig. 6.4a). The screw is oriented 25° upwards (Fig. 6.4b) and 15°–25° medially (Fig. 6.4c).

A 2.5-mm drill is used with the adjustable drill guide as described above. The anticipated length of the drill hole is 30–35 mm.

6.1.2.1.3
Upper Thoracic Spine from T1–T3 (Fig. 6.5) (See Chap. 7.2.2, Pedicle Fixation)

Upper thoracic screws are placed in the pedicles rather than in the articular mass. The point of entry is just below the rim of the upper facet joint 3 mm lateral to the center of the joint near the base of the transverse process (Fig. 6.5a). The screws should be angled 7°–10° toward the midline (Fig. 6.5b) and 10°–20° caudally (Fig. 6.5c).

6.1.2.1.4
Occiput Screws (Fig. 6.6)

Screws can be placed safely in the occiput but this requires a careful understanding of the occipital anatomy. Screws should not be placed above the inion to avoid damage to the intracranial sinus. The bone present in the midline allows strong screw purchase 2–3 mm lateral from the midline the occipital cortex becomes thin (Fig. 6.6a). Drilling and screw placement must avoid injury to the cerebellum although dural lacerations with CSF leak are not uncommon and are dealt with by screw insertion into the drill hole.

In the midline of the occiput a 2.5-mm drill is used with an adjustable drill guide initially set at 8 mm and increased by 2-mm increments until the far cortex is penetrated. The oscillating drill is used to prevent soft tissue from wrapping around the

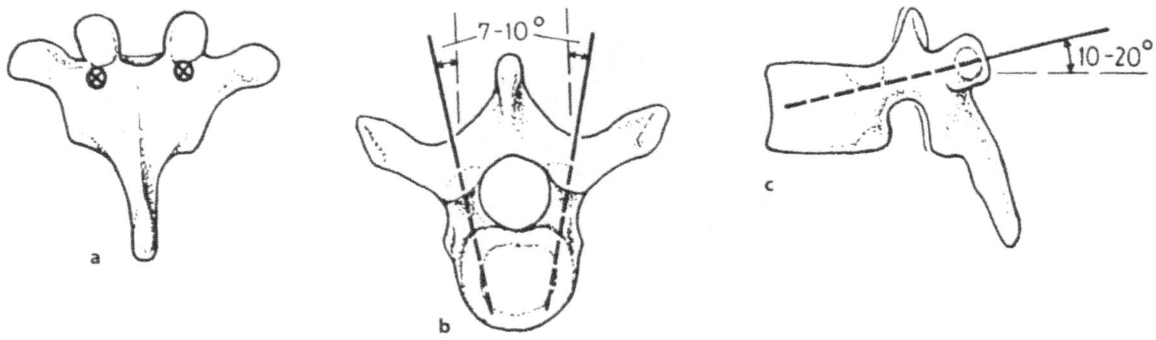

Fig. 6.5 Upper thoracic screws in T1–T13
a Entry point below the rim of the upper facet joint 3 mm lateral to the center of the joint
b Screw direction 7°–10° towards the midline
c Screw direction 10°–20° caudally in the sagittal plane

drill (Fig. 6.6b). The thickness of the cortex *lateral to the midline is only 5–7 mm* and care must be taken in using the drill. After each drilling procedure, the hole is checked for penetration with a depth gauge, and when penetration of the distal cortex has occurred the depth is measured (Fig. 6.6c). A 3.5-mm cortical tap is used and must include the far cortex (Fig. 6.6d); the 3.5-mm screws are then inserted (Fig. 6.6e).

6.1.2.2 3.5-mm Cervical Titanium Plate

6.1.2.2.1 *Plate Fixation in the Middle and Lower Cervical Vertebrae (C2–C7) (Fig. 6.6)*

Principle

The posterior plating technique provides stable tension band fixation in flexion, increasing stability in rotation, and buttressing in extension.

Indications

- Ligamentous and/or osseous lesions of the posterior complex without significant damage of the vertebral body.
- Uni- or multisegmental instability.
- Instability associated with deficiency of the posterior elements from laminectomy or fractures, e.g.,
  - Trauma
  - Tumor
  - Failed anterior fusion

Advantages

- Superior stability compared with wiring techniques.
- Can be used in the presence of lamina and spinous process fractures.

Disadvantages

- Potential for neurovascular damage.
- Ideal screw placement may be compromised by the spacing of the holes.
- Demanding surgical technique.

Surgical Technique (Fig. 6.7)

A midline posterior approach is performed. It is essential to identify the levels to be fused with radiographs. Subperiosteal preparation of the laminae and lateral masses is carried out. The entry points and directions have been previously described. The most cranial and caudal vertebrae of the selected area of fusion are drilled, K-wires inserted into the drill holes (Fig. 6.7a) and the small titanium template with hole spacings of 8 mm and 12 mm is used to assess whether the 8-mm or 12-mm plate will fit the proximal and distal drill holes (Fig. 6.7b): the template is also contoured to create the cervical lordosis. The chosen titanium plate is contoured to match the template and applied to the spine. The proximal and distal holes are measured through the titanium plate (Fig. 6.7c); *only the near cortex is tapped* (Fig. 6.7d). Prior to screw insertion, the posterior surface of the facet joints is decorticated and packed with autogenous cancellous bone graft. The plate is fixed to the lateral masses cranially and caudally with 3.5-mm cancellous screws in the drill holes (Fig. 6.7e). The intervening lateral masses are now drilled in the correct direction, the depth measured and the near cortices tapped and the appropriate length screws inserted (Fig. 6.7f).

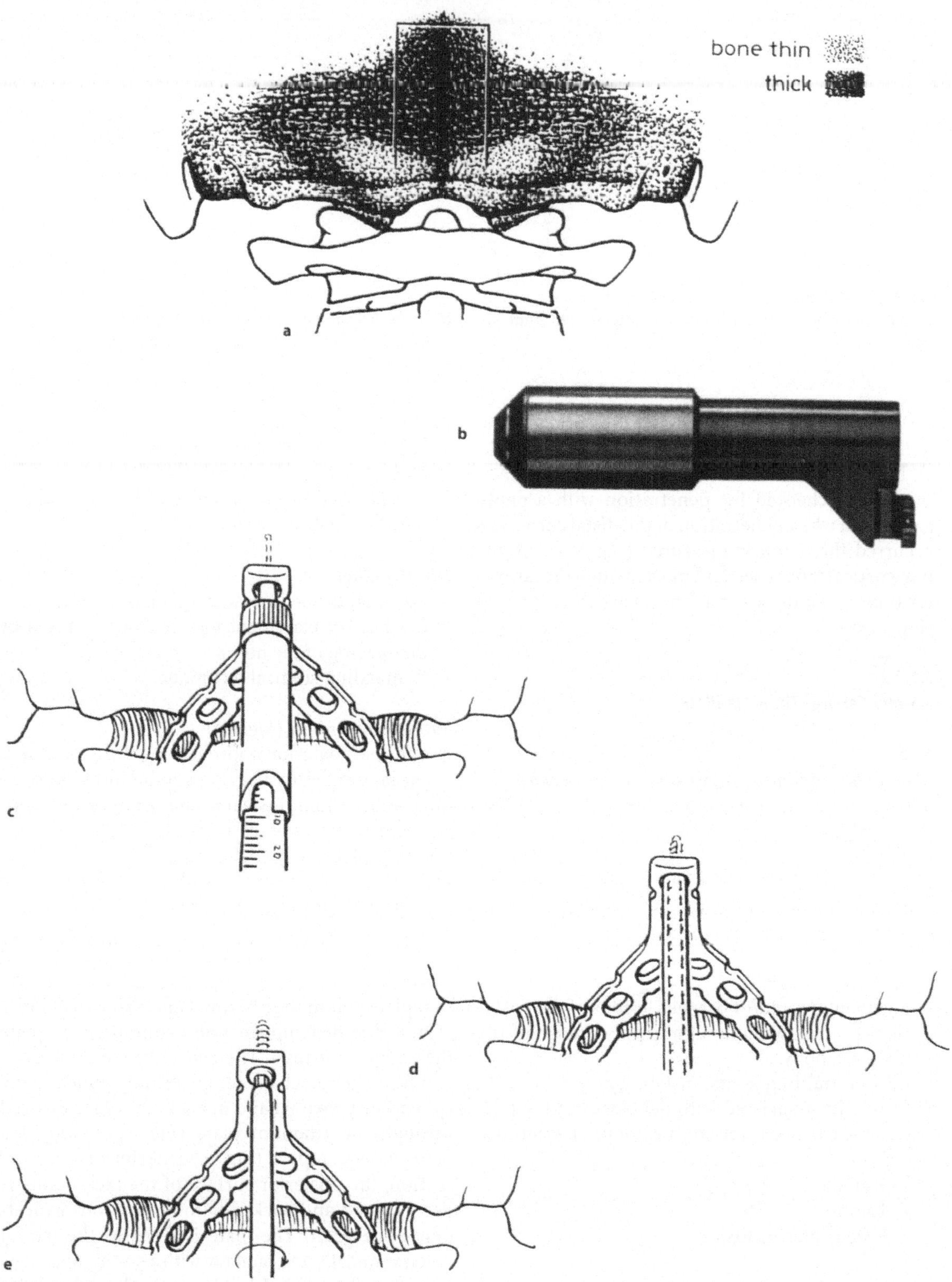

Fig. 6.6 Occiput screws
a Optimal location for screw placement into the occiput
b Drill is used with an oscillating drill attachment
c Measuring depth
d Tapping of near cortex
e Insertion of the screw with the appropriate screwdriver

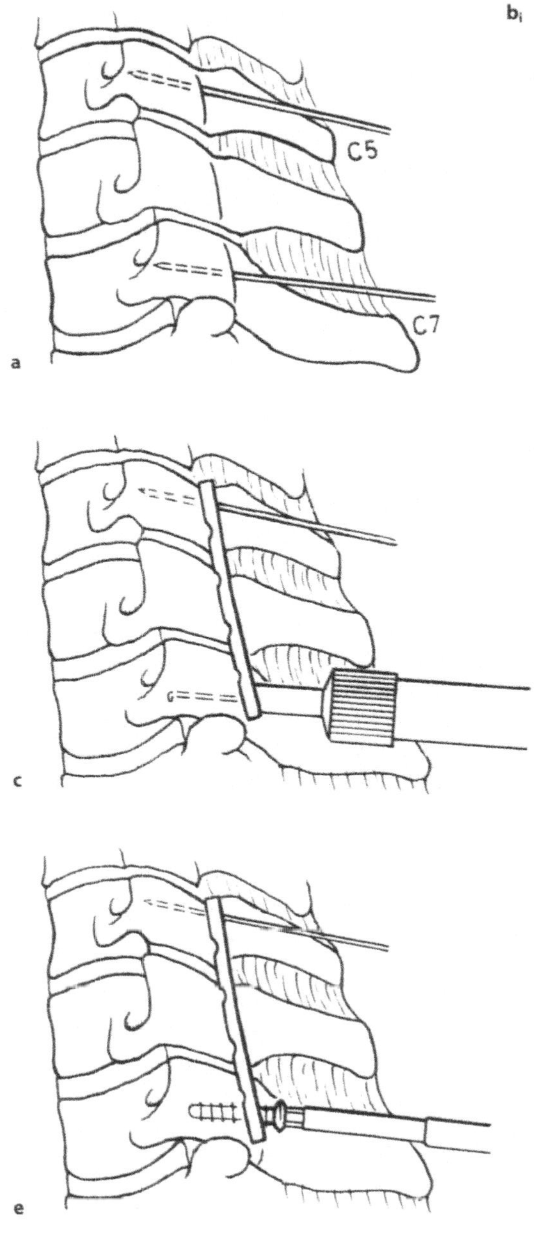

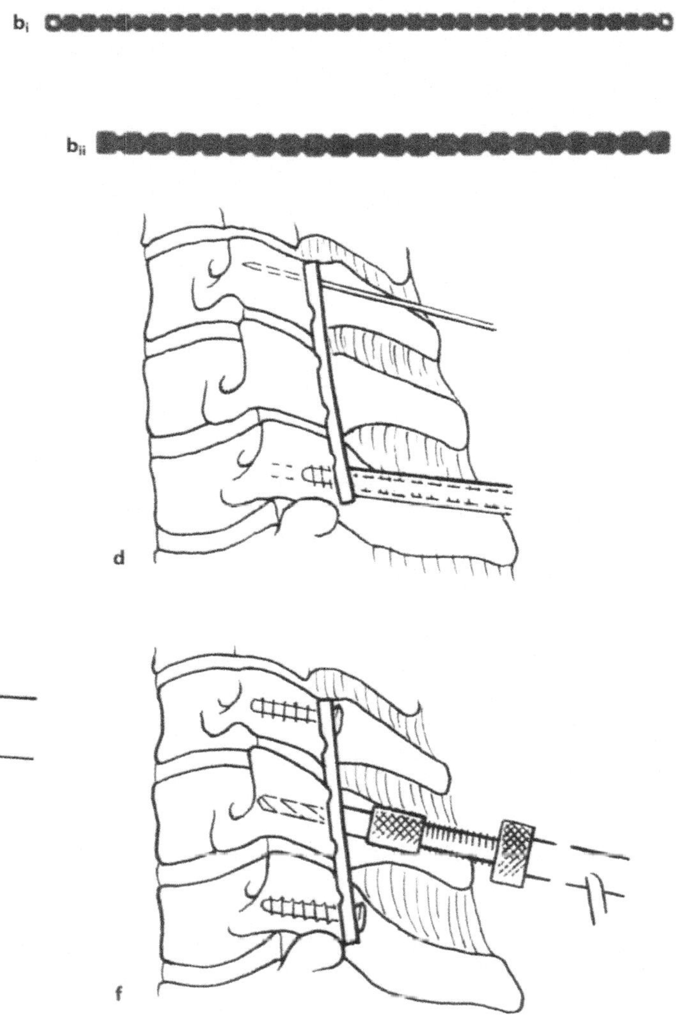

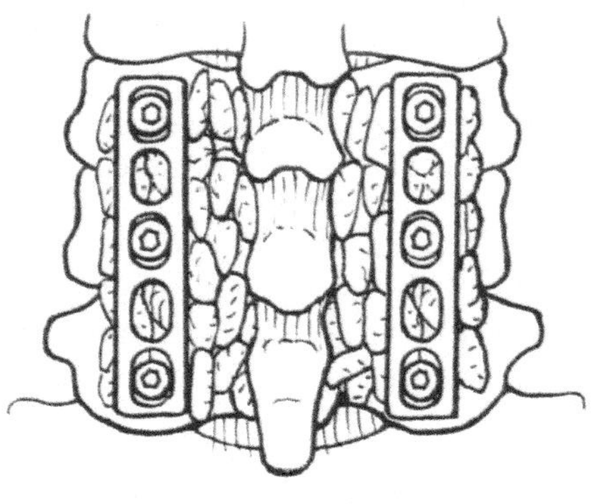

Fig. 6.7 3.5-mm cervical titanium plate: C2–C7
a The most cranial and caudal vertebrae are drilled, and K-wires are inserted into the drill holes
b The small titanium template with hole spacings of 8 mm (i) and 12 mm (ii) is used to assess whether the 8-mm or 12-mm plate will fit the proximal and distal drill holes
c (The proximal and distal holes are measured through the contoured titanium plate (matching the template)
d (Only the near cortex is tapped
e (The plate is fixed to the lateral masses cranially and caudally with 3.5-mm cancellous screws after decorticating the posterior surface of the facet joints and packing with cancellous bone graft
f (The intervening lateral masses are now drilled in the correct direction, the depth measured and the near cortices tapped and appropriate-length screws inserted
g (The laminae and spinous processes are decorticated with a burr and cancellous bone graft applied

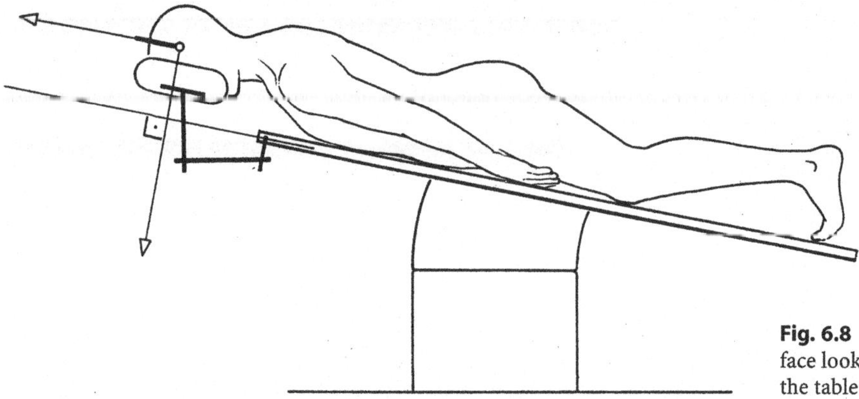

Fig. 6.8 Positioning with the patients face looking horizontally, in relation to the table

The process is then repeated on the contralateral side; the laminae and spinous processes corresponding to the area of fixation are decorticated with a burr and cancellous graft is applied (Fig. 6.7g).

Postoperative Care
A cervical orthosis is worn for 6–12 weeks depending upon the pathology. It can be removed for hygiene purposes. Isometric muscle exercises are begun immediately following surgery.

6.1.2.2.2
Occipitocervical Plate Fixation (Figs. 6.8, 6.9)

Principle
The function of the plate to the occiput is mainly as a buttress and partially as a tension band.

Indications
- Occipitocervical instability.
  - traumatic
  - congenital
- Cranial settling or basilar invagination.
- Pseudarthrosis of atlanto-axial arthrodesis.

Advantages
- Rigid stability afforded by the plating technique eliminates the use of a postoperative halo-jacket.
- Maintenance of reduction during arthrodesis.

Disadvantages
- Technically demanding and potential for neurovascular injury.
- Poor purchase of occipital screws due to thin cortex, when not put in an optimal position.
- Incorrect head position.

Technique
N.B. It is important when positioning the patient at the beginning of the operation that the face is looking horizontally (Fig. 6.8).

Two Parallel Notched Plate (Standard) (Fig. 6.9)
A midline incision is used from the inion to C3. Subperiosteal dissection is performed, the occiput is cleared up to 4 cm from the midline on both sides, and the C1 lamina is exposed only 2 cm laterally in order to prevent damage to the vertebral artery with arches over C1 more laterally: the C2 lamina and spinous processes are also cleared of soft tissue. A drill hole is placed into C2/C1 using the Magerl transarticular technique (see Fig. 5.4); alternatively if this is not possible as a result of distorted anatomy, a C2 pedicle screw is inserted as previously described (Fig. 6.4). The 3.5-mm templates are contoured to measure and to accommodate the occiput/cervical angle and to assess the correct length of the required plate. The template should allow fixation to C2 and three holes of fixation in the occiput (Fig. 6.9a).

The plate can be extended into the lower cervical spine if required.

The appropriate spacing in the template is chosen (8 or 12 mm) so that the plate hole is over the C2/C1 drill hole and if extended distally the lower hole must be in the middle of the lateral mass of C3 (Fig. 6.9a). To facilitate placement of the plate, a small amount of the lamina of C2 usually requires removal.

The 8-mm or 12-mm plate is applied to the spine, and the depth of the C2/C1-drilled hole is measured (Fig. 6.9c). *The near cortex and joint surfaces are tapped* and the correct length 3.5-mm cancellous screw inserted (Fig. 6.9d). The remaining holes in the plate are now drilled. The three occipital holes are drilled with a 2.5-mm flexible drill (Fig. 6.9e). Care must be taken when drilling the occiput, lateral

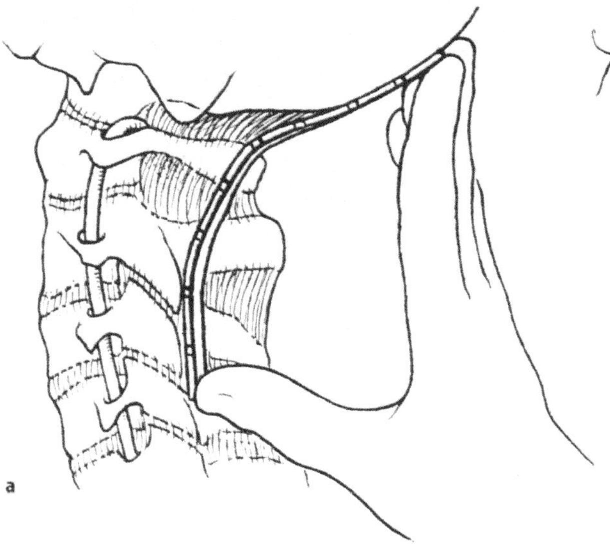

a

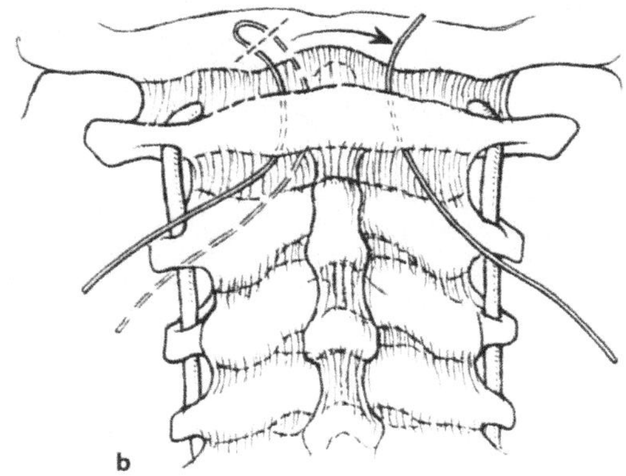

b

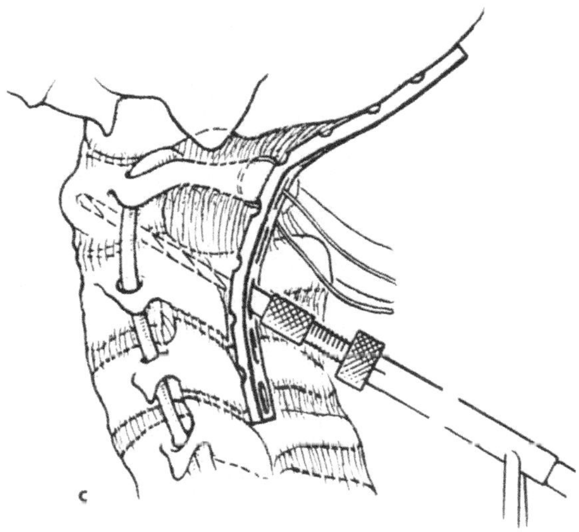

c

Fig. 6.9 Occipitocervical plate fixation: two parallel notched plates (standard).

a The template is contoured to fit the occipital and cervical spine. The appropriate spacing of either 8 mm or 12 mm is chosen. The hole must fit over the C_2/C_1-drilled hole and the distal end hole must be central over the lateral masses.

b A sublaminar wire can be placed beneath either side of the C_1 arch.

c A transarticular hole is drilled into the C_2/C_1 masses using a 2.5-mm drill and the length of the C_2/C_1 screw is measured.

d The appropriate titanium plate is contoured and applied to the spine and a 3.5-mm cortical screw is inserted through the plate. The wires are placed through a hole in the plate.

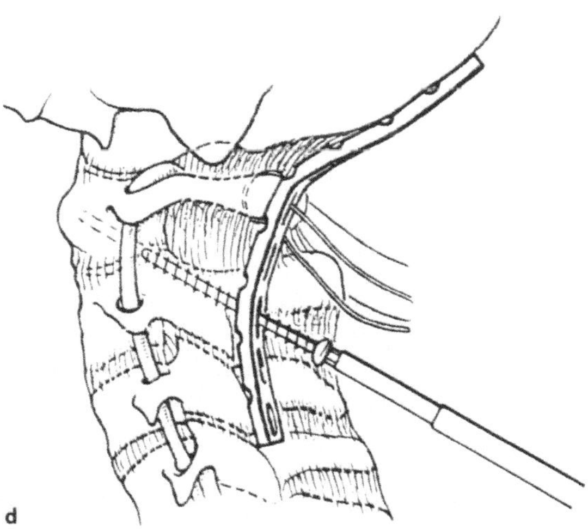

d

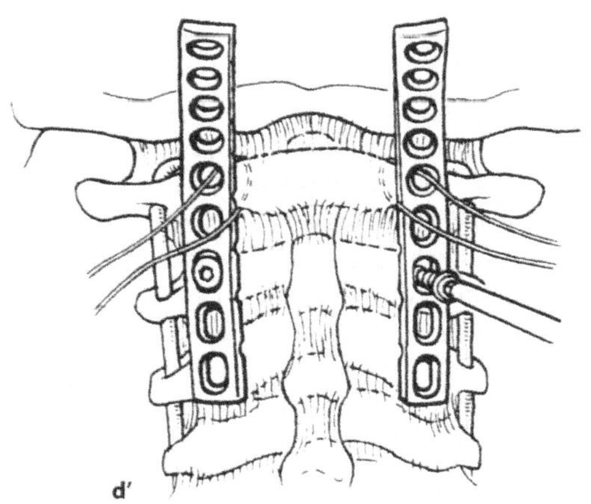

d'

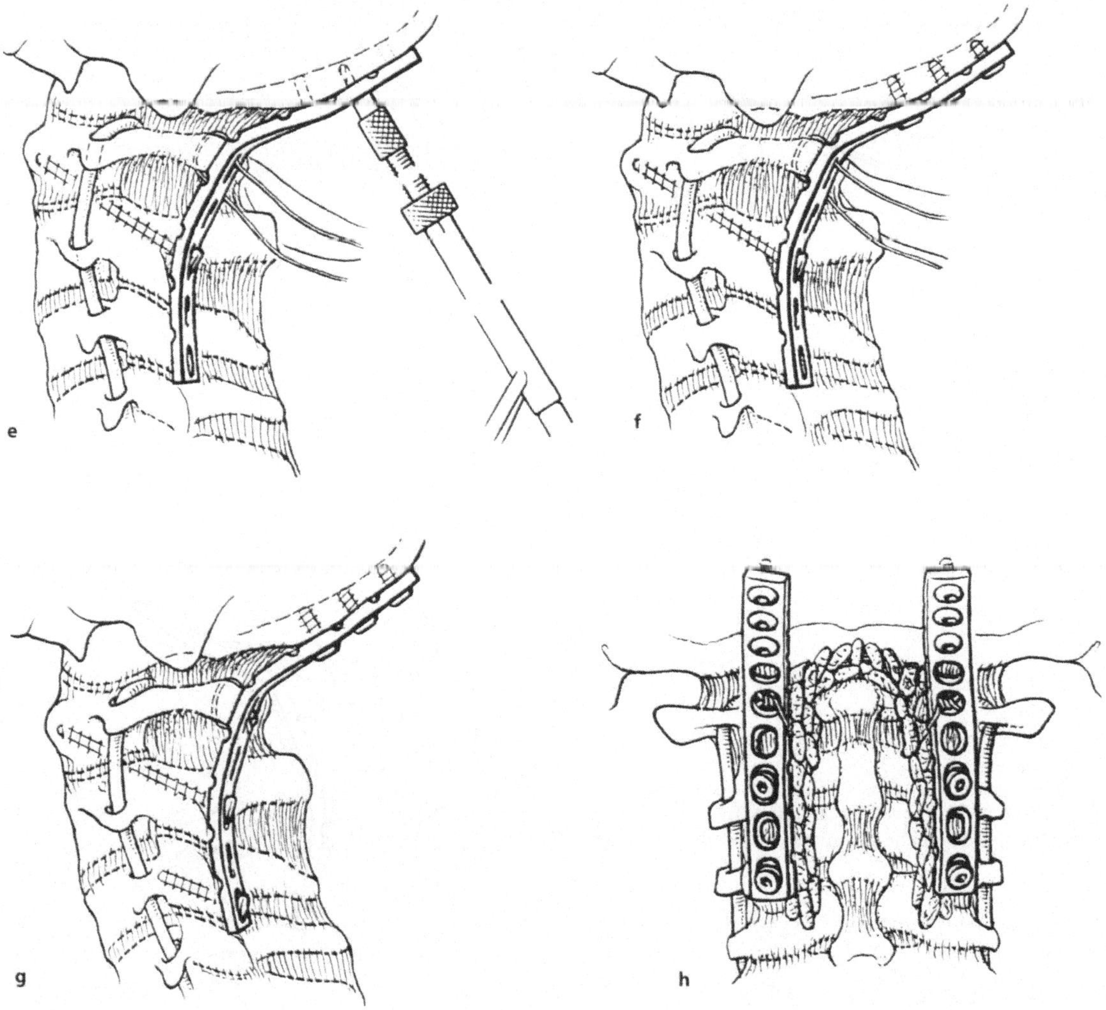

(Fig. 6.9)
e The occiput is drilled, (if necessary with a flexible drill sleeve)
f The occiput is tapped and the screw inserted
g The additional cervical segments are instrumented with screws if necessary
h A bone graft is applied after decorticating the lamina and the occiput with the burr

to the midline, since the depth is between 5 and 8 mm only. The hole is tapped *by hand.* The depth is measured and the appropriate 3.5-mm cortical screw is inserted (Fig. 6.9f). The caudal screws are inserted through the plate into the lateral mass as previously described (Fig. 6.9g).

The procedure is repeated on the contralateral side. The occiput, spinous processes and laminae are decorticated using a burr. Cancellous bone is packed over the decorticated areas of bone (Fig. 6.9h).

If there is significant subluxation of C1 on C2, then a sublaminar wire can be placed beneath either side of the C1 arch (Fig. 6.9b). The wires are placed through a hole in the plate and tightened (Fig. 6.9d–f); this will prevent anterior subluxation of C1.

Y-Notched Plate

As an alternative to the two parallel notched reconstruction plate, a Y-shaped notched reconstruction plate can be used (Fig. 6.10); this allows the occipital holes to be placed in the midline, allowing increased purchase on the occipital bone (Fig. 6.6a). The appropriate-length plate for the cervical spine can be cut and the parallel limbs of the plate can be closed or open to meet the desired anatomy of the cervical masses with the plate benders.

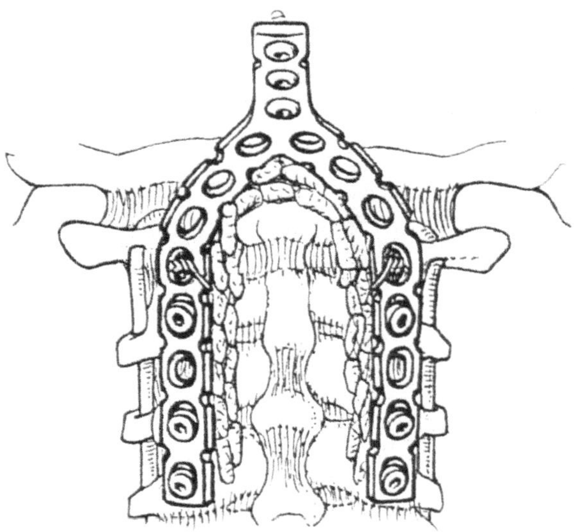

Fig. 6.10 Occipitocervical plate fixation: Y-shaped notched reconstruction plate as an alternative fixation device

Postoperative Care
Usually a cervical orthosis is only applied for 6–12 weeks postoperatively depending on the type of pathology treated and stability reached. The orthosis can be removed for the daily hygiene and isometric muscle exercises are started postoperatively.

6.1.2.2.3
Cervicothoracic Plate Fixation (Fig. 6.11)

Principle
This posterior plating technique provides a stable tension band.

Indications
Instability at the cervicothoracic junction
- Fracture at C7/T1.
- Multisegmental fracture.
- Tumor.
- Multisegmental chronic inflammatory disease in particular ankylosing spondylitis and rheumatoid arthritis.

Advantages
- Easy access to the cervical thoracic junction.
- No need for sternotomy or thoracotomy.
- Stability easier to achieve with a tension band technique.
- Good anchorage in the thoracic pedicles.

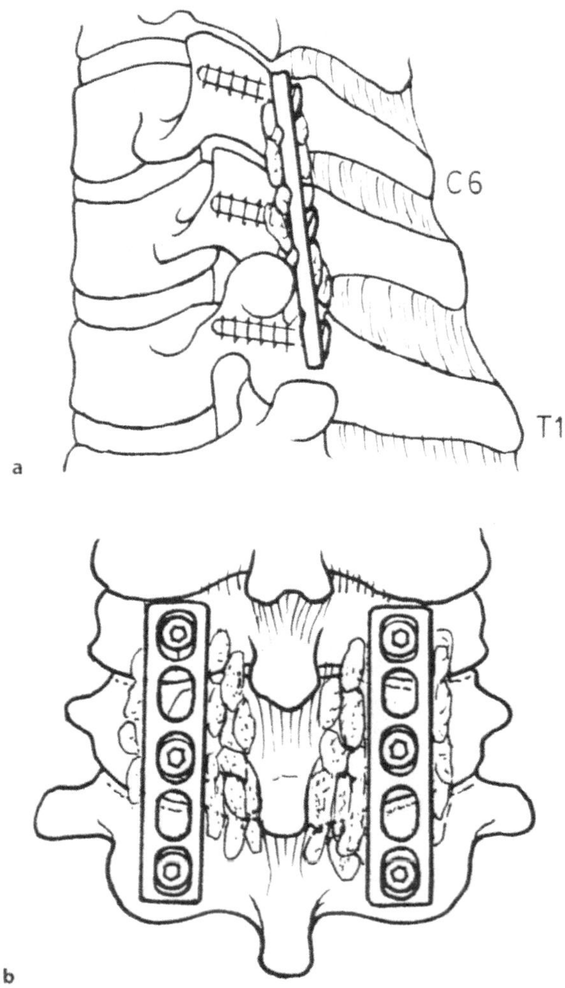

Fig. 6.11 Cervicothoracic fixation with titanium plate. Both plates are tightened with the screws. Bone graft is then applied to the decorticated laminae at the cervico-thoracic junction (procedure as decribed in Fig. 6.7)

Disadvantages
- Difficulty in alignment of plate.
- Technically demanding.
- Small screws into thoracic pedicles.

Technique
The upper level of cervical fixation is chosen and confirmed by radiographs, and the lateral mass of the vertebra is drilled and tapped as previously described. The most caudal pedicles of the thoracic spine are drilled with a 2.5-mm drill to a length of 20–24 mm as described in Chap. 7.2.2.. K-wires are placed in the drill holes of the thoracic pedicles and the cervical lateral masses and an appropriate 8-mm or 12-mm reconstruction template is then chosen,

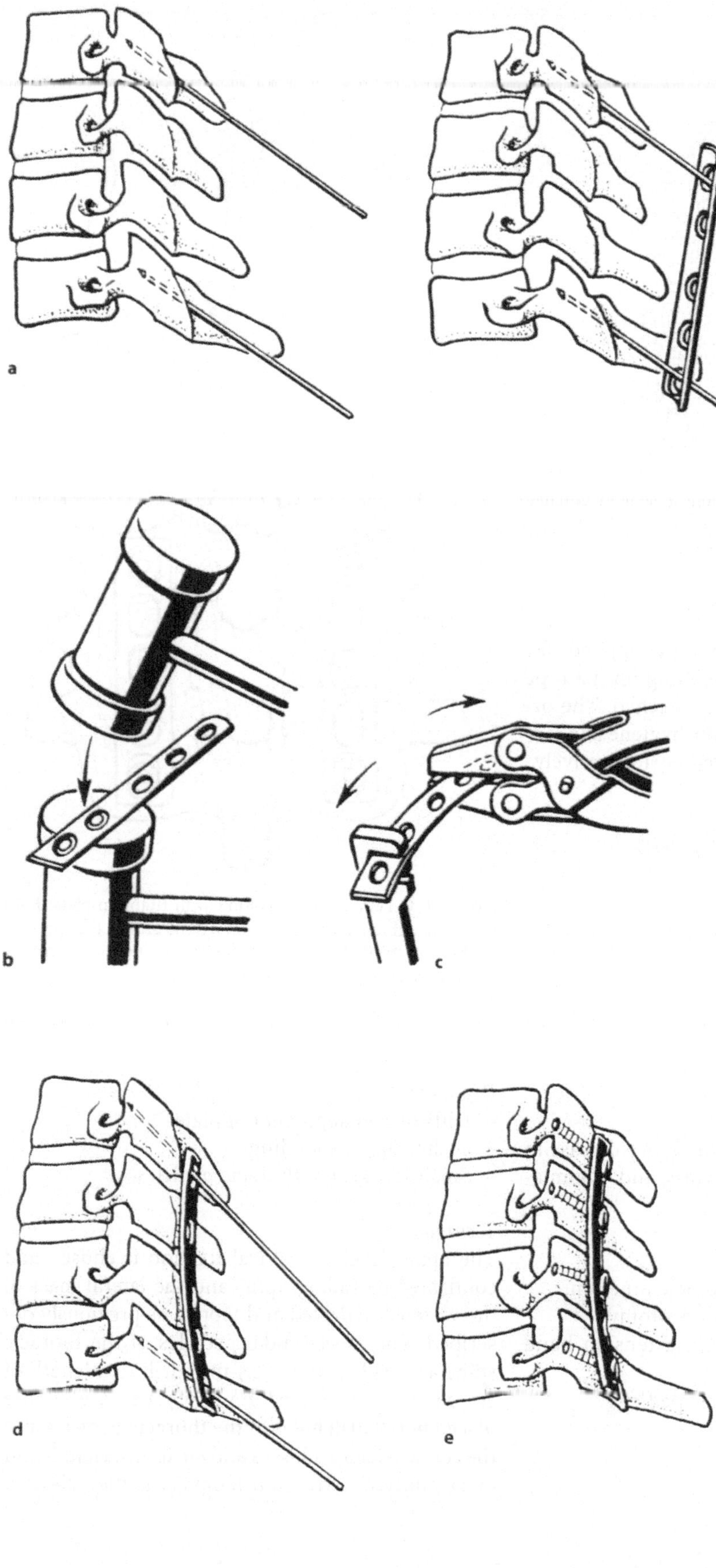

Fig. 6.12 Posterior plate fixation with one-third tubular plate
a Kirschner wires are inserted in the lateral masses of the end vertebrae. The entry points and direction are the same as for the notch-plates
b The appropriate length of the one-third tubular plate is chosen and hammered flat
c The plate is contoured
d The plate is positioned over the protruding K wires
e The Kirschner wires are then individually removed and replaced by 3.5-mm cortex screws in the usual way

which fits over the cranial K-wires and is contoured to create a normal cervicothoracic kypholordosis (Fig. 6.11a).

The appropriate 8-mm or 12-mm titanium cervical plate is placed over the upper and lower K-wires onto the spine. If required, the posterior portion of the facet joints in the fusion can be decorticated and packed with cancellous bone (Fig. 6.11b). The plate is first fixed to the uppermost cervical vertebrae with the lateral mass screw and then the thoracic pedicle screws are inserted. The intervening cervical lateral masses are then drilled, measured, tapped and fixed with 3.5-mm bicortical screws. The spinous processes and laminae are decorticated with a burr and cancellous bone graft added (Fig. 6.11b).

Postoperative Management
A cervicothoracic orthosis is worn for a period of 6–12 weeks. The orthosis can be removed to wash.

6.1.2.3 One-Third Tubular Plate Fixation (Fig. 6.12)

As an alternative to the 3.5-mm reconstruction plate, the one-third tubular plate may be used.

Principle
The posterior plating provides stable tension band fixation in flexion, increasing stability in rotation, and buttressing in extension.

Indication
- Ligamentous and/or osseous lesions of the posterior complex without significant damage of the vertebral body. The lesions may be uni- or multisegmental.

Advantages
- Superior stability compared with the wiring technique.
- Can be used in the presence of laminar and spinous processes fractures.
- Requires no special instrumentation.

Disadvantages
- Ideal screw placement may be compromised by the spacing of the holes.

Surgical Technique
Kirschner wires are inserted in the lateral masses of the end of the vertebra (Fig. 6.12a). The entry points and direction are the same as for the other posterior plates. A one-third tubular plate of appropriate length is chosen, hammered flat (Fig. 6.12b), contoured (Fig. 6.12c) and positioned over the protruding Kirschner wires (Fig. 6.12d) to check whether the end holes of the plate correspond to the entry points of the Kirschner wires. If they do not, the entry points will have to be altered accordingly. The Kirschner wires are then individually moved and replaced by 3.5-mm cortex screws in the usual way (Fig. 6.12e). Care must be taken when perforating the anterior cortex of the lateral mass. If more than one motion segment is to be included, the end screws are not fully tightened, so that the plate can be adjusted and the remaining screws inserted. As the anatomic landmarks are hidden by the plate, check the entry point and direction of the drill in these holes with the image intensifier. The remaining screws are then introduced and all are tightened. The laminae are decorticated and a cancellous bone graft applied.

Postoperative Care
The patient wears a firm collar for 10–12 weeks. The collar can be removed for daily care and after 6 weeks; it need no longer be worn while resting.

6.1.2.4 Hook Plates (Fig. 6.13)

Hook plates are used for posterior stabilization and fusion over one or two cervical motion segments (area of application: C2–C7). They are available in different lengths with either one or two holes (Fig. 6.13).

Principles
A spondylodesis with hook plates is a prestressed construct which is inherently stable. Any resistance to compression is due to the intervertebral joints and the interspinous H graft. These form a triangle in the horizontal plane. The compression force is provided by the plate when the screws are tightened. The spondylodesis is stable in all planes, since the resulting compression force lies within the triangle (Fig. 6.14).

Indications
- Discoligamentous instability due to subluxation or dislocation.
- Additional stabilization following anterior fusion in grossly unstable situations.
- Treatment of an anterior pseudarthrosis.

Advantages
- The primary stability achieved with the hook plate fixation is superior to that of interbody fusions and posterior cerclage wiring.

Figs. 6.13–6.18 Posterior hook plate fixation

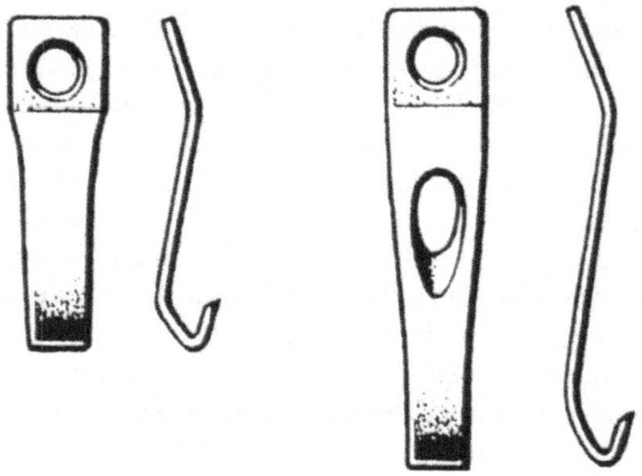

Fig. 6.13 Hook plates are available in different lengths with either one or two holes

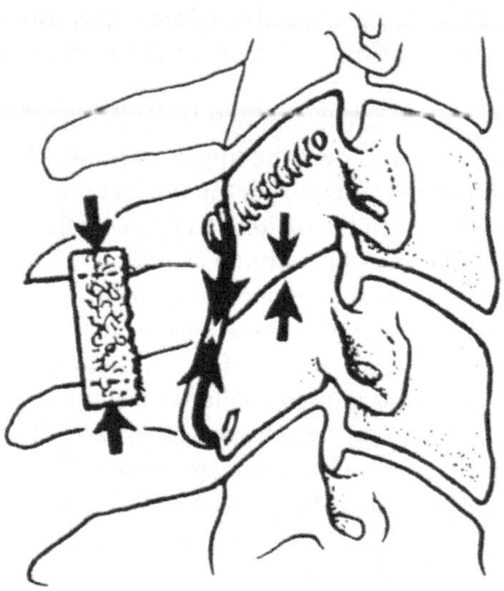

Fig. 6.14 The spondylodesis is stable in all planes since the resulting compression force lies within the triangle formed by the facet joints and the interspinous graft

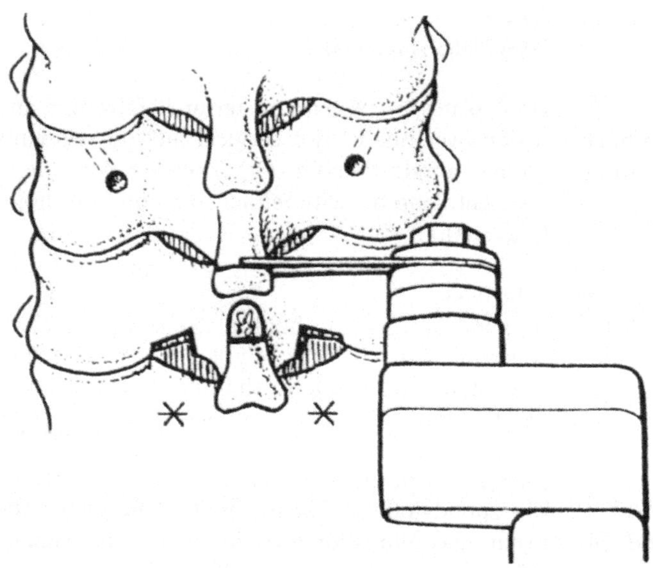

Fig. 6.15 Hook and graft bed. In order to prevent the hooks from sliding into the intervertebral joints, corresponding notches are cut into the lamina medial to the joints (*).The site of the graft is prepared, using an oscillating saw

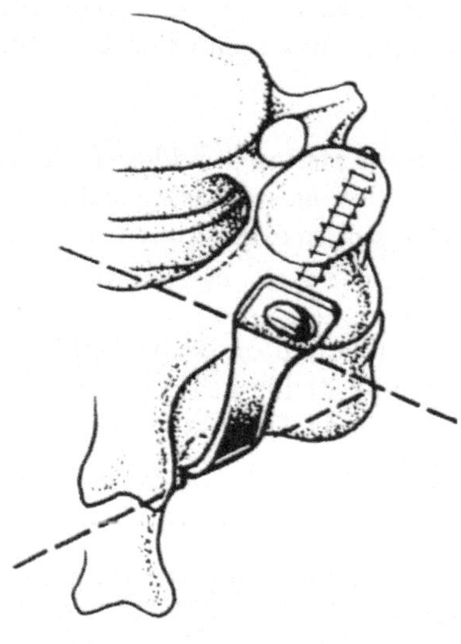

Fig. 6.16 Contouring of the plates by torque and bending to match the posterior aspect of the lamina as well as the articular process

- There is less danger of injuring the vertebral anterior nerve root than in posterior fusions using plates with screws inserted sagittally.
- There is less danger or injury to the dura or spinal cord than in sublaminar wiring.

Disadvantage

Technically more demanding than wiring procedures.

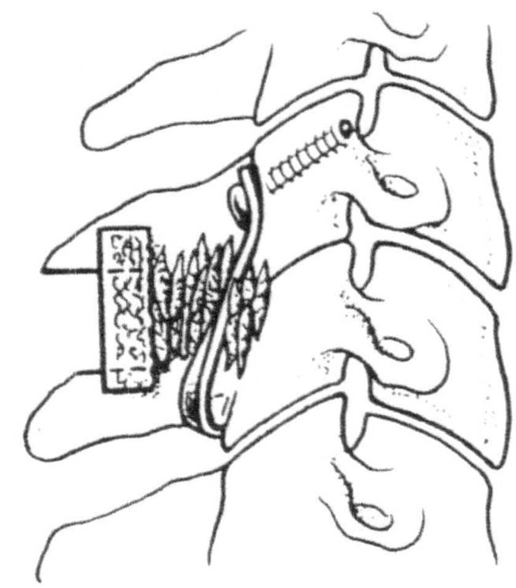

a

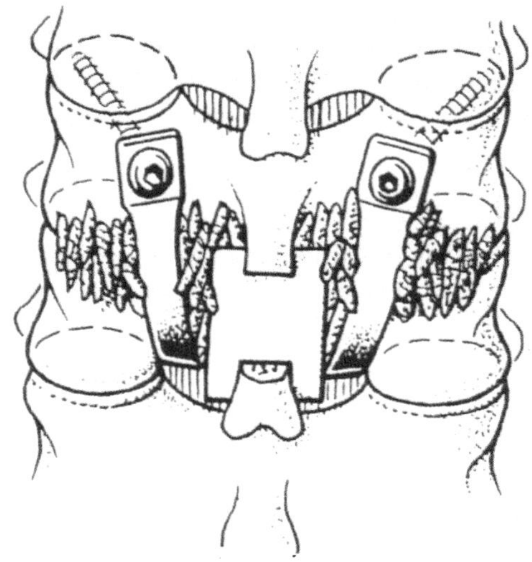

b

Fig. 6.17 Stabilizing one motion segment. H-graft is inserted. The contoured hook plates are placed into the prepared notches, and 3.5-mm cortex screws are inserted

a Lateral view
b Posterior view
Finally, the cancellous bone graft is applied between the laminae and across the facet joints

Surgical Technique

Hook and Graft Bed. In order to prevent the hooks from sliding into the intervertebral joints, corresponding notches are cut into the lamina medial to the joints. The site of the H graft is prepared using an oscillating saw (Fig. 6.15). The lower notch must not be too deep in order to avoid a fracture of the spinous process.

Stabilizing One Motion Segment (Fig. 6.16). The plates are contoured by torque and bending to match the posterior aspect of the lamina as well as the articular mass (Fig. 6.16). A cortico-cancellous H-graft is inserted between the spinous processes with the vertebrae in the neutral position. The contoured hook plates are placed into the prepared notches, and 3.5-mm cortex screws are inserted (Fig. 6.17a, b). In a very small articular mass, 2.7-mm cortex screws may be used.

Tightening the screws sandwiches the H graft. If a hook begins to lift out, the curvature of the hook should be increased. With two-hole plates, it is possible to secure the hook by inserting a short screw into the lower lamina, but this is rarely necessary. Finally, a cancellous bone graft is applied between the laminae and across the facet joints (Fig. 6.17a, b).

Stabilizing Two Motion Segments (Fig. 6.18). With the long hook plates, two motion segments may be bridges (Fig. 6.18). The middle spinous process is removed. The upper screw canals, hook notches and graft bed are prepared and the plates appropriate in length are chosen and centered. They should be about 2 mm shorter to allow compression. The H-graft is inserted, the plates applied and the upper screws inserted. They are tightened until some compression results. This is followed by drilling of the lower screw holes, parallel to the screws above. The

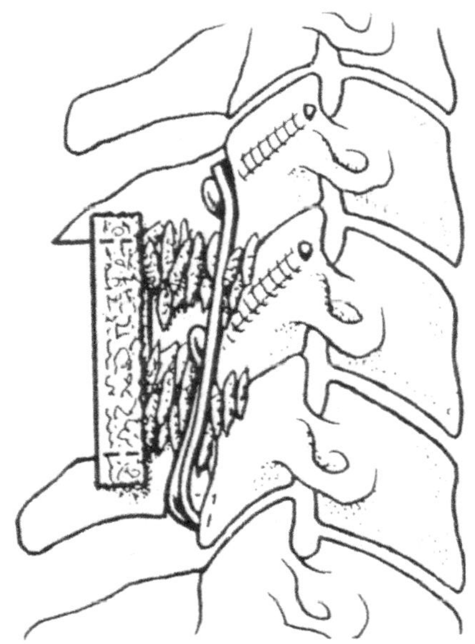

Fig. 6.18 Stabilizing two motion segments. With the long hook plates, two motion segments may be bridged. The middle spinous process is removed

drill is placed eccentrically through the upper part of the plate holes. First, the lower screws are fully tightened, then the upper screws again. With this technique, compression is achieved in both motion segments.

Postoperative Care
A firm collar is worn for 6–8 weeks. It may be removed for daily care and, after 3 weeks, when resting.

6.1.3 Cervical Spine Titanium Rod System (Cervifix)

Principle
The Cervical Spine Rod System is a modular tension band system for posterior fixation of the occipitocervical spine, upper and lower cervical spine, and upper thoracic spine. A choice of clamps and hooks are fixed on a 3.5-mm titanium rod by means of set screws. 3.5-mm bone screws can be optimally positioned through the clamps in any desired direction and on each motion segment. If desired, locking screws may be used. For fixation to the occiput, a rod with one end shaped like a reconstruction plate has been designed. A cross-linking device may also be used to connect both rods and protect the spinal cord in cases of extensive laminectomy. The rod can be directly connected to the larger diameter rods of the Universal Spine System (USS) with a special connector.

Indications
- Occipitocervical and upper cervical spine instabilities (rheumatoid arthritis, anomalies, posttraumatic conditions, tumors, infections).
- Instabilities in the lower cervical spine (traumatic instabilities, tumors, iatrogenic instabilities following laminectomy, etc.).
- Degenerative and painful post-traumatic conditions in the lower cervical spine.
- Anterior fusions requiring additional posterior stabilization.

Advantages
- Allows optimal screw insertion at all levels instrumented.
- Allows optimal bone grafting.
- Allows postoperative magnetic resonance imaging (MRI).
- Can be connected to other rod systems, such as the USS.

Disadvantages
- Destruction of the vertebral bodies with loss of stability in compression cannot be treated by a posterior approach alone. Such instabilities require a reconstruction of the anterior column. CerviFix can be used for additional posterior stabilization.
- More expensive than posterior plate fixation.

6.1.3.1 Implants and Instruments

Implants and instruments are shown in Fig. 6.19.

6.1.3.2 Occipitocervical Stabilization

Surgical Technique
The patient is placed in a prone position. If the spine is unstable, reduction of C1 on C2 is checked under fluoroscopy immediately after positioning the patient: if necessary, closed reduction is performed. A posterior midline incision is performed. The occiput, posterior ring of the atlas, the posterior elements of C2, spinous processes, vertebral arches, and articular masses of those lower cervical spine vertebrae to be included in the fusion are exposed subperiosteally. If transarticular screw fixation C2/C1 is necessary, the isthmus of C2 must be exposed on both sides. A template is contoured in such a way that its cranial end lies adjacent to the midline and is situated just caudal to the occipital protuberance, and the rod passes over the lateral rims of the articular processes of the levels to be incorporated in the fusion (Fig. 6.20a). The occipital rod is cut and bent according to the template. If necessary, a residual C1–2 dislocation is reduced under image intensification. Firstly the holes for the transarticular screws in C1–2 are drilled (Fig. 6.20b) (see Chap. 5.2, Transarticular screw fixation C2/C1). In order to provisionally stabilize C1/C2, the drill bit is left in place on one side while instrumenting the opposite side.

The most caudal screw hole in the vertebrae to be stabilized is now drilled using the Magerl technique for the lower cervical spine (Fig. 6.20c). All planned clamps are provisionally mounted and slightly fastened on the rod, which is now positioned over the vertebrae. The C2/C1 transarticular screw is inserted first through its appropriate lateral mass clamp (Fig. 6.20d). Next, the most caudal screw of the assembly is inserted (Fig. 6.20e). The occipital screw holes are drilled through the plate (Fig. 6.20f) and the screws inserted (care must be taken to place the

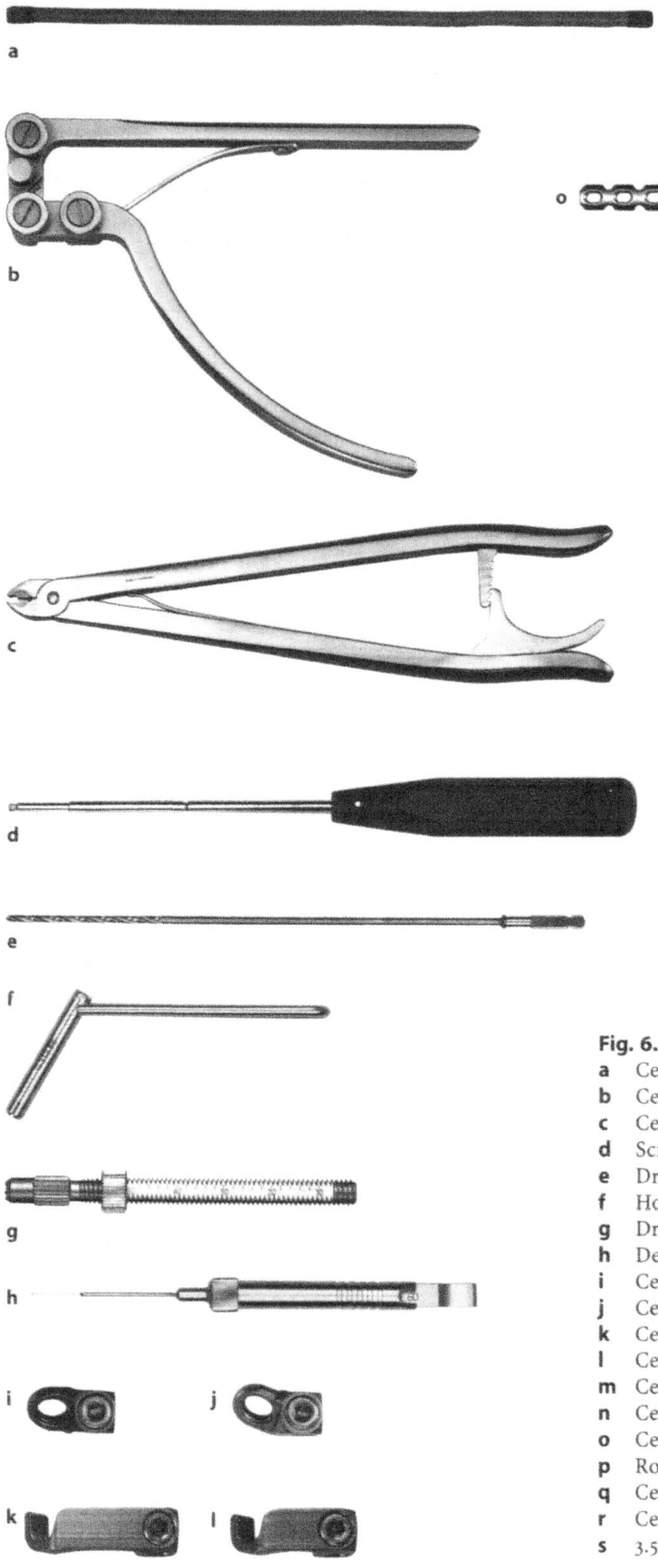

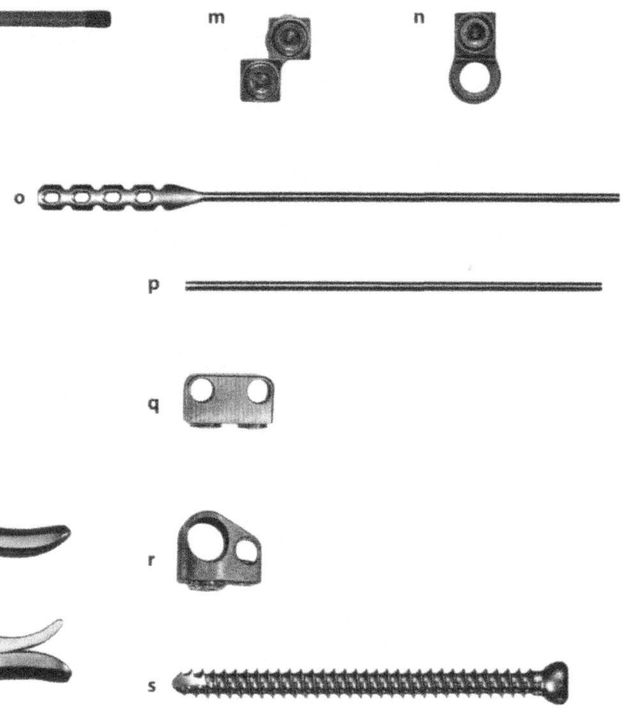

Fig. 6.19 Implants and instrumentation.
a CerviFix rod template
b CerviFix bending pliers
c CerviFix holding forceps
d Screwdriver, hexagonal, small, self-holding
e Drill bit, 2.5 mm diameter
f Holder for drill guide inserts
g Drill guide insert 2.7, calibrated
h Depth guage for 2.7
i CerviFix C2 clamp
j CerviFix C3/C7 clamp
k CerviFix hook, large
l CerviFix hook, small
m CerviFix lamina clamp
n CerviFix pedicle clamp
o CerviFix occiput rod
p Rod 3.5 mm diameter
q CerviFix parallel connector 3.5/3.5
r CerviFix parallel connector 3.5/6
s 3.5 mm cortex screw, self-tapping

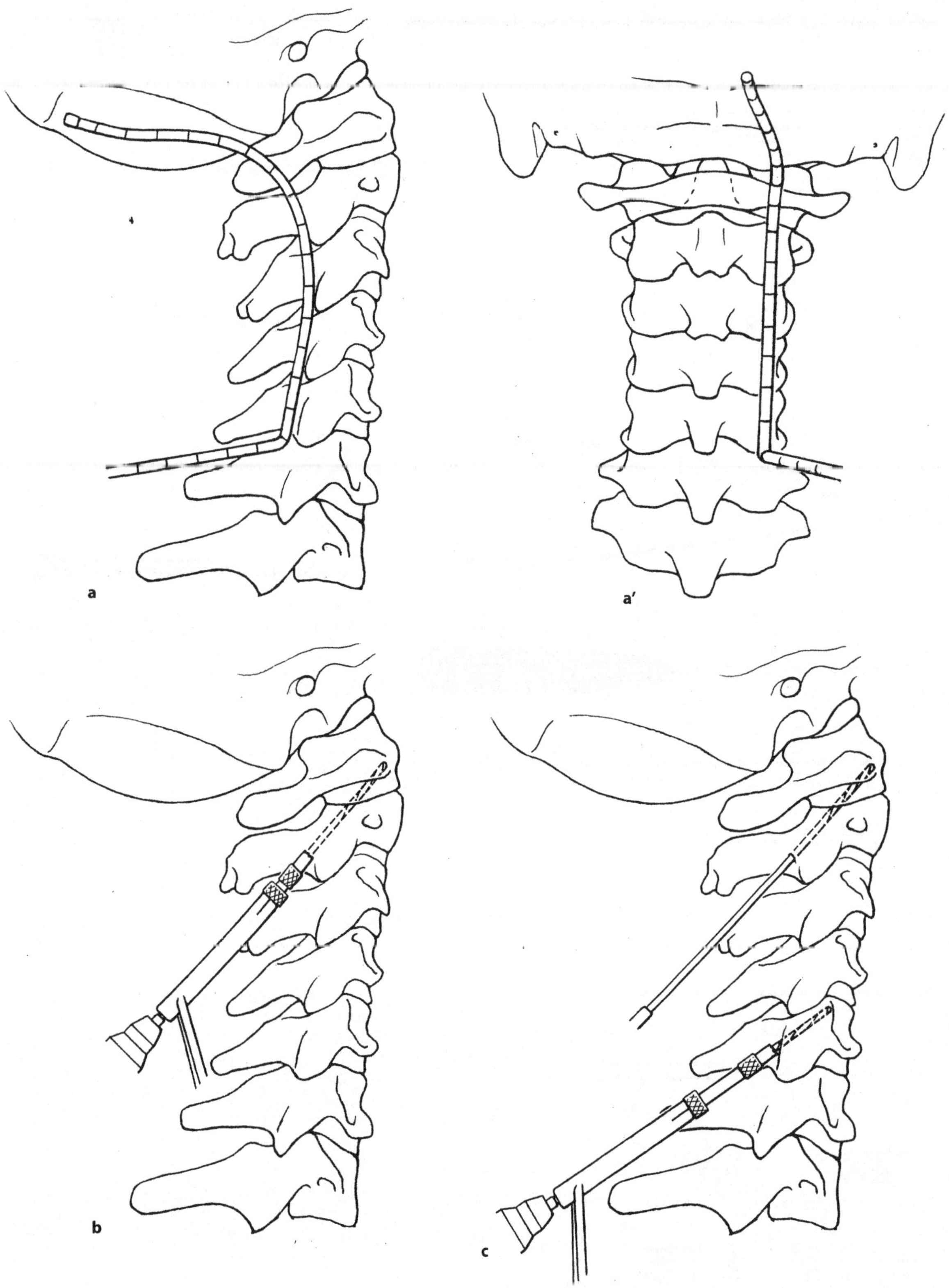

Fig. 6.20
a Siting of the template applied to C5, lateral and posterior views
b Drilling of the C1/C2 transarticular screw
c Drilling of the distal cervical screw, leaving a drill in the C2/C1 drill hole

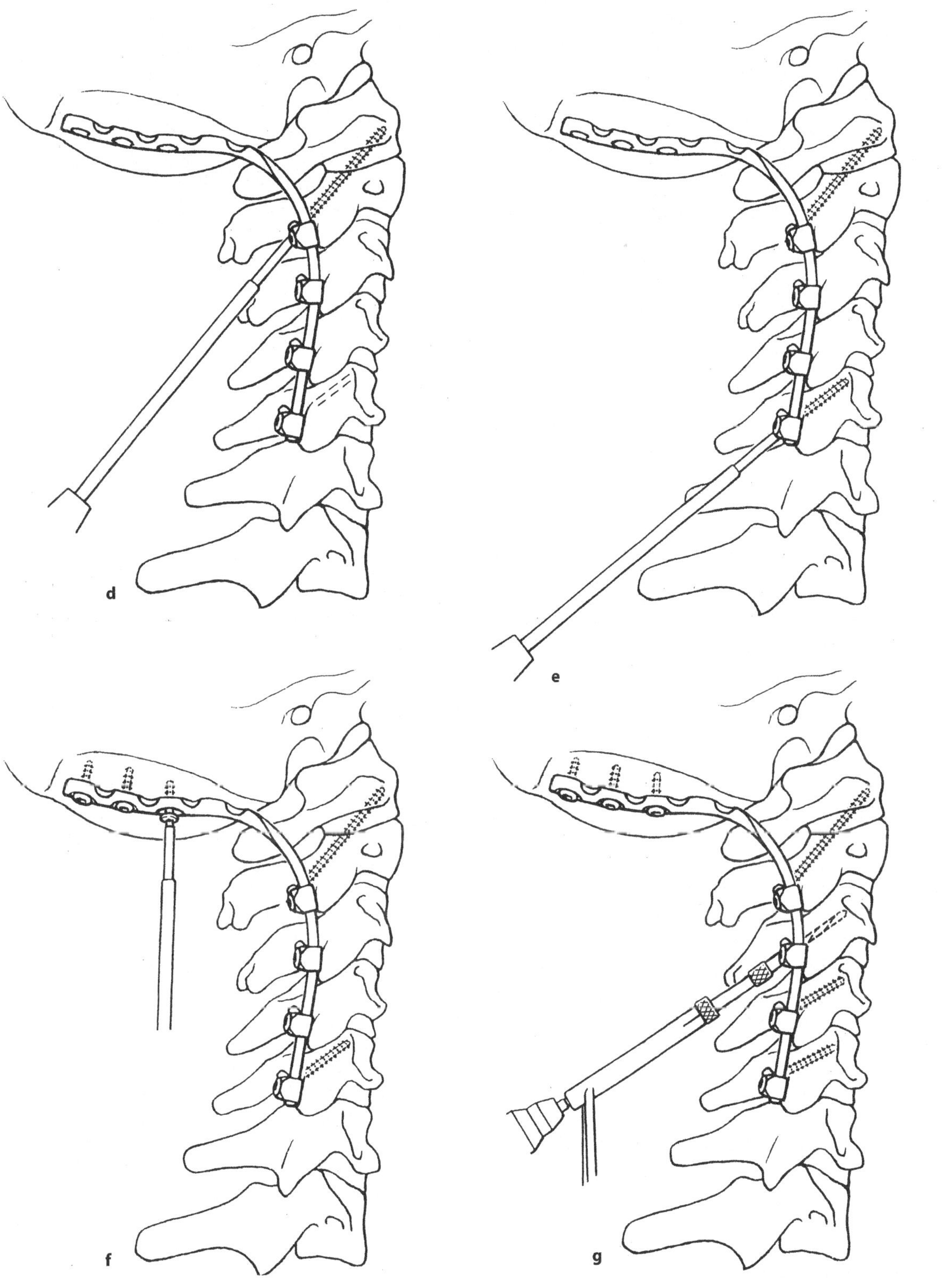

(Fig. 6.20)
d Insertion of the C2/C1 screw through its corresponding clamp
e The most caudal screw is inserted
f Drilling of the occipital screw holes and insertion of the screws
g Insertion of the screw in the lateral masses through the clamp

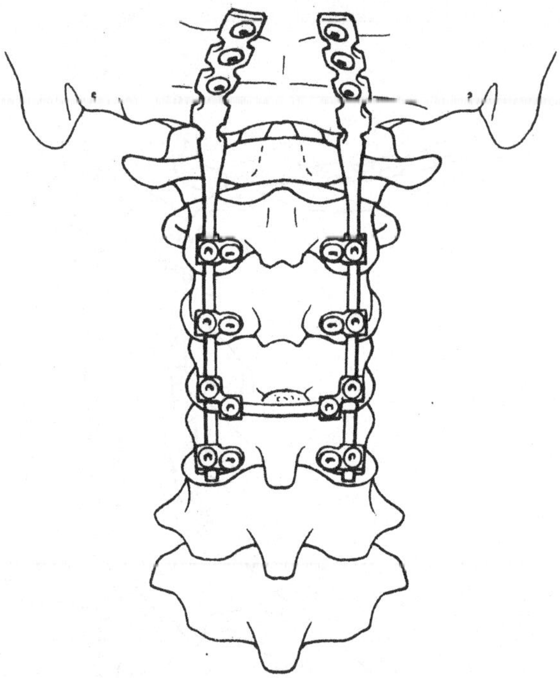

(Fig. 6.20)
h Application of the cross-link

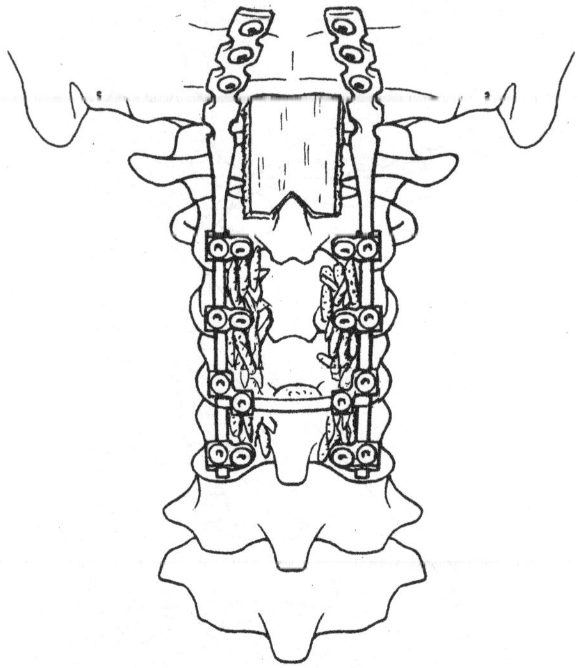

i Both plates and rods in place with application of cancellous bone graft and a cortico-cancellous graft at the occipito-cervical junction (occiput-C5)

cranial end of the plate as close as possible to the midline of the skull, in order to provide the best possible purchase). The intermediate clamps are positioned in the appropriate portion on the lateral masses and the holes are drilled, the depth measured and the screws inserted (Fig. 6.20g; see Sect. 6.1.2, Plate Technique). The other side is instrumented in a similar manner. A cross-link is applied (Fig. 6.20h). Cancellous bone graft is applied over the decorticated laminae and articular masses (Fig. 6.20i). Between the occiput and the spinous process of C2, a cortico-cancellous bone graft is inserted acting as a buttress.

Postoperative Care
A Philadelphia collar is worn for a period of 6–12 weeks depending on the underlying pathology. It may be removed for daily care and while resting.

6.1.3.3
Cervicothoracic Fixation from C2 to Th2 (as for Occipitocervical Fixation)

Surgical Technique
The patient is placed in the prone position. A midline incision is performed. The spinal processes, laminae and articular masses of the vertebrae to be included in the fusion are exposed subperiosteally. The screw holes for the most cranial and most caudal clamps are drilled using the Magerl technique for the cervical spine (Fig. 6.21a; see Sect. 6.1.2) and the transpedicular technique for the upper thoracic spine (see Sect. 8.2.2).

The rod is cut and slightly contoured in lordosis. All planned clamps (or hooks) are mounted on the rod. The most caudal screw followed by the most cranial screw is inserted (Fig. 6.21b). If slight posterior compression (lordosis) is desired, the cranial clamp is brought closer to the caudal one and fixed to the rod before inserting the bone screw: the cranial screw will cause intersegmental compression and lordosis when tightened. The intermediate screw holes are drilled through the clamps and the screws inserted (Fig. 6.21c). After extensive laminectomies, the dura may be protected by laminar substitute connecting both longitudinal rods. Cancellous bone graft is placed on the articular masses.

Postoperative Care
The cervical spine is immobilized for 8 weeks in a Philadelphia collar, which can be removed while resting.

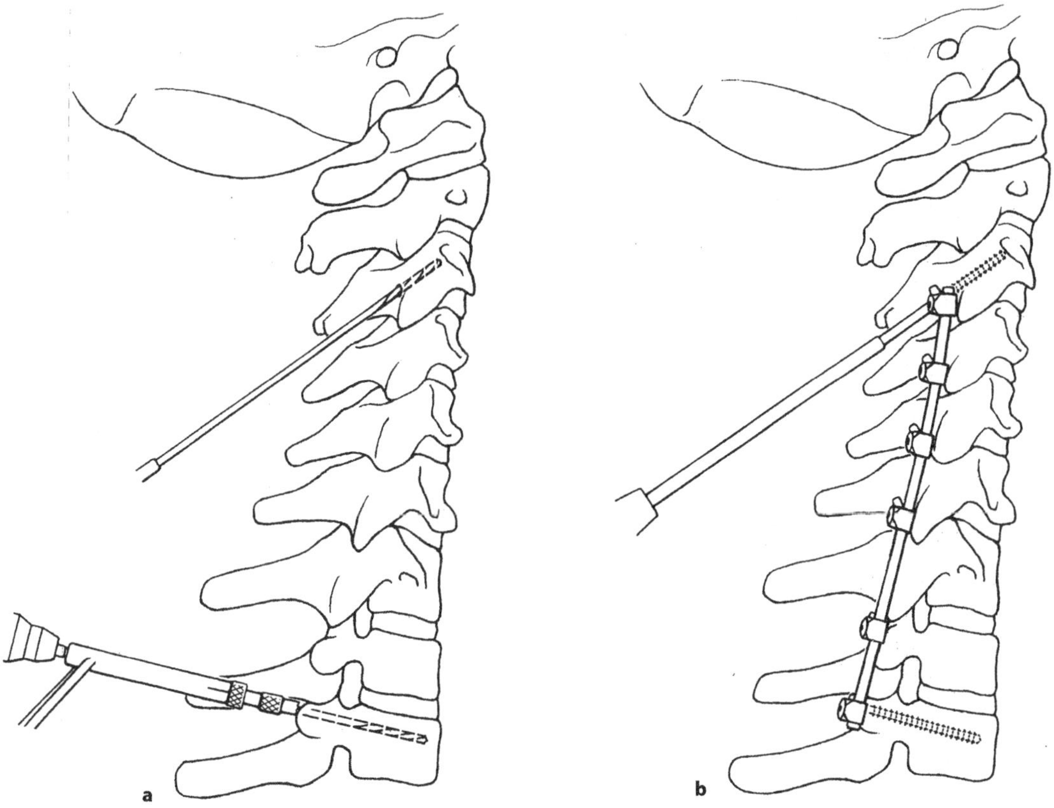

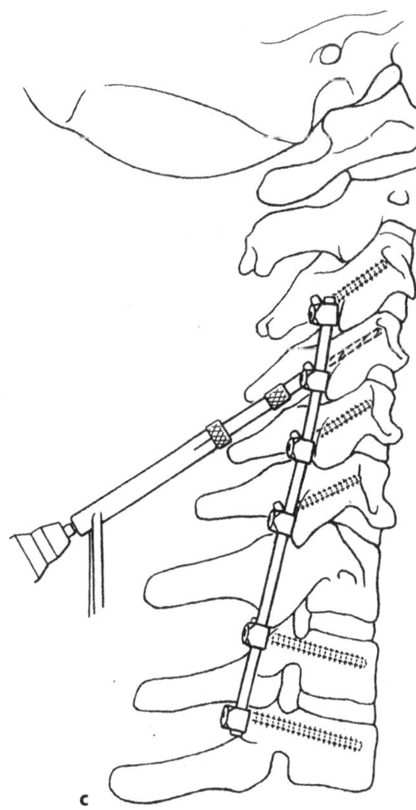

Fig. 6.21 Cervical and upper thoracic spine, C2 – Th2
a Drilling of the most caudal and cranial lateral mass holes
b Insertion of the proximal and distal screws into the lateral masses
c Insertion of the remaining lateral mass screws

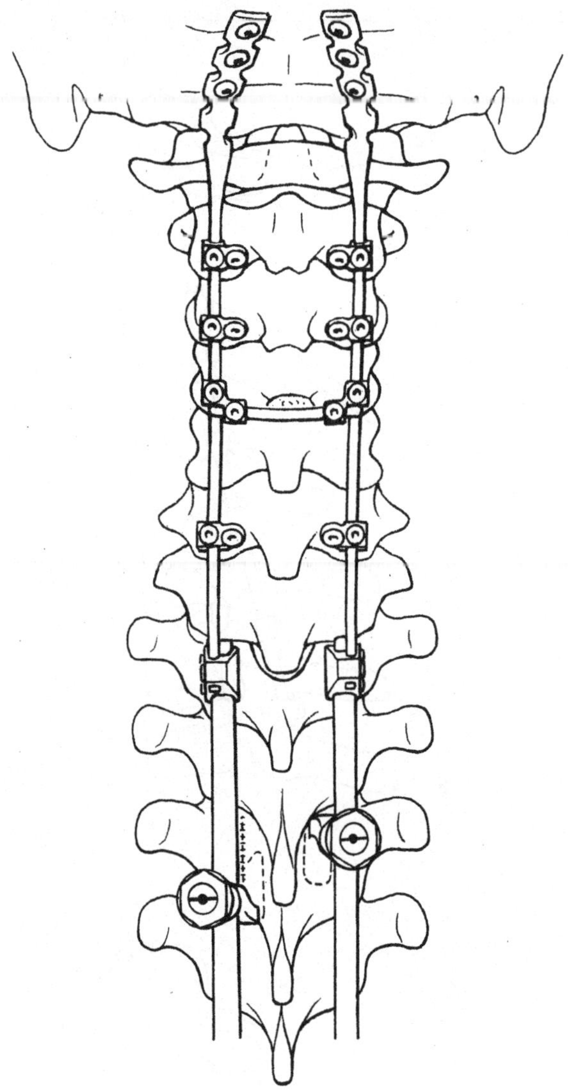

Fig. 6.22 Connection of the cervical spine rod system to the 6-mm USS rod system

6.1.3.4
Connection of the Cervical Spine Rod System to the 6-mm USS Rod (Occipitocervical Fixation)

In long constructs, the cervical spine system can be connected to the 6-mm USS rod system with a special connector (Fig. 6.22).

6.2 Anterior Techniques

6.2.1 Plating Techniques

Principle
Anterior plate fixation is used to increase the stability of the anterior column following grafting techniques. The plate functions as a tension band in extension and as a buttress plate in flexion.

Indications
- To support the anterior column when instability persists, particularly when associated with loss of height of the vertebral body following a severe wedge and compression or burst fracture.
- Following partial or total vertebrectomy, for decompression of the spinal cord.

6.2.1.1 *Standard H Plate* (Fig. 6.23)

Advantages
- Less instrumentation.
- More versatility regarding screw direction.
- Eccentric screw placement allows for compression of the graft.
- 2,7 mm and 3,5 mm cortex screws possible.

Disadvantages
- The screws have to penetrate the posterior cortex of the vertebral body with potential risk to the spinal cord. (The oscillating attachment for the drill should be used for this technique.)
- Screw loosening with anterior migration can occur.
- No intrinsic stability of the fixation system (no fixed angle between screws and plate).

Surgical Technique
An anterior approach is used. It is essential to know the sagittal diameter of the vertebral body to prevent overpenetration of the posterior cortex with the drill. In the majority of cases, the disk or vertebral bone at the site of injury has been removed prior to fusion, and at this stage the depth of the vertebral body is measured with the depth gauge (Fig. 6.24a). Before applying the plate, an anterior interbody fusion is performed using either a tri-cortical graft or spacer. The graft should be wedge shaped to maintain the cervical lordosis (Fig. 6.24b). The special drill guide with an inside diameter of 2.7 mm is set to the previously measured depth of the vertebral body and the length of the protruding 2.5-mm drill measured with a ruler (Fig. 6.24c). Ensure that the nut on the drill guide is tightly locked (Fig. 6.24d). Before drilling, a plate of suitable length is placed onto the anterior aspect of the vertebral bodies and held with a clamp. Using the preset special drill guide, the hole is drilled through the plate hole (Fig. 6.24e) and the length is checked with the depth gauge (Fig. 6.24f). If the posterior cortex has not been penetrated, then the special drill guide is adjusted to allow a further 1 mm of drilling. This is repeated until the posterior cortex of the vertebral body has been penetrated and must be done with great care to prevent injury to the contents of the spinal canal.

Only the anterior cortex of the vertebral body is tapped with the 3.5-mm tap (Fig. 6.24g). The appropriate-length 3.5-mm cortex screw is inserted. A similar procedure is performed with the other screw

a
b
c
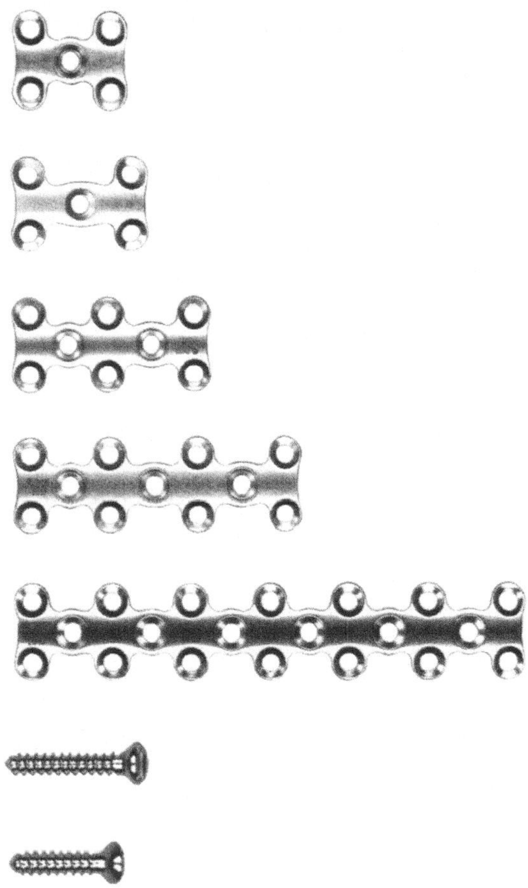

Fig. 6.23 Standard H-plate
a Cervical spine H-plates
b 2.7 mm cortex screw
c 3.5 mm cortex screw

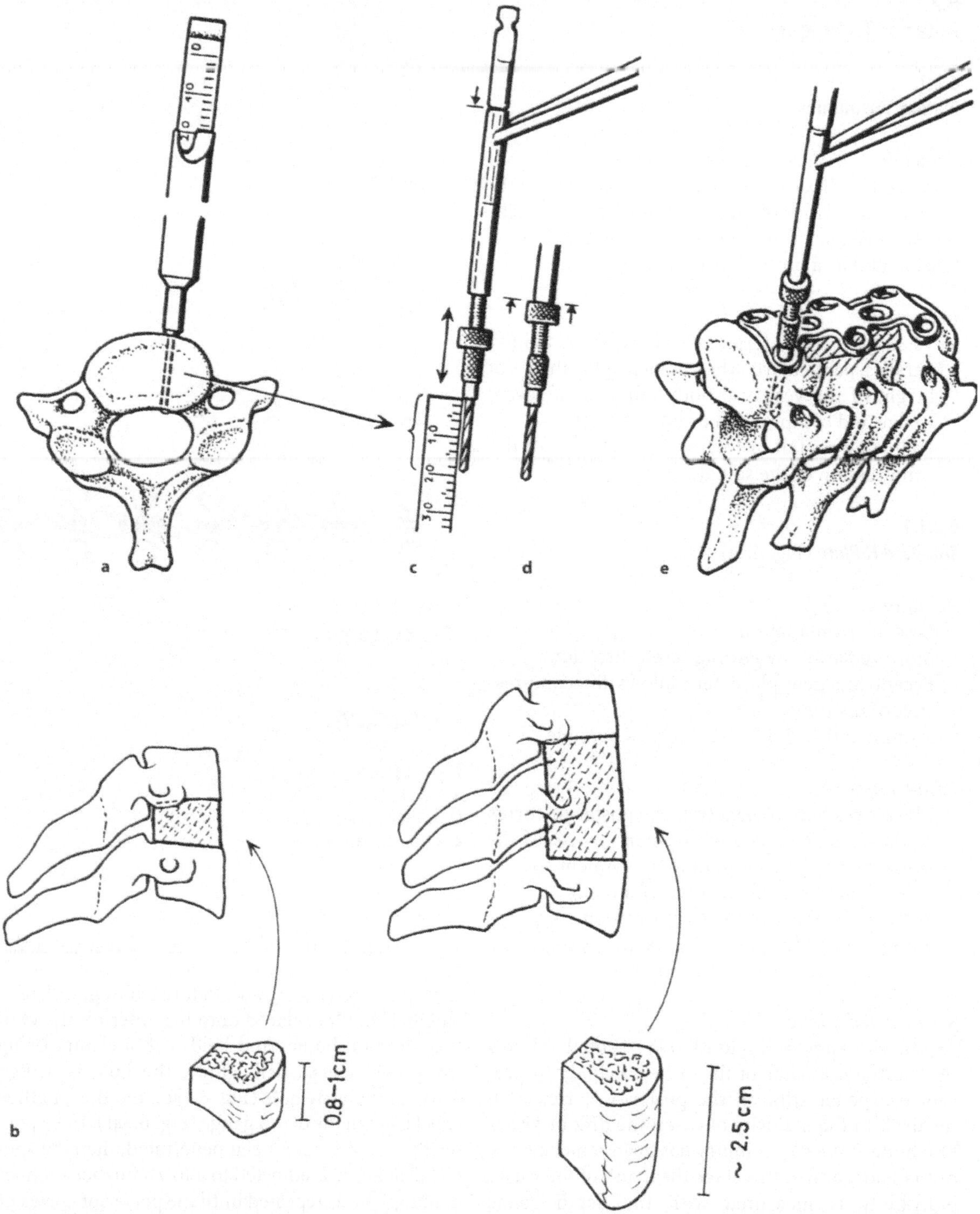

Fig. 6.24 Technique

a The depth of the vertebral body is measured with the depth gauge through the intervertebral space after removal of the disk

b Insertion of the wedge-shaped tricortical graft in order to maintain the lordosis in the sagittal plane

c The length of the protruding 2.5 mm drill is measured with a ruler (14–16 mm)

d It is ensured that the nut on the drill guide is tightly locked

e Using the present special drill guide, the hole is drilled through the plate hole

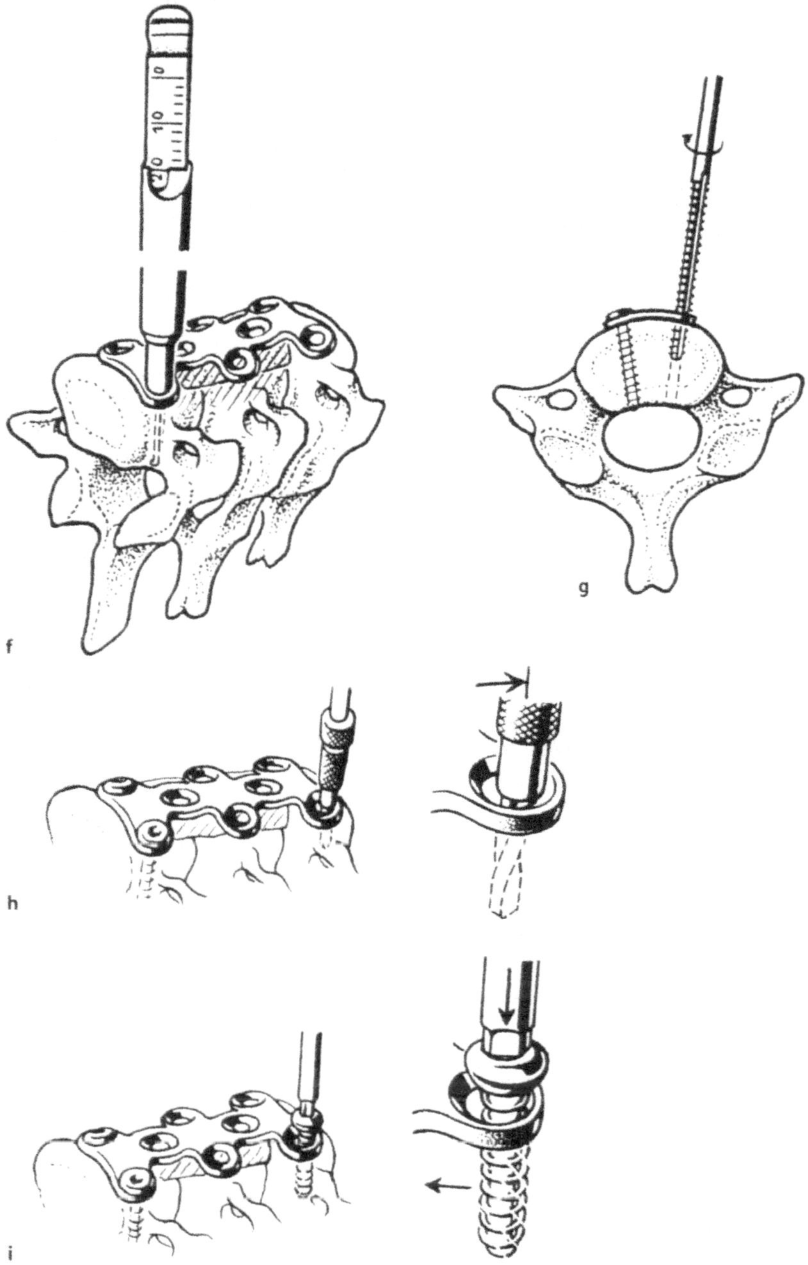

(Fig. 6.24)
f The length is checked with the depth gauge
g The anterior cortex of the vertebral body is tapped with the 2.5-mm tap
h Drilling eccentrically to allow compression of the graft
i Insertion of the eccentrically placed screw, which causes compression

holes. The drill holes can be eccentrically drilled (Fig. 6.24h) to allow axial compression on the vertebral graft and to enhance stability when tightening the screws (Fig. 6.24i).

Postoperative Care
A collar is worn for 6 weeks but may be removed for daily care.

6.2.1.2
Titanium Cervical Spine Locking Plate (CSLP)
(Figs. 6.25, 6.26)

Principle
The anterior titanium cervical spine locking plate system acts as a buttress plate in the stabilization of the anterior vertebral column.

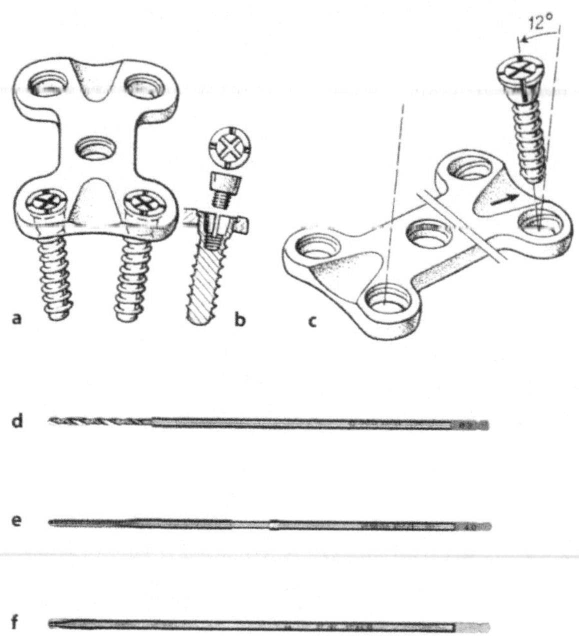

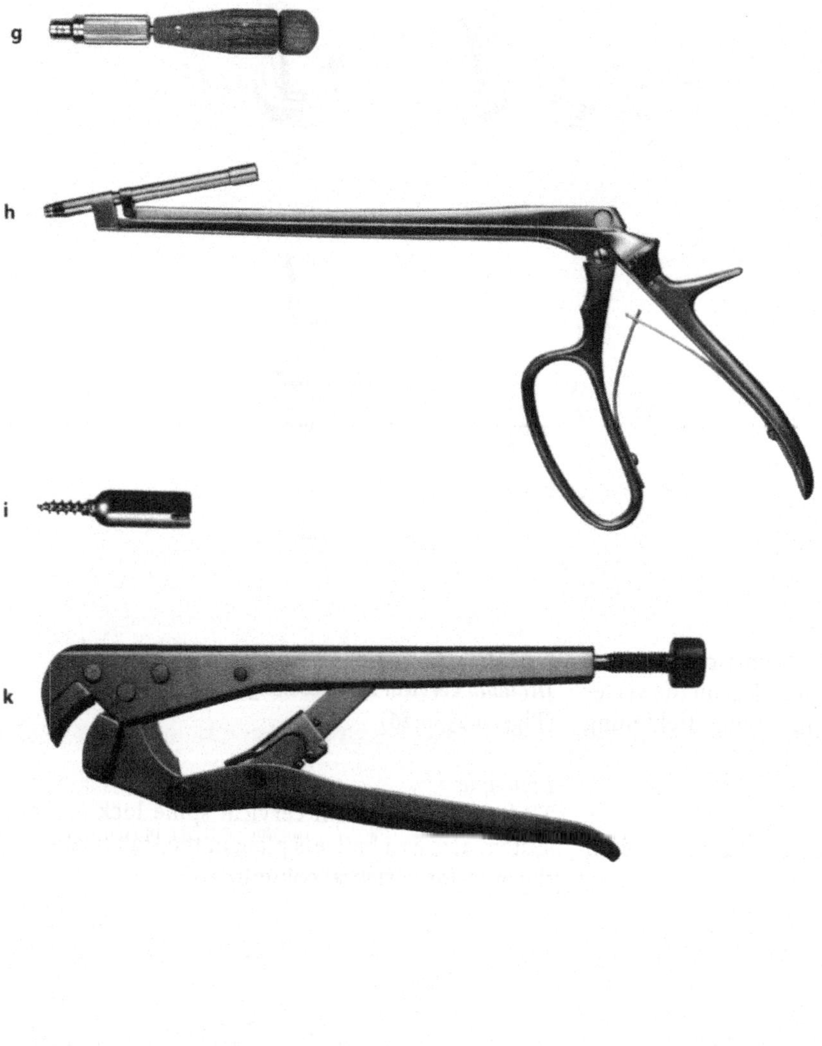

Fig. 6.25 Anterior plating techniques: cervical spine locking plate (CSLP) system. Implants and instruments.
a The screw-head is cross-split just above the start of the thread
b It can, therefore, be locked into the plate hole by means of a conical expansion bolt
c The direction of the screws in the plate. The arrow is used to ensure the plate is applied in the correct alignment. If the plate is applied at the cervicothoracic junction, the direction of the screw holes on this occasion pointing downwards, enabling the instruments to be used without impingement on the sternum
d Drill bit with stop, 3.0 mm diameter
e Tap for cervical spine
f Screwdriver shaft 4.0/4.35, cruciform, self holding
g Handle with quick coupling
h Drill guide 3.0, self-holding
i Fixation pin, temporary
k Bending pliers

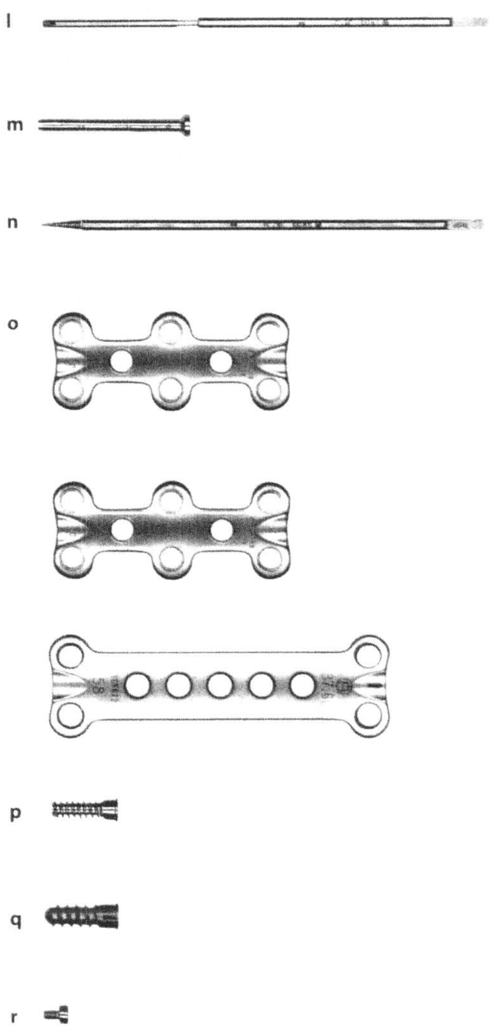

(Fig. 6.25)
l Screwdriver shaft 1.8, cruciform
m Holding sleeve
n Extraction screw, conical
o Cervical spine locking plates 4.0/4.35
p 4.0 mm solid expansionhead screw
q 4.35 mm cervical spine solid expansionhead screw
r 1.8 mm locking screw

Advantages
- The screws do not penetrate the posterior wall of the vertebral body.
- The locking of the screw heads into the cylindrical holes provides intrinsic stability.
- Locking prevents migration of the screw anteriorly.

Disadvantages
- The alignment of the screw holes in relation to the plate is fixed and can lead to occasional difficulties in screw placement.
- No axial compression is possible.

Implants and Instruments (Fig. 6.25a-c)
The expansion head of the screw is cylindrical with a rim stop and has a diameter of 4.5 mm. The screw head is cross-split just above the start of the thread (Fig. 6.25a,b) and can, therefore, be locked into the plate hole by means of a conical expansion bolt (Fig. 6.25b). The standard screws are 14 mm long with a thread diameter of 4.0 mm (Fig. 6.25p). Screws of 12 mm are available for patients of small stature and 16-mm screws for large patients or osteopenic patients. Appropriate drills and taps are available and are color coded along with the appropriate-screw lengths. The diameter of the screw holes is 4.5 mm and the plate thickness 2.0 mm. The direction of the screws in the plate must be appreciated: the cranial screws point 12° superiorly and 10° medially while the remaining screws are directed 10° medially (Fig. 6.25c). The cranial portion of the plate has a small arrow to identify the correct alignment of the plate (Fig. 6.25c).

When inserting the plate low in the cervical spine, especially into Th1 or occasionally into Th2, the plate can be placed with the arrow pointing downwards, which allows the lower screws to be inserted. This downward angulation allows the use of the instruments and screw which, otherwise, would abutt against the sternum. A smaller plate which has a lesser radius is available for patients of small stature. There is a wide range of plate sizes to allow application to the cervical and the upper thoracic spine. The titanium plasma spray-coated screws give a rough surface, increasing the area of contact. The original hollow screws which allowed ingrowth of bone have been changed to solid screws to facilitate screw removal.

Surgical Technique
The spine is approached anteriorly through a transverse incision at the appropriate level. Since the disks are angled in the horizontal plane such that their direction changes from caudal to cranial as

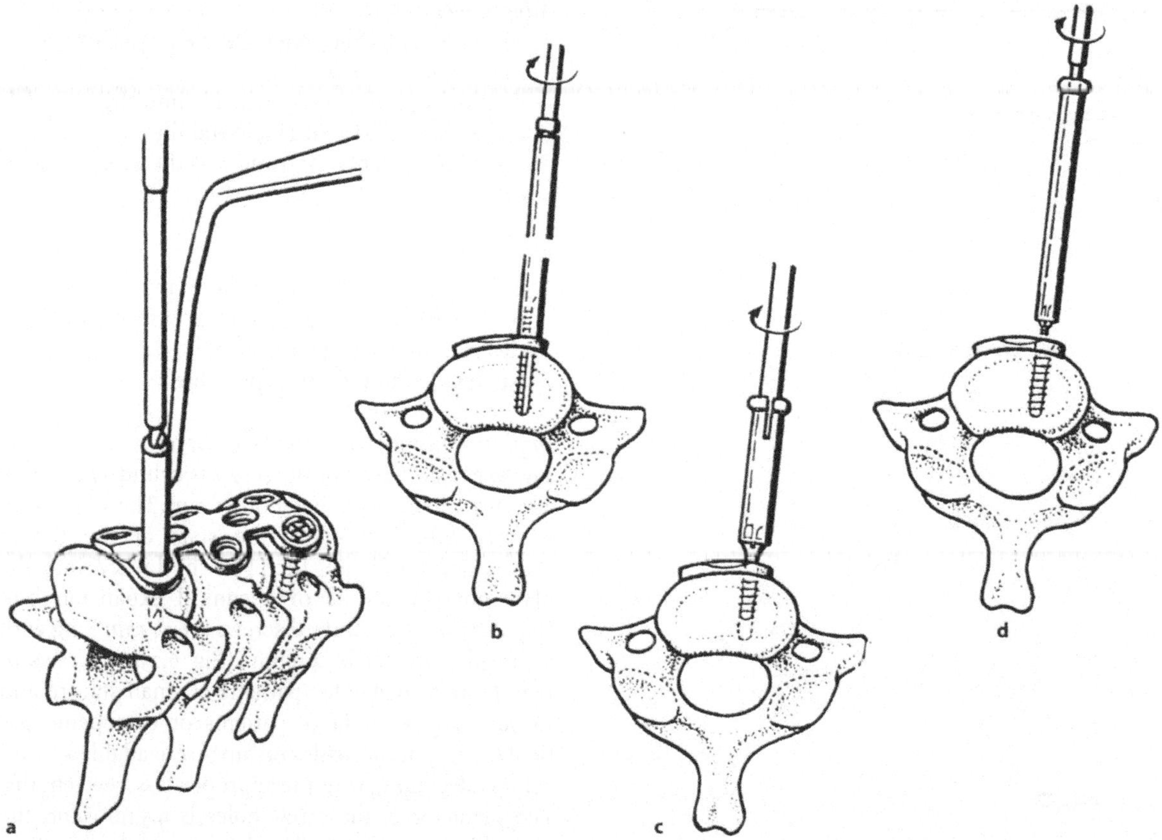

Fig. 6.26 Surgical technique
a The drill has a stop which allows only 14 mm penetration into the vertebral body
b The soft tissue protector is used when tapping the thread, and the tap also has a stop to prevent overpenetration
c The two split leaves disengage when tightened but remain on the screwdriver for ease of removal
d When the small screw is driven in, it expands the head of the larger screw and locks it into the plate

they extend from anterior to posterior, the plate size is selected to ensure that the screws penetrate the upper region of the vertebral bodies. This will prevent the screws from entering into the intervertebral disk above and below the level which requires fusion. Overriding of a normal disk by the plate must be avoided.

The plate is positioned and held with the self-holding drill-guide (Fig. 6.25h) and the first screw hole drilled with the aid of a special drill guide. While stabilizing the plate temporarly with a fixation pin located in a plate hole diagonally opposite the self-holding drill guide (Fig. 6.25i). The drill has a stop which allows only 14 mm penetration into the vertebral body (Fig. 6.26a). The soft tissue protector is used when tapping the thread, and the tap also has a stop to prevent overpenetration (Fig. 6.26b) *(note: do not carry on tapping after you reached the safety stop).*

The screws are applied using the crosshead screwdriver. A screw is taken from the screw tray with the Selfholding Screwdriver and inserted at the given angle. The screw should at first not be fully tightened because this could cause the opposite side of the plate to tilt (Fig. 6.26c).

The other screws are then inserted in the same manner, first the screw diagonally opposite, and then the others. When the last screw has been inserted, all screws should then be tightened in such a way that the screw heads are completely sunk in the plate. The plate is finally locked in place by the insertion of a small screw with a conical head. The small screw is held on the screwdriver by a split sleeve in the same way as the previously used screw. When the small screw is driven home, it expands the head of the larger screw and locks it into the plate (Fig. 6.26d).

Postoperative Care
A collar is worn for 6 weeks but may be removed for daily care.

CHAPTER 7

Stabilization Techniques: Thoracolumbar Spine

For stabilization of the thoracolumbar spine, anterior, posterior and combined techniques are used.

7.1 Anterior Techniques

7.1.1 Plate Techniques

7.1.1.1 Fixation with the Large Dynamic Compression Plate (DCP)

Principle

Anterior plate fixation is used to enhance stability of the anterior column following grafting techniques. The plate functions as a tension band in extension and as a buttress plate in flexion. From the practical point of view, it can be fixed to the front or the lateral aspect of the vertebral body without any difference in stability (Fig. 7.2).

Indications

- To support the anterior column when instability persists, particularly in association with loss of height of the vertebral body following a severe wedge compression or burst fracture.

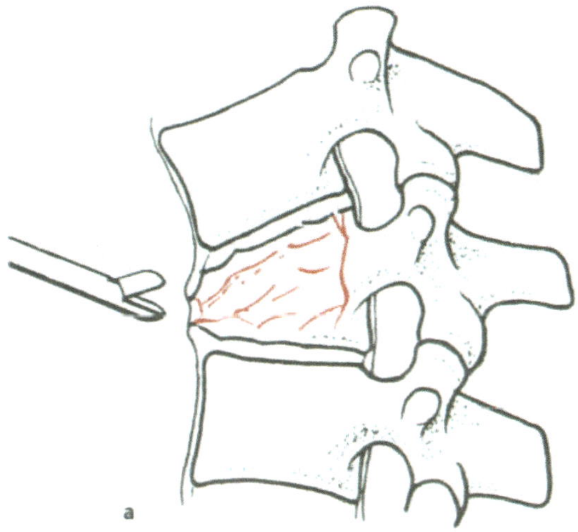

a

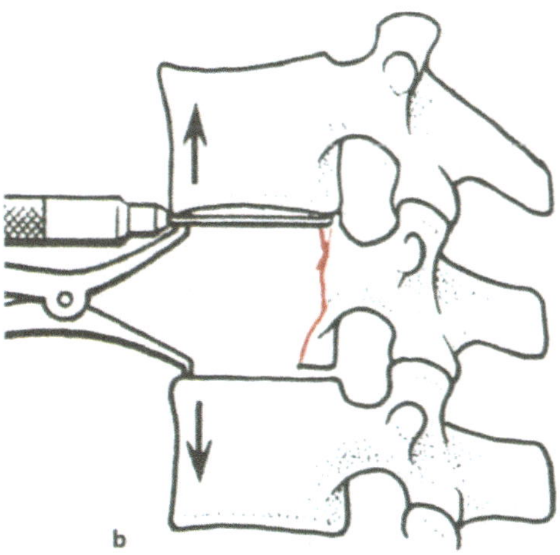

b

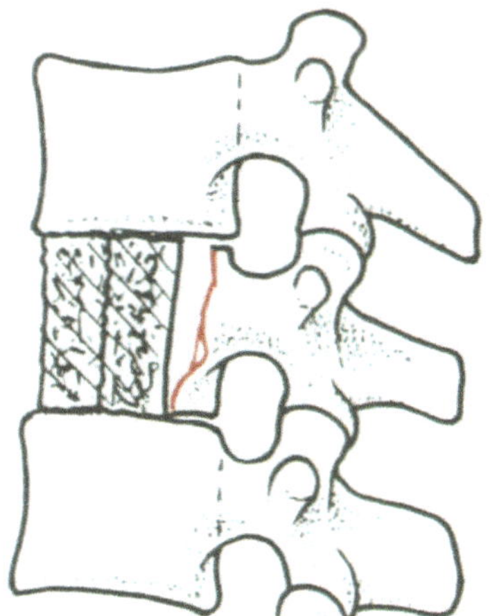

c

Fig. 7.1 Anterior fixation with the broad DCP in the thoracolumbar spine
a The fragments of the fractured vertebral body and the disks are removed
b The depth of the vertebral body is measured with the depth gauge, and the intervertebral defect is distracted with a bone distractor
c The anterior column is reconstructed with one to three corticocancellous iliac bone grafts

- Following partial or total vertebrectomy for decompression of the spinal cord especially in spinal tumors.

Advantages
- Short segment fixation.
- Relatively easy technique.

Disadvantages
- Loosening of the screws due to poor fixation in cancellous bone.
- Backing out of screws, especially if the plate is placed in the front of the vertebral body.
- No fixed angle between the screws and the plate.

Implants and Instruments
A stainless steel broad DCP (femur plate) and 4.5-mm cortical and/or 6.5-mm cancellous screws are used.

Surgical technique
A standard approach is made to expose the anterior vertebral column. The segmental vessels are ligated. Before applying a plate, the anterior column is reconstructed with a tricortical iliac bone graft and supplemented with cancellous bone (Fig. 7.1c).

Anterior Placement of the Plate. After removal of th appropriate disks (Fig. 7.1a), the depth of the verte bra is measured with the depth gauge (Fig. 7.1b) The special 3.2-mm drill guide is used and adjuste so the appropriate length of drill will penetrate th vertebra and the length of the protruding drill i measured with a ruler. The femoral plate thicknes is 4 mm and is added to the measured depth. Th broad DCP of appropriate length is applied to th anterior aspect of the vertebral body and fixed wit 4.5-mm screws (Fig. 7.2a). If the bone is porotic, th 6.5-mm cancellous bone screws may be used, partic ularly in the end holes.

When considering anterior application of th plate, the risk of grave complications inherent in thi placement must be taken into account. Its use in thi situation may only be indicated in exceptional cir cumstances such as metastatic tumors with a shor life expectancy. Implant loosening, especially back ing out of screws, may cause erosion of the esopha gus, aorta or vena cava.

Lateral Placement of the Plate. An appropriate length broad DCP is placed on the lateral aspect o the vertebral body. The plate is applied using stan dard AO methods (Fig. 7.2b). The advantage of thi technique is that one keeps away from the aorta an vena cava, especially should a screw become loos and back out.

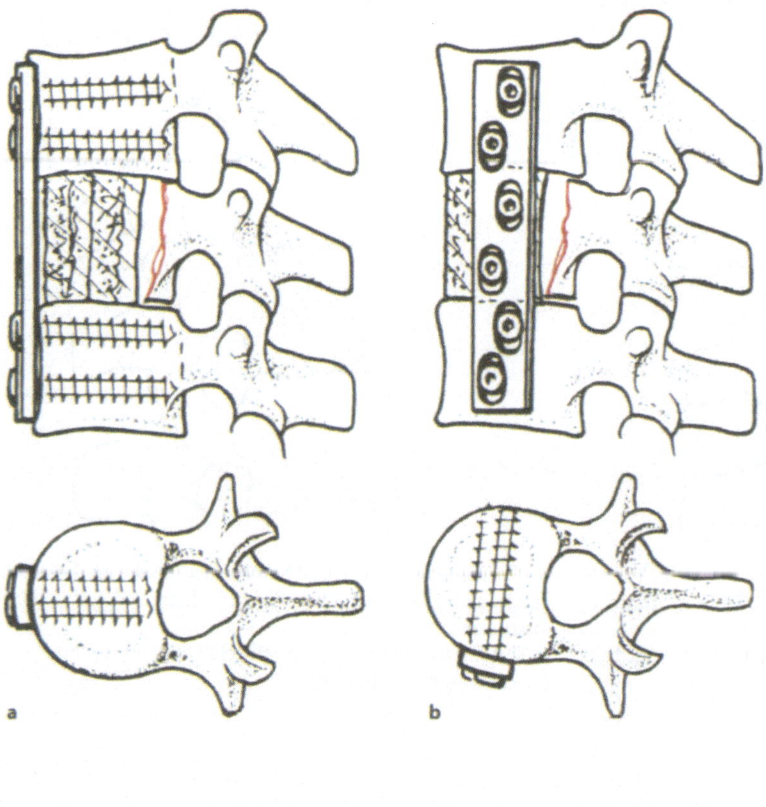

Fig. 7.2 Anterior or lateral placement of the plate
a Application of the broad DCP of appropriate length to the anterior aspect of the vertebral body and fixation with 4.5-mm screws
b Application of the plate, using standard AO techniques, to the lateral aspec of the spine

Postoperative Care

The patient is mobilized with an appropriate thoracolumbar support for 12 weeks. The support may be removed for daily care and, after 6 weeks, when resting.

7.1.1.2
Anterior Titanium Thoracolumbar Locking Plate

Principle

The Anterior Titanium Thoracolumbar Locking Plate (ATLP) system is designed to secure and stabilize the anterior column of the spine and act as a buttress plate. The ATLP allows direct compression across the graft site and provides stable fixation of the anterior column of the spine. The AO/ASIF long spinal instruments for anterior surgery facilitate this procedure.

Indications

- To support the anterior column when instability persists, particularly in association with loss of height of the vertebral body following a severe wedge compression or burst fracture.
- Following partial total vertebrectomy for decompression of the spinal cord especially in spinal tumors.

Advantages

- Short segmental fixation.
- Allows compression across the graft.
- Maintains the sagittal plane.
- Fixed angle between the screws and the plate.
- Screw locks into the plate.
- Magnetic resonance imaging (MRI) compatible.

Disadvantages

- Fixed position of screws into the vertebral body.
- Screw direction critical.
- Cannot be used above Th8/Th10.

Implants and Instruments (Fig. 7.3)

Surgical Technique

Preoperative planning plays an important role in the preparation for surgery. Titanium ATLP system X-ray templates are available to assist in selecting the appropriate range of plate sizes. The decision on which side to approach the patient is based on the vascular anatomy and spinal pathology.

If a disk excision or a vertebrectomy has been performed (Fig. 7.4a), the vertebral body spreader is used to restore the normal sagittal profile (Fig. 7.4b, c). The height is maintained by the use of a tricortical graft or substitute vertebral body (Fig. 7.5). The threaded drill-guide is attached to the center hole of the plate. This drill-guide is attached to the threaded drill-guide applicator and functions as a plate-holder (Fig. 7.6). The plate is positioned anterolaterally on the posterior one-third of the vertebral body. Take care to ensure that all screws will be placed into the vertebral body. In most surgical procedures, either the whole disk or a partial/total vertebrectomy has been performed and the position of the posterior cortex of the vertebral body can be visualized. If in doubt, a lateral radiograph should be taken to ensure appropriate placement of the screws so that no screw violates the spinal canal.

The first temporary fixation hole is made using the 2.5-mm three-fluted drill bit with stop and the 2.5-mm-long DCP drill guide through the DCP hole (Fig. 7.6a). The DCP drill guide has an arrow on the drill barrel that must pointed toward the graft site to achieve compression. The 2.5-mm drill bit has an automatic stop at 30 mm which corresponds to the length of the temporary screws.

A 4.0-mm titanium cancellous bone screw is used with a long-handled small hexagonal screwdriver

Figs. 7.3–7.6 Anterior Titanium Thoracolumbar Locking Plate

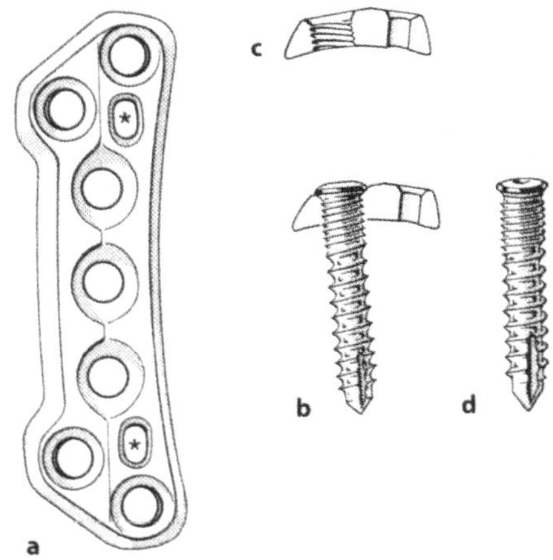

Fig. 7.3 Instruments and implants
a The plate is precontoured to conform to the shape of the anatomy
b Screws are triangulated for improved resistance to construct pullout. Screws are countersunk into the plate to provide a low profile
c Screws incorporate a machine thread section which locks the screw to the plate to prevent backout. Plates and screws are available in a wide variety of sizes to accommodate variations in anatomy
d Self-tapping screws have a cancellous pitch
* DCP holes

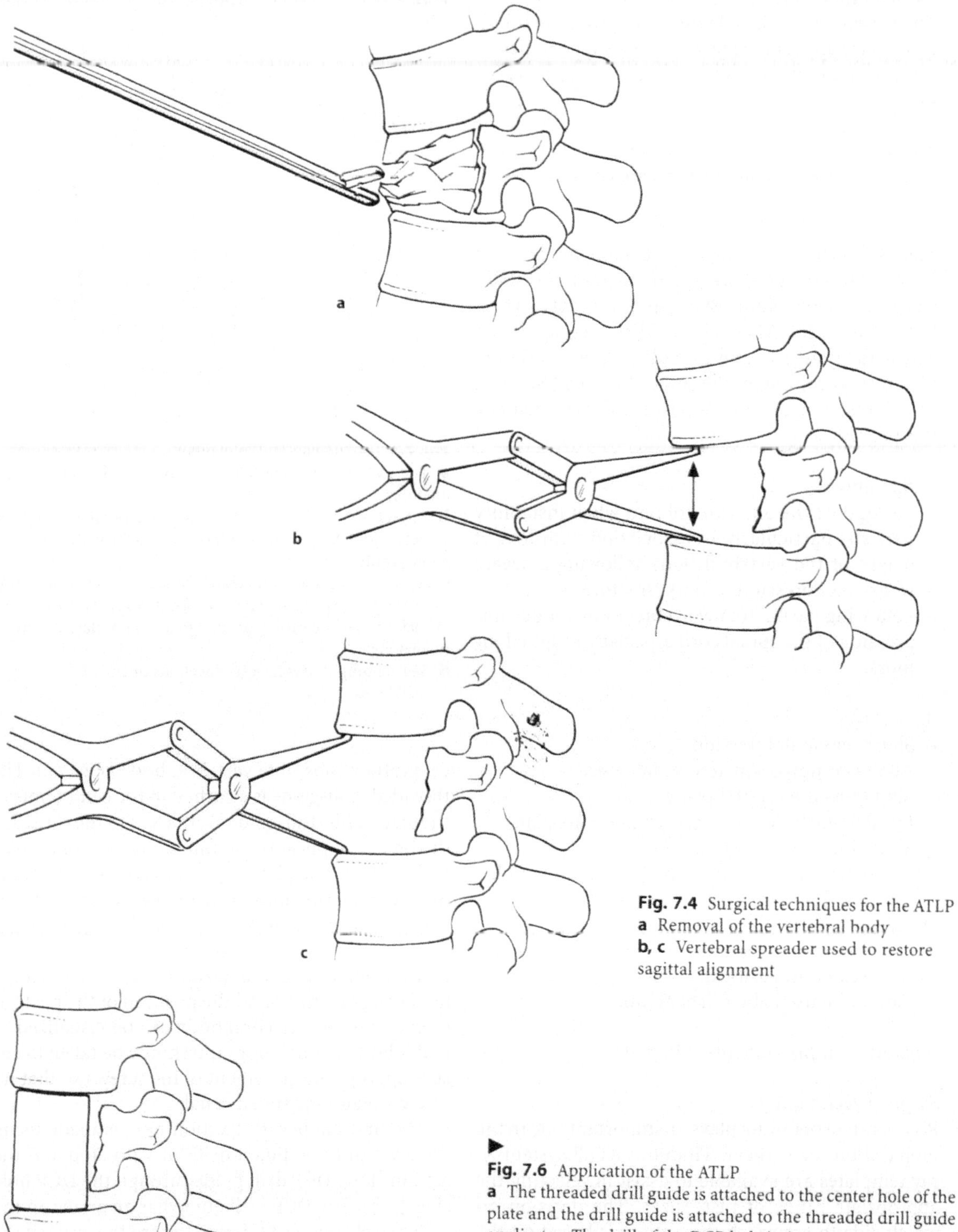

Fig. 7.4 Surgical techniques for the ATLP
a Removal of the vertebral body
b, c Vertebral spreader used to restore sagittal alignment

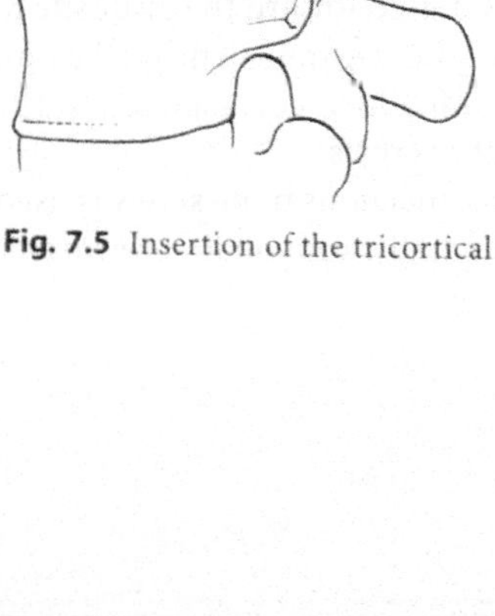

Fig. 7.5 Insertion of the tricortical bone graft

▶
Fig. 7.6 Application of the ATLP
a The threaded drill guide is attached to the center hole of the plate and the drill guide is attached to the threaded drill guide applicator. The drill of the DCP hole in its appropriate guide
b Insertion of the 30-mm screw with the long-handled small hexagonal screwdriver and tightening of the second screw, thus placing the graft under compression prior to final plate fixation
c Application of the threaded drill-guide onto the posterior hole

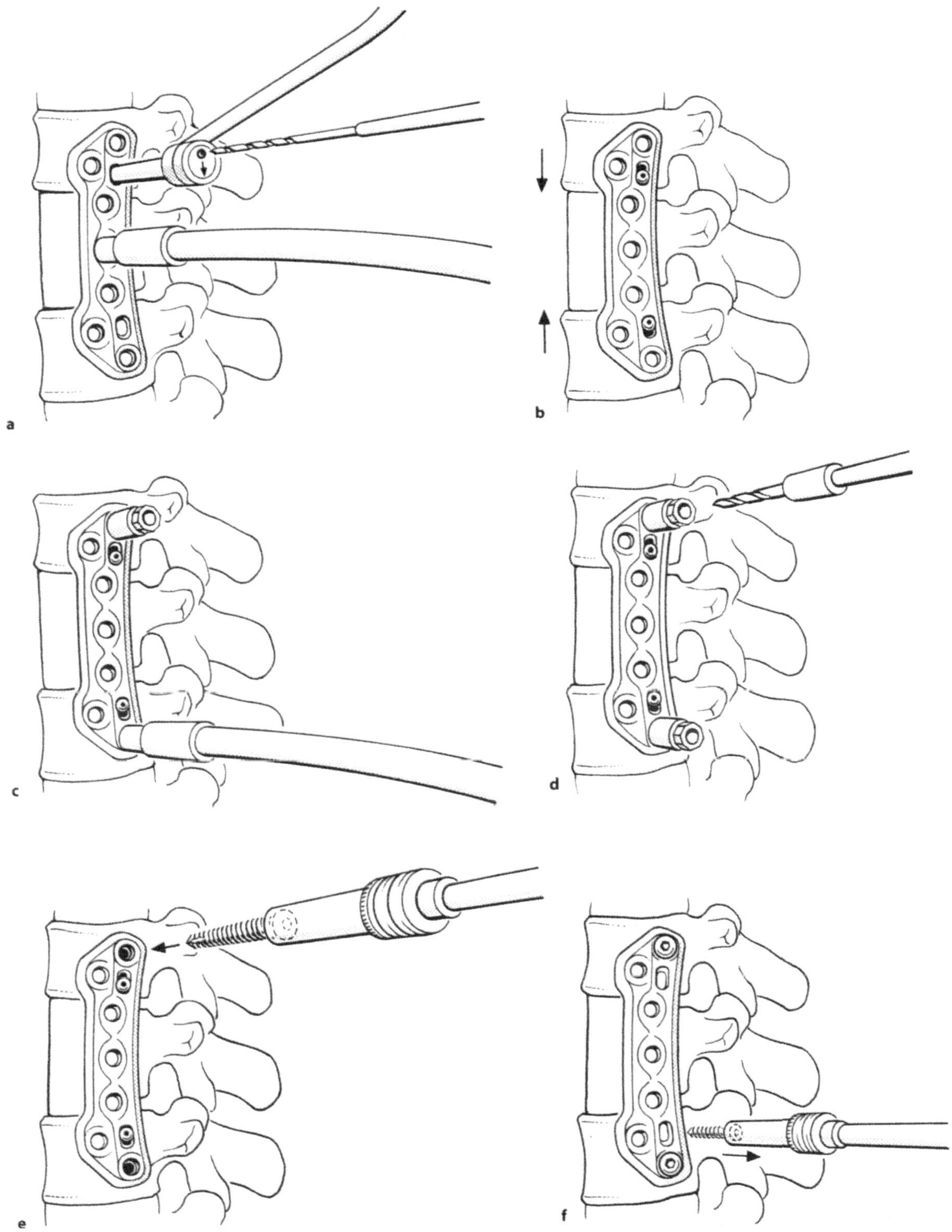

d Drilling through the preassembled drill guide with the 5.0-mm flexible drill bit with stop
e Insertion of the 7.5-mm anterior titanium locking screw using the long hexagonal screwdriver and sleeve. The screw must be inserted perpendicular to the plate to ensure that the screw will lock into the plate
f Removal of the temporary 4.0-mm cancellous bone screw
(Fig **g**, **h** see p. 88)

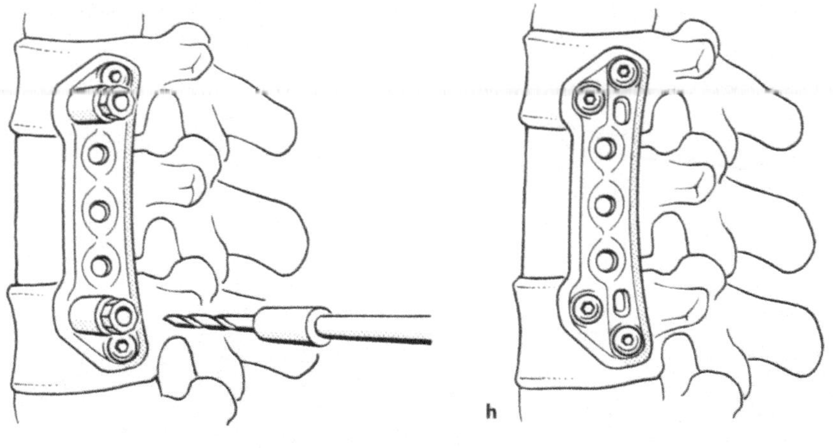

g h

(Fig. 7.6)
g Anterior holes drilled with 5.0-mm flexible drill bit and drill-guide
h The plate with screws inserted

and holding sleeve. Do not completely tighten the screw. Place the secondary temporary screw in the same manner. The screws are now sequentially tightened to place the graft under compression prior to final plate fixation (Fig. 7.6b).

The threaded drill-guide applicator is used to remove the threaded drill-guide from the center hole and place the threaded drill guide in one of the posterior holes. Place the second threaded drill guide in the other posterior hole, again using the threaded drill guide applicator (Fig. 7.6c). These drill-guides ensure perpendicular placement of the drill bit relative to the plate.

Drill the posterior holes through the preassembled threaded drill guides using the 5.0-mm flexible drill-bit with stop (Fig. 7.6d). Since purchase in the opposite cortex is not necessary, the drill bit has an automatic stop at 30 mm to prevent overdrilling. If the bone is osteoporotic, then the purchase of the screw to the opposite cortex may be necessary; in this case, the length of the screw is determined by measuring by using the AO depth gauge using the tip to abut against the far cortex.

Remove the threaded drill-guides with the threaded drill-guide applicator. Insert the appropriate-length 7.5-mm titanium anterior spinal locking screws using the long large hexagonal screwdriver and holding sleeve (Fig. 7.6e). The screws must seat completely into the plate to secure the locking mechanism of the screw. Special care should be taken to retract properly the surrounding soft tissue so that there is no movement of the screw from its perpendicular position as it is inserted into the plate.

The 4.0-mm titanium cancellous bone screws which served as temporary fixation must now be removed (Fig. 7.6f). The compression of the graft site will be maintained by the permanent 7.5-mm locking screws. Failure to remove the temporary screws will inhibit the insertion of the anterior locking screws.

Insert the threaded drill-guides into the anterior holes using the threaded drill-guide applicator. Drill the anterior holes through the preassembled threaded drill-guides using the 5.0-mm flexible drill bit with stop as before (Fig. 7.6g). Remove the threaded drill-guides with the threaded drill-guide applicator. Insert the 7.5-mm locking screws with the long large hexagonal screwdriver and holding sleeve. Special care should be taken to retract properly the surrounding soft tissue so that there is no movement of the screw from its perpendicular position as it is inserted into the plate. Once again, the screws must seat completely into the plate to secure the locking mechanism of the screw (Fig. 7.6h).

7.1.2
Rod Systems

7.1.2.1
Fixation with the Anterior USS (See also Chap. 9)

7.1.2.1.1
Anterior Construct

Instruments and Implants (Fig. 7.7)
The Universal Spine System (USS) can be used to reconstruct or stabilize the anterior column. The construct will allow compression across the graft site and it will also act as a buttress plate.

Indication
- Similar to the other constructs in this section.

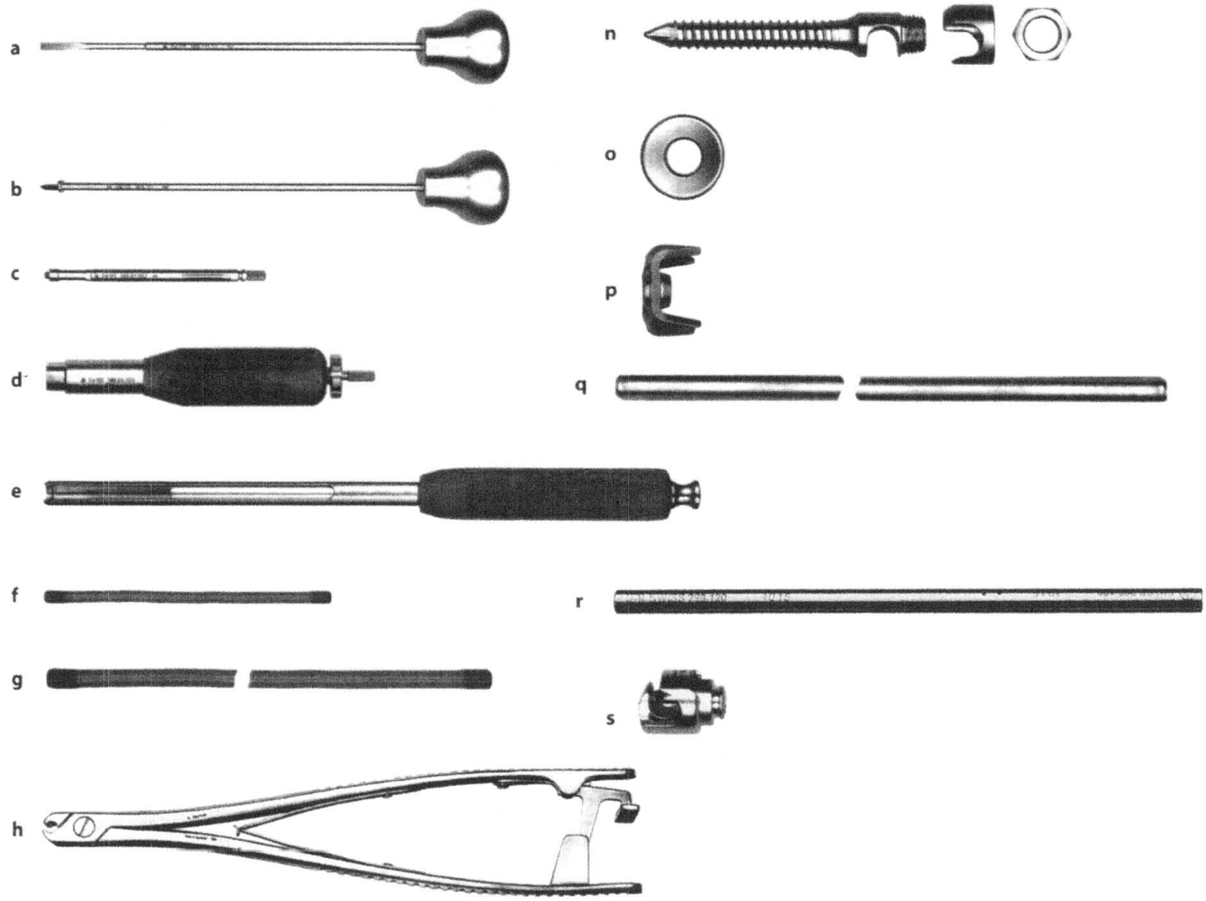

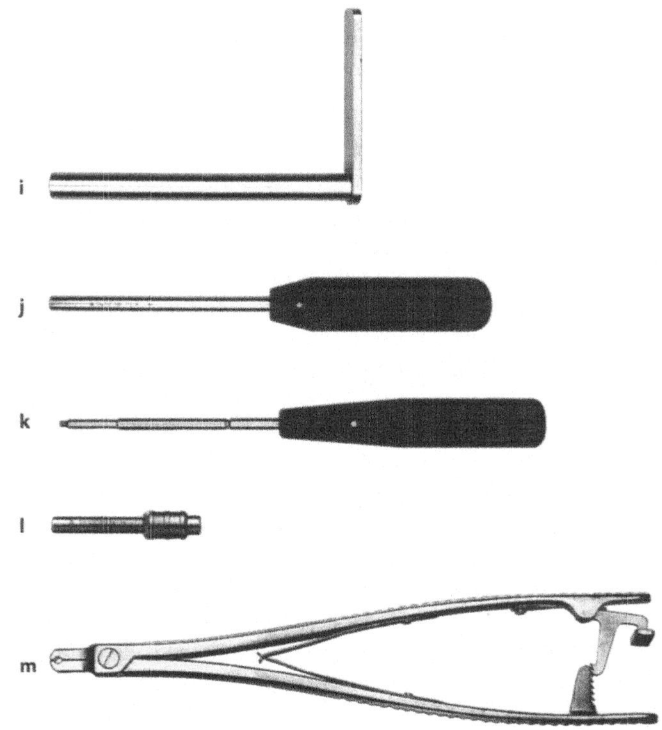

Fig. 7.7 *a–m* Instruments, *n–s* Implants
- **a** USS pedicle probe 3.8 mm diameter
- **b** USS pedicle awl
- **c** USS hook and screw holder
- **d** USS universal handle
- **e** USS pusher for angled USS washers
- **f** USS bending template for USS rods 6.0 mm diameter, 150 mm
- **g** USS bending template for USS rods 6.0 mm diameter, 400 mm
- **h** USS holding forceps for USS rods 6.0 mm diameter
- **i** USS socket wrench 11 mm
- **j** USS socket wrench 6 mm
- **k** Screwdriver, hexagonal, small with groove
- **l** USS holding sleeve
- **m** USS holding forceps for USS rods 3.5 and 4.5 mm diameter
- **n** USS pedicle screw, side-opening, 5, 6 and 7 mm diameter
- **o** USS washer for screws, 5, 6 and 7 mm diameter
- **p** USS staple for screws 5,6 and 7 mm diameter
- **q** USS rod 6 mm diameter, hard
- **r** USS rod 3.5 mm diameter for USS cross-link system
- **s** USS cross-link system

Figs. 7.8, 7.9 The USS anterior construct

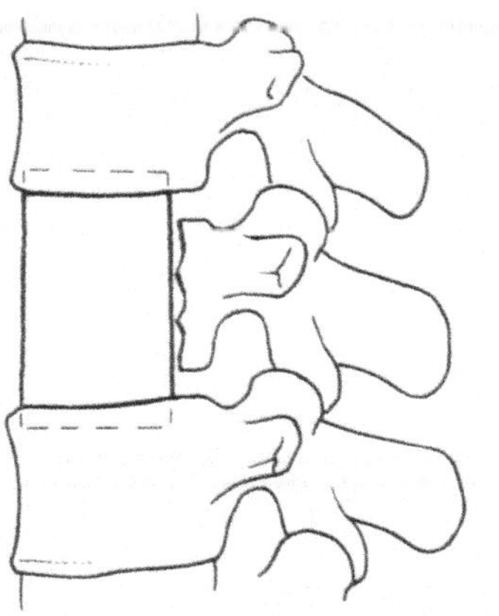

Fig. 7.8 Placement of the spacer – tricortical graft or cage (see Fig. 7.5)

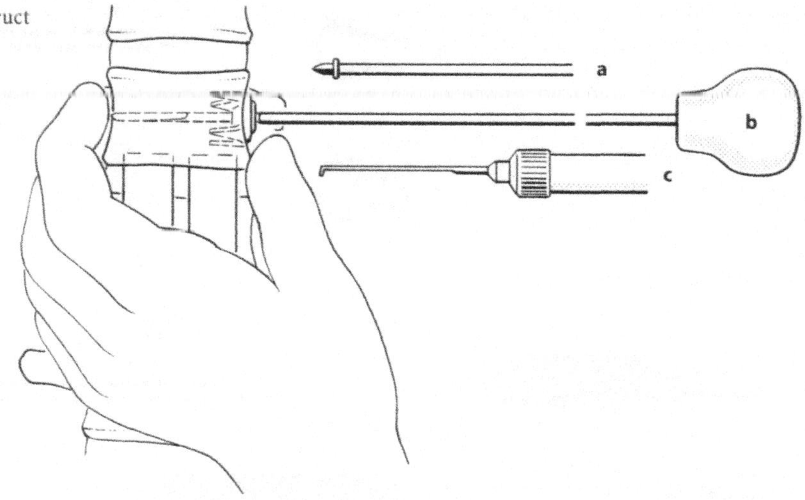

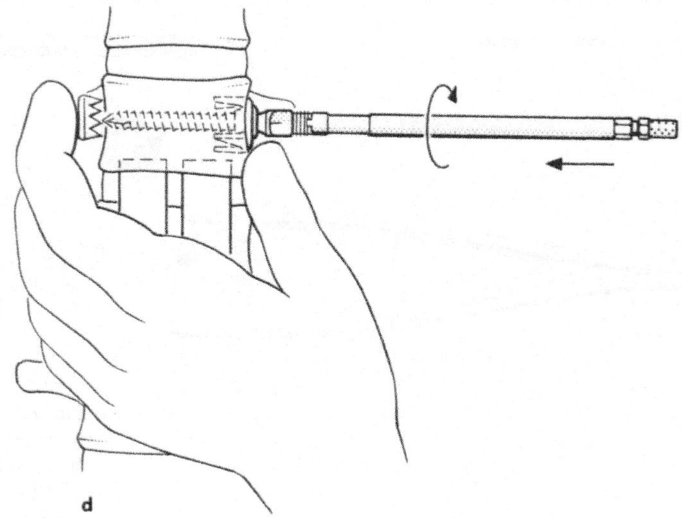

Fig. 7.9
a Penetration of the cortex with the sharp awl
b Opening of the direction for the screw with the blunt awl. This must not penetrate the spinal canal
c The depth is measured
d A staple is positioned over the set screw hole and the appropriate-length 6-mm titanium USS screw is inserted with a plastic washer when penetrating the far cortex

Advantages

- Ease of application.
- Allows compression across the bone graft.
- Maintains the sagittal plane.
- MRI compatible.

Disadvantage

- Higher profile than the ATLP or Ventrofix.

Surgical Technique

The spine is exposed and after treating the pathology, the sagittal plane is restored as described earlier in this section with either a bone graft or spacer (Fig. 7.8, see also Fig. 7.4). The standard 6-mm titanium USS screws are used. The first screws are placed toward the posterior aspect of the vertebral body near the base of the pedicle and should be parallel to the back of the posterior wall of the vertebral body. The entry point is made with the sharp awl (Fig. 7.9a). The blunt awl is then inserted into the vertebral body parallel to the posterior cortex of the vertebral body. It is useful to aim the tip of the awl at the tip of the index finger which has been placed at the planned exit point (Fig. 7.9b). If the quality of the bone is poor, the far cortex should be penetrated. The depth is measured (Fig. 7.9c), a staple positioned and the appropriate-length 6-mm titanium USS screw inserted (Fig. 7.9d). When penetrating the far cortex, a plastic washer can be used in order to stabilize the screw better in the porotic vertebral body.

A similar procedure is performed in the caudal vertebra. The length of the 6-mm hard rods is determined with the template (Fig. 7.9e). The two rods attached to the parallel connector are now fixed to the

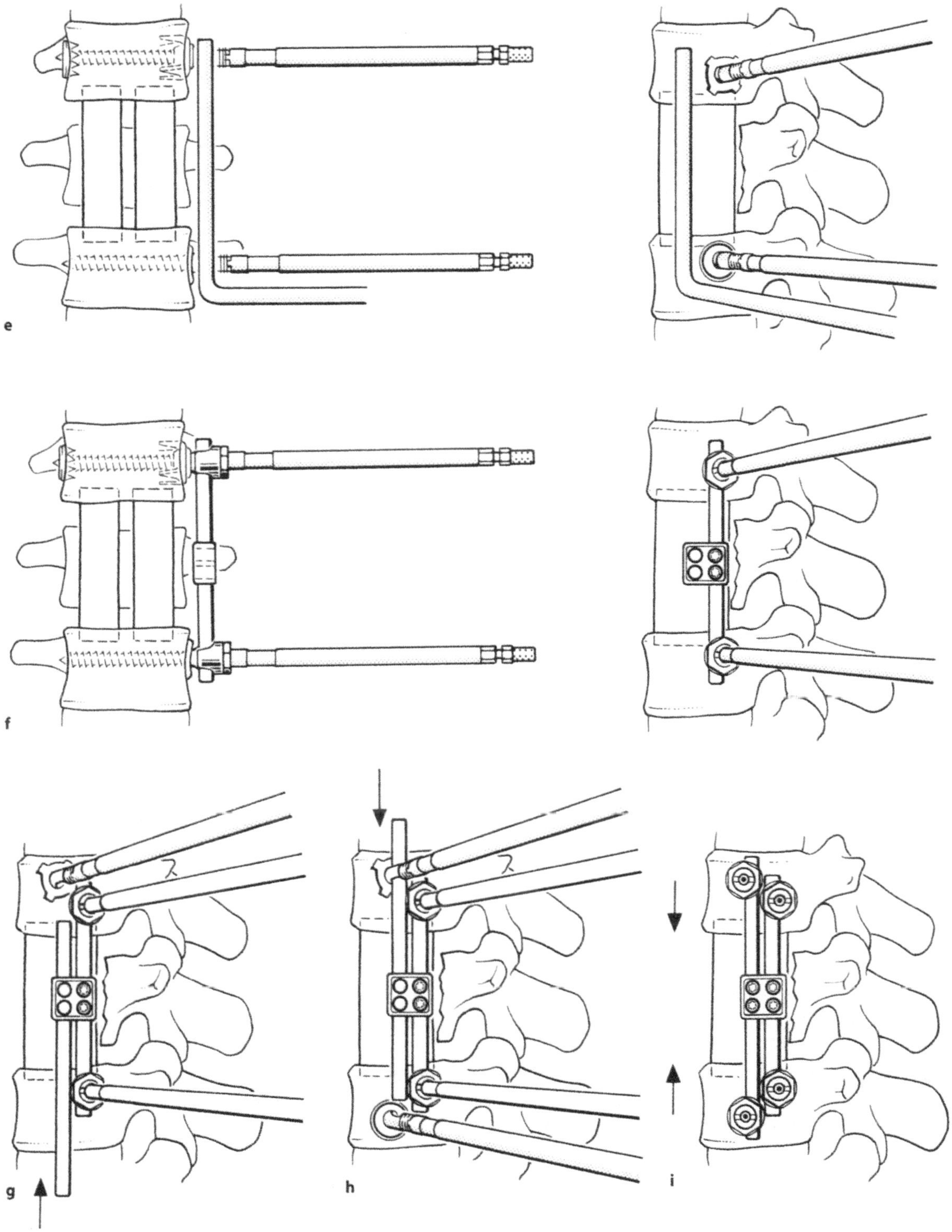

(Fig. 7.9)
e A template rod is used to assess the required length of the 6-mm hard titanium rods
f The correct-length rods and parallel connector are attached to the posterior screws
g The anterior 6-mm rod is slid distally and the cranial 6-mm screw is inserted
h The 6-mm rod is now moved proximally and the distal 6-mm screw is inserted
i Compression is applied to the graft via compression clamp and the distal screws are tightened

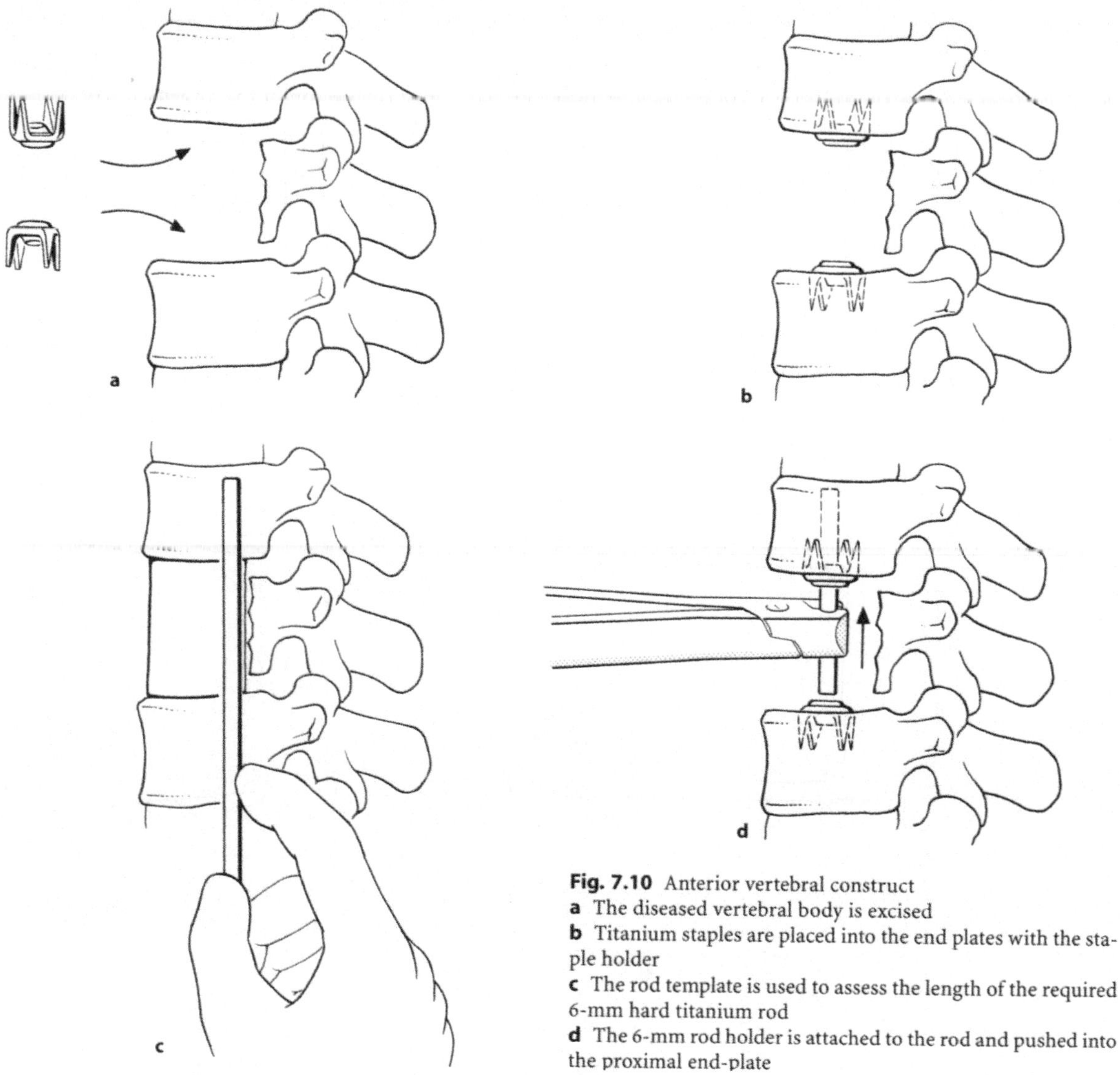

Fig. 7.10 Anterior vertebral construct
a The diseased vertebral body is excised
b Titanium staples are placed into the end plates with the staple holder
c The rod template is used to assess the length of the required 6-mm hard titanium rod
d The 6-mm rod holder is attached to the rod and pushed into the proximal end-plate

posterior screw and held with the sleeves and nut (Fig. 7.9f). The anterior rod is slid distally and the 6-mm-diameter USS screw opening prepared as described above and the screw inserted so that the opening of the screw aligns with the rod (Fig. 7.9g). The rod is then slid proximally and the distal screw inserted (Fig. 7.9h). Compression is now applied by locking the parallel connector to the rods. The proximal screw should be locked to the rods. The compression clamp is used to apply compression to the graft (Fig. 7.8i). The distal rods are then locked to the pedicle screws.

7.1.2.1.2
Anterior Vertebral Body Construct (Fig. 7.10)

Indication
This technique is *only* used to reconstruct vertebral bodies which have been destroyed by malignant tumors.

Contraindication
Multilevel disease requiring more than two vertebral excisions.

Surgical Technique
The dorsal vertebrae are removed (Fig. 7.10a). The titanium staples are embedded into each normal

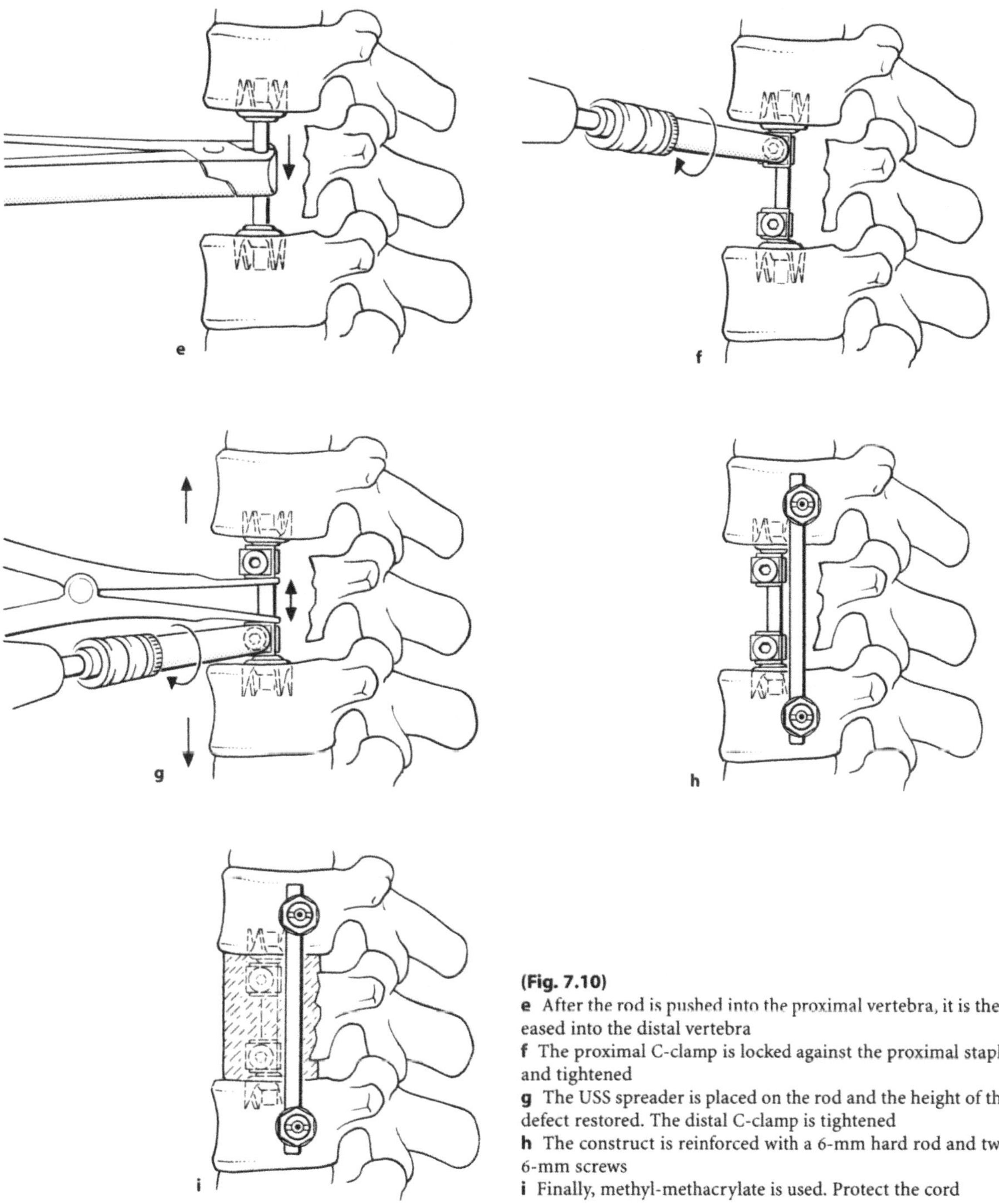

(Fig. 7.10)

e After the rod is pushed into the proximal vertebra, it is then eased into the distal vertebra

f The proximal C-clamp is locked against the proximal staple and tightened

g The USS spreader is placed on the rod and the height of the defect restored. The distal C-clamp is tightened

h The construct is reinforced with a 6-mm hard rod and two 6-mm screws

i Finally, methyl-methacrylate is used. Protect the cord

end-plate (Fig. 7.10b). A rod template is used to assess the length of the 6-mm hard rod, which should protrude into a third of each vertebral body (Fig. 7.10c). The 6-mm rod holder is attached to the rod and pushed into the proximal end-plate; if difficulty is encountered, start the entry hole with the sharp awl. The rod is pushed into the proximal vertebral body (Fig. 7.10d) and then eased into the distal vertebral body (Fig. 7.10e). C-clamps are placed loosely onto the rod so that they abut against the proximal and distal staple. The proximal C-clamp is locked (Fig. 7.10f). The USS spreader is placed onto the rod and between the C-clamps and the height of the space is restored. The distal C-clamp is now locked (Fig. 7.10g). This construct is reinforced with a 6-mm hard rod and two 6-mm pedicle screws. The technique of insertion is described in the previous section (Fig. 7.10h). The defect is now packed with methyl-methacrylate. However, it is important that, before applying the cement, the cord is protected with a sheath of collagen substitute. A blunt elevator is also used to ensure the cement does not extrude onto the cord (Fig. 7.10i).

7.1.2.2 Fixation with the Anterior Titanium Rod System (VentroFix)

Principle
The anterior rod system acts in a similar manner to the plate systems.

Indications
- To support the anterior column when instability exists particularly in association with loss of height of the vertebral body following a severe wedge compression or burst fracture.
- Following partial or total vertebrectomy.

Advantages
- Short segment fixation.
- Allows distraction and compression of the defect.
- Maintains the sagittal plane.
- Fixed angle between clamps and screws.
- Screws locked onto clamps.
- MRI compatible.

Disadvantage
- Direction of screws critical.

Implants and Instruments
Implants and instruments are shown in Fig. 7.11.

7.1.2.2.1 Double-Rod Clamp Configuration

This construct is used when the whole vertebra is available for the insertion of the screws. The implants consist of two 6-mm USS bars of appropriate length. Two double-rod clamps with the holes for the screws placed diagonally and locking screws are used.

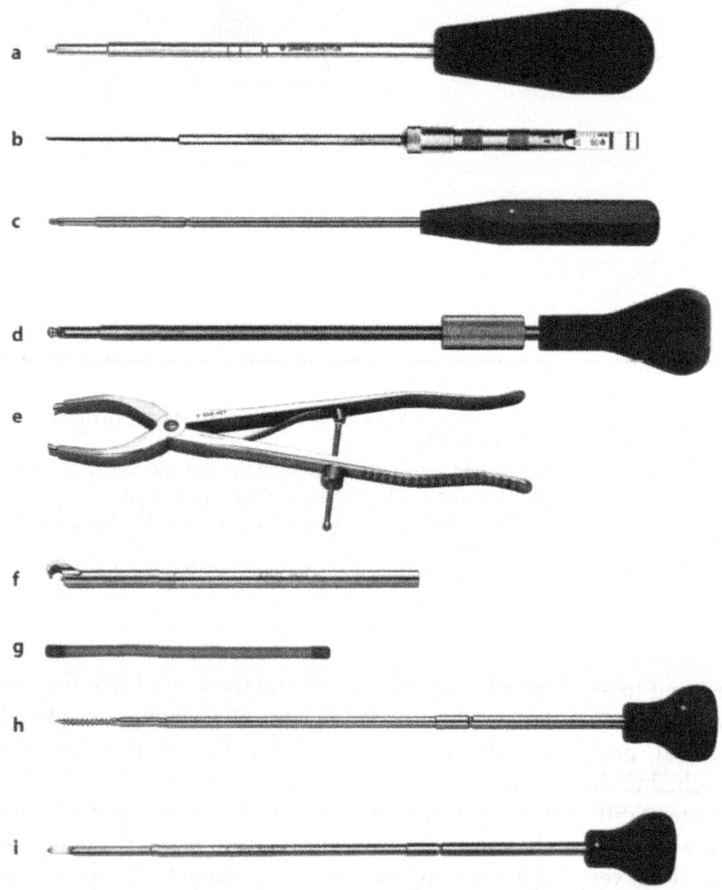

Fig. 7.11 VentroFix: implants and instruments
a Screwdriver, hexagonal, large
b Depth guage
c Screwdriver torx T15
d Positioner, self-holding
e Compression forceps
f Compression support
g USS bending template
h Fixation pin
i Awl 4.9 mm diameter

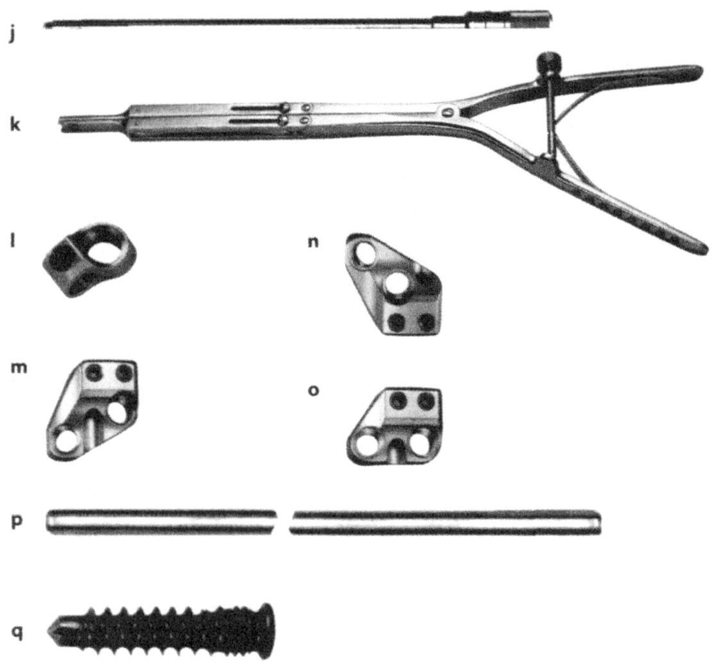

(Fig. 7.11)
j Drill sleeve for Awl 4.9 mm diameter
k Spreader forceps, parallel
l VentroFix single clamp
m VentroFix double rod clamp, right cranial
n VentroFix double rod clamp, left cranial
o VentroFix fracture clamp
p USS rod
q Locking screw 7.5 mm diameter, self-tapping

Assembly of the Montage (Fig. 7.12)
The correct length 6-mm USS rods are placed into the clamps, the set screws over the incomplete holes are tightened (Fig. 7.12a) and the length protruding adjusted to allow compression of the graft (Fig. 7.12b). The construct is ready for use.

Surgical Technique (Fig. 7.13–7.21)
A standard approach is made to expose the anterior vertebral body. If a vertebrectomy has been performed, the column is reconstructed with either a tricortical graft or a titanium cage. The anterior column defect is distracted with a spreader (Fig. 7.13) and a graft inserted (Fig. 7.14). A template is used to measure the appropriate-length 6-mm rod (Fig. 7.15). The double-clamp montage is assembled (see above) and the drill guides with integrated fixation pin are attached to the posterior hole of each clamp (Fig. 7.16a). The montage is held at both ends with the long drill-guides/fixation pins. The fixation pins should not be exposed at this stage.

The assembled montage is placed onto the anterior vertebral column (Fig. 7.16b). The superior and inferior end plates are trimmed to ensure the clamps lie in direct contact with the vertebral body. The self-tapping 2.5-mm fixation pins are exposed and inserted into the posterior holes of the clamps and tightened to ensure close approximation of the implant against the vertebral body (Fig. 7.17a). *Ensure the direction of the drill holes does not penetrate the spinal canal.* At this stage it is necessary to ensure the height of the anterior column is correct and the sagittal plane has been restored. *A lateral radiograph is absolutely essential.*

A third drill-guide with integrated awl is attached to the anterior hole of one clamp (Fig. 7.17b). Breach

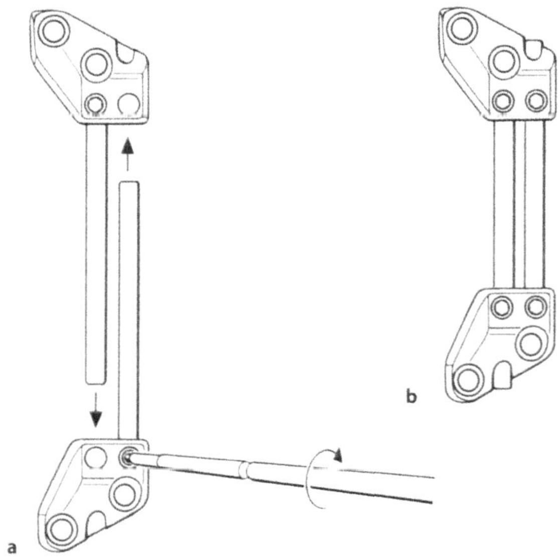

Fig 7.12 Assembly of the montage
a Appropriate length 6-mm USS rods placed into clamps; set screws over the incomplete holes are tightened
b Protruding length adjusted

Figs. 7.13–7.21 Surgical technique

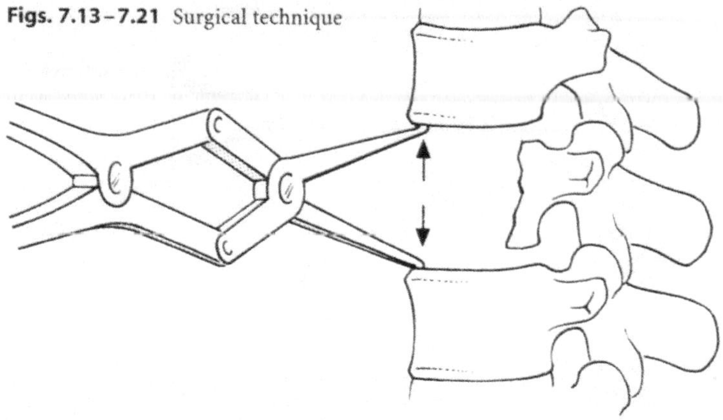

Fig. 7.13 Distraction of the anterior column defect with a vertebral spreader

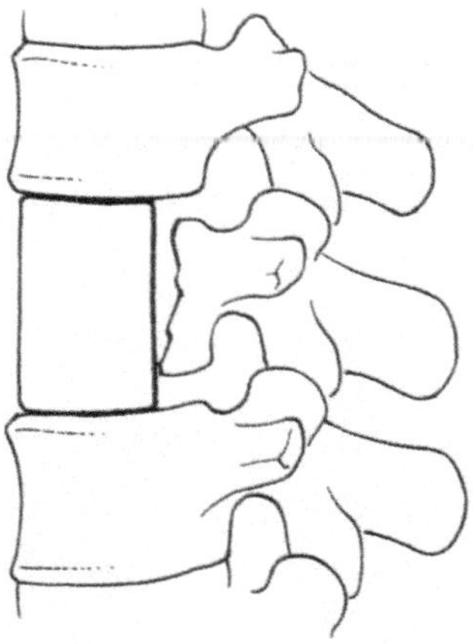

Fig. 7.14 Insertion of the tricortical graft

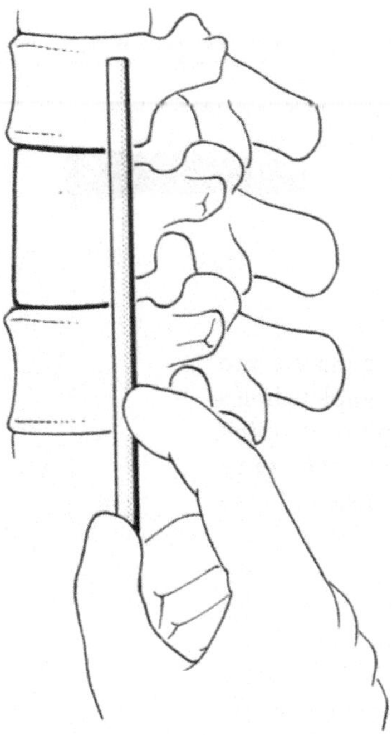

Fig. 7.15 Template applied to assess the length of the definite length of the USS rods

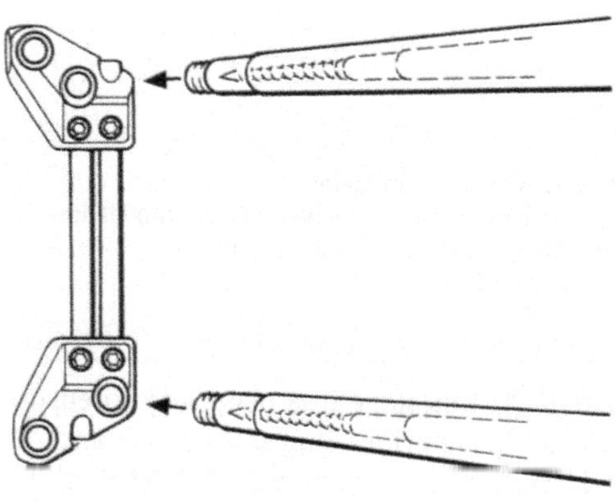

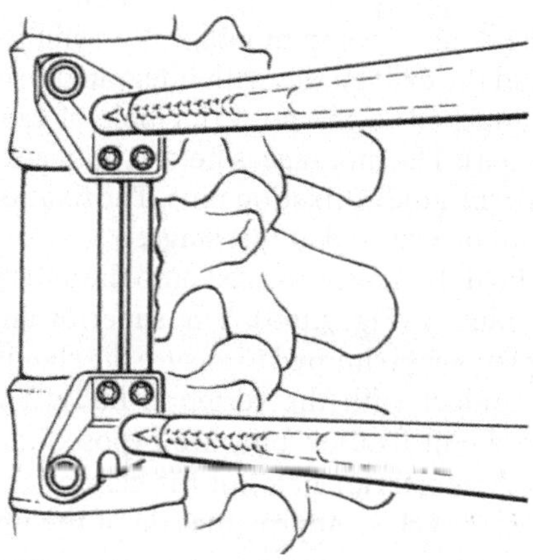

Fig 7.16
a Drill-guide/fixation pins are attached to the clamps

b VentroFix placed on the vertebral column

Fig. 7.17
a Insertion of the fixation pins
b Drill-guide/awl is attached to anterior hole of one clamp
c Insertion of the awl to open the cortex
d Measuring the depth of the hole

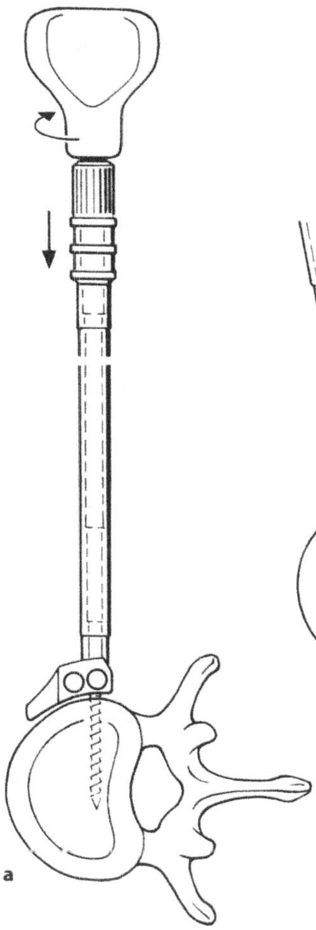

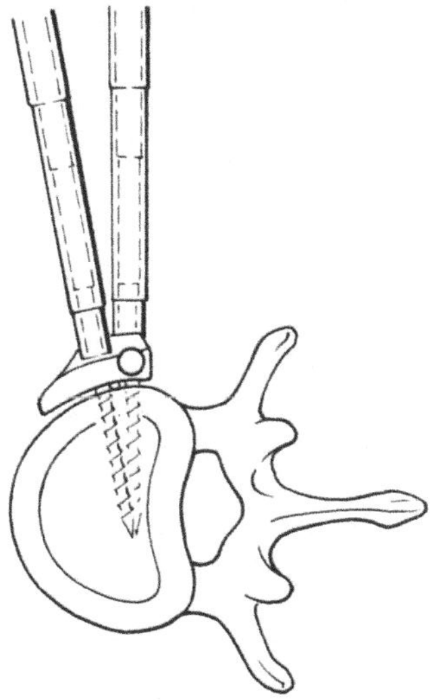

a

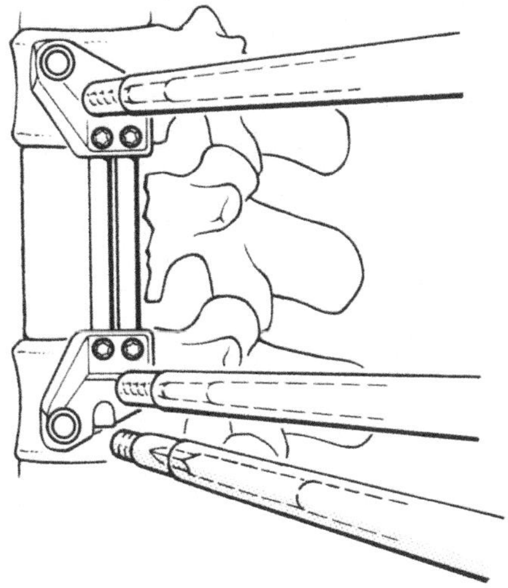

b

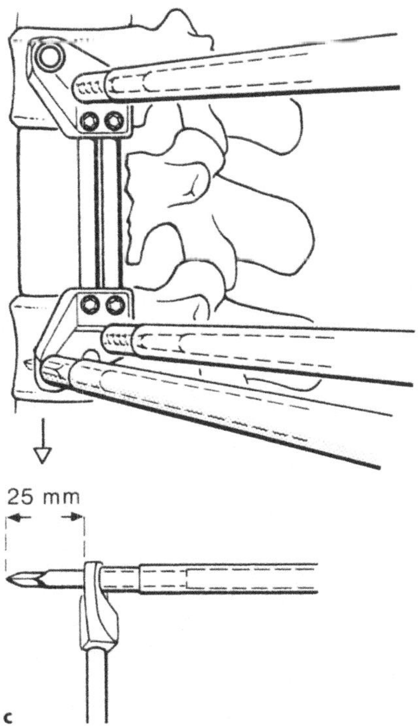

c

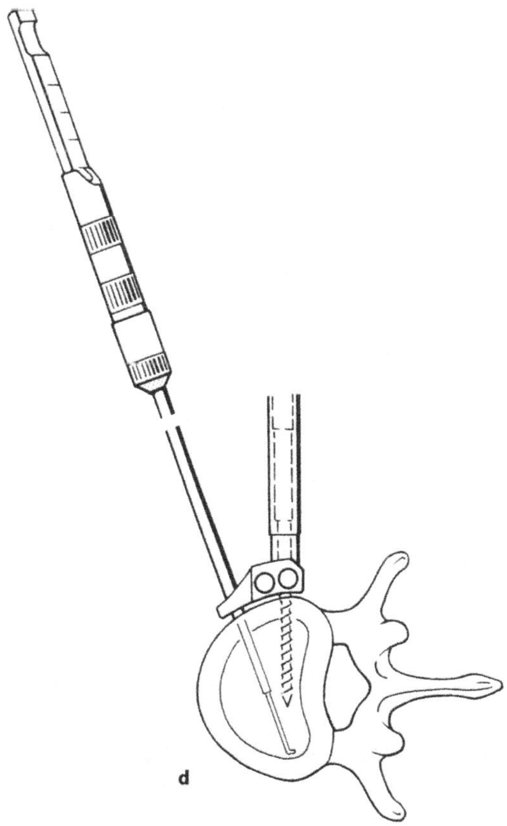

d

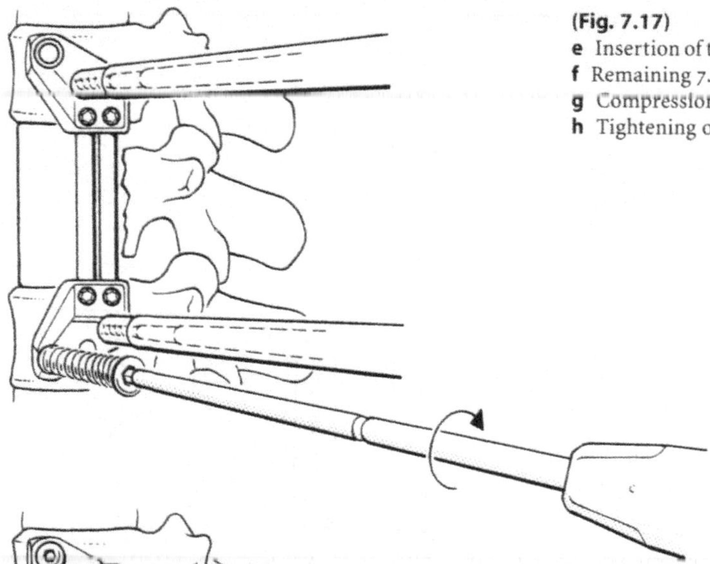

e

(Fig. 7.17)
e Insertion of the 7.5-mm titanium self-tapping locking screw
f Remaining 7.5-mm screws are inserted
g Compression of the graft
h Tightening of set screws

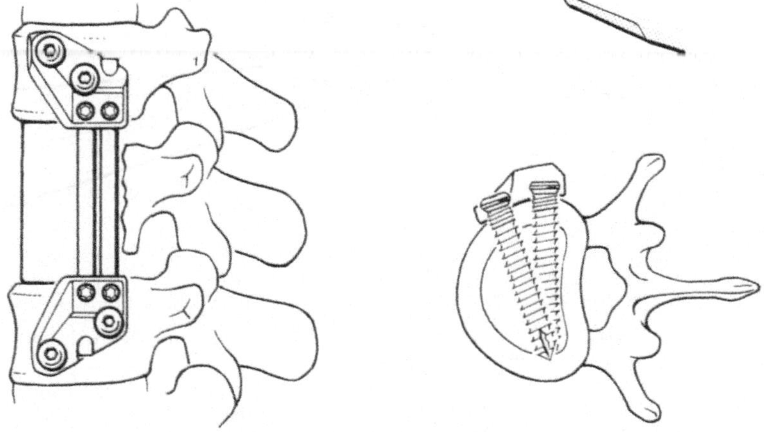

f

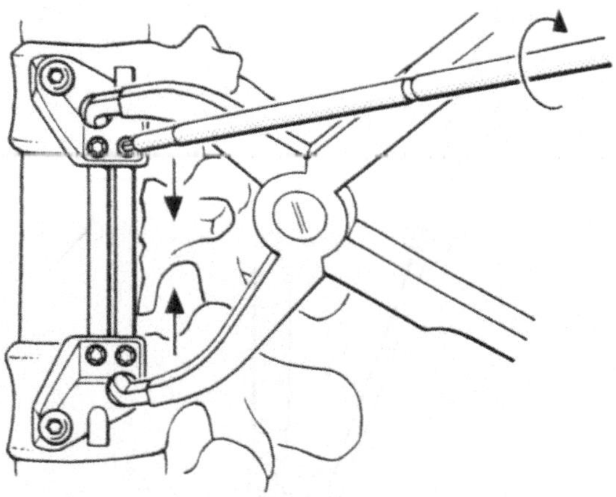

g

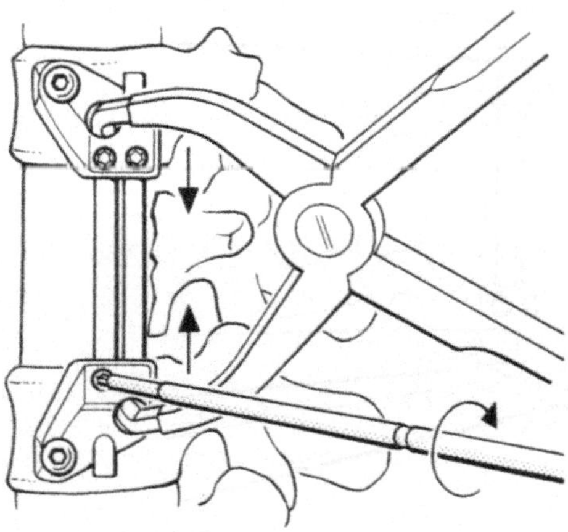

h

the drill through the anterior hole using the awl (Fig. 7.17c). Remove the drill-guide and awl. The assembly is held in place with the fixation pins.

Since purchase in the opposite cortex is not necessary, the awl has a stop at 25 mm to prevent overdrilling. If the bone is osteoporotic, then purchase of the screw to the opposite cortex may be necessary. In this case the length of the screw is determined by measuring with the AO depth-gauge using the tip to abut against the far cortex (Fig. 7.17d).

Insert the appropriate-length 7.5-mm titanium locking screw, first using the self-holding positioner and then the large hexagonal screwdriver (Fig. 7.17e). The screw is self-tapping. The anterior hole of the other clamp is drilled in a similar manner and the second anterior screw is inserted. After removal of the fixation pins and penetration of the awl through the posterior hole of each clamp, the posterior 7.5-mm titanium screws are inserted (Fig. 7.17f).

The implant is compressed by using the VentroFix compression forceps (Fig. 7.17g) and the set screws are tightened (Fig. 7.17h). (If the distance between the clamps is too long to use the compression forceps alone, the compression support is attached to the posterior rod.) This technique maintains a sagittal profile of the spine.

7.1.2.2.2
Fracture Clamp Configuration

Advantage
- Preservation of a disk space if the distal portion of the vertebral body is intact.

Surgical Technique
The application of this montage is the same as for the double clamp, the only difference being that the holes in the distal clamp are transverse and not offset in an oblique way (Fig. 7.18).

7.1.2.2.3
Single-Clamp – Double-Rod Configuration

Principle
The indications and concepts are the same as for the above clamps.

Advantages
- Independent positioning of the screws on the vertebral body.

Implants and Instruments
The implants consist of four single clamps, one parallel connector and two appropriate-length 6-mm rods (Fig. 7.19).

Assembly of the Montage
The montage is assembled. The set screws of the clamps are lightly tightened and the ones of the parallel connector firmly tightened!

Surgical Technique
The technique is similar to that for the double-clamp technique (Fig. 7.20a, Fig. 7.16). The length of the rods is determined with a template. The two anterior clamps are held with the drill sleeves with an integrated fixation pin. The montage is placed on the vertebral column after reconstruction (see above), the clamps adjusted to the desired position and the set screws of the posterior clamps firmly tightened.

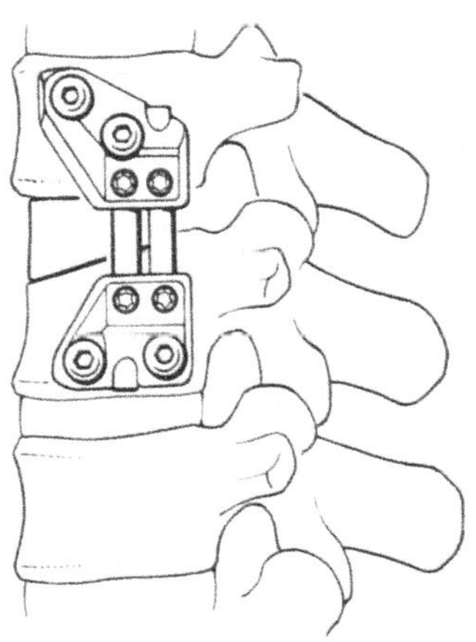

Fig. 7.18 Double-rod construction with fracture clamp

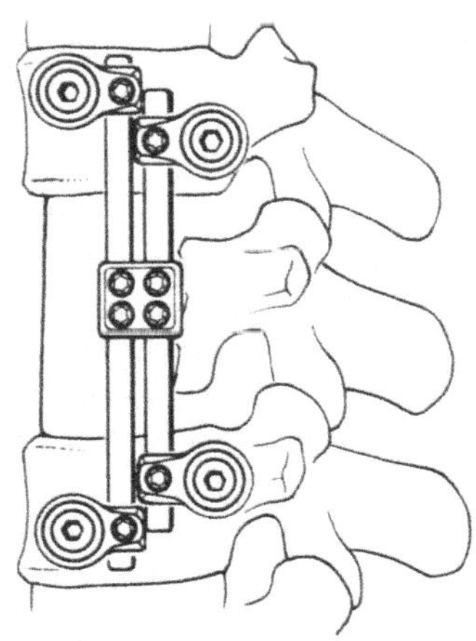

Fig. 7.19 Single-clamp – double-rod construction

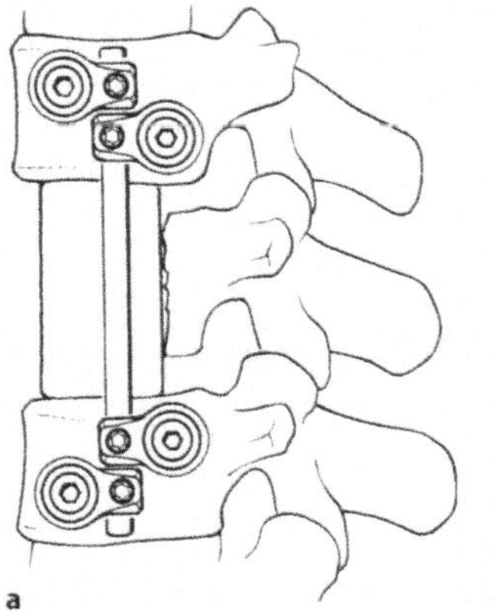

a

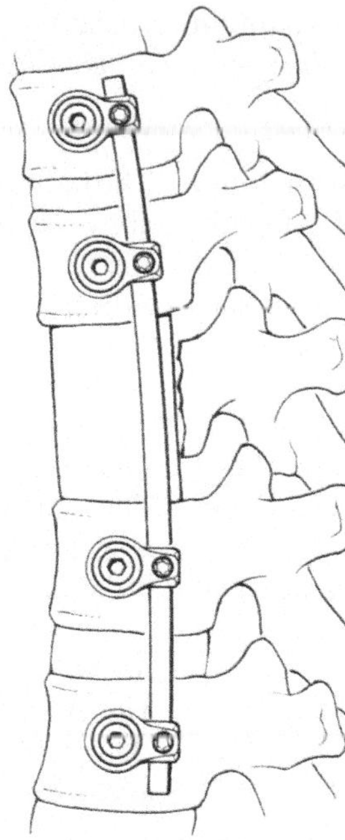

b

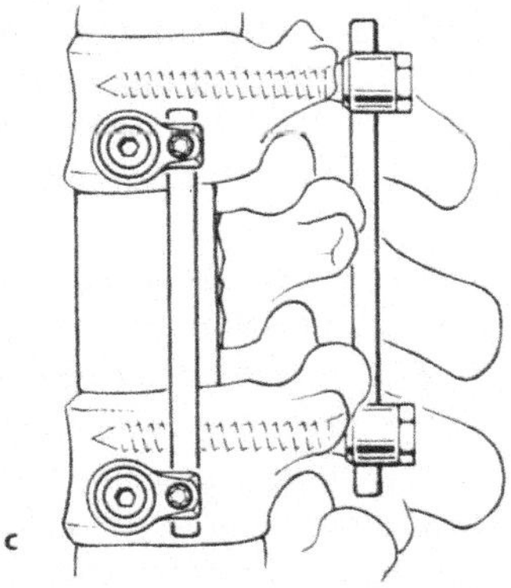

c

Fig. 7.20 Single-clamp – single-rod construction
a Single-rod – double-clamp construct
b Single-rod – single-clamp construct
c Single-rod – single-clamp construct in combination with posterior fixation

Both fixation pins are exposed and inserted to hold the implant on the vertebral bodies. *Ensure the direction of the drill holes is such that they do not penetrate the spinal canal.* At this stage, it is necessary to ensure the height of the construct is correct and the sagittal plane has been preserved; *a radiograph is absolutely essential.* The anterior clamps are adjusted to the desired position and the set screws firmly tightened. The drill sleeve with integrated awl is attached to one anterior clamp. Breach the drill through the anterior hole using the awl and insert the appropriate 7.5-mm locking screw. The hole of the second anterior clamp is drilled in a similar manner and the second anterior screw is inserted. After removal of the fixation pins and penetration of the awl through the posterior hole of each clamp, the posterior locking screws are inserted.

To apply compression loosen the two distal set screws and compress between the parallel connector and distal clamps with the VentroFix compression forceps and tighten the set screws.

7.1.2.2.4
Single-Clamp – Single-Rod Configuration

The construct should not be used alone in the lumbar spine and thoracolumbar junction, because it has poor rotational stability. It may, however, be used in the thoracic spine or to supplement fixatio or anterior reconstructions in the metastatic diseas (Fig. 7.20a,b). For correct placement the rod may b bent (Fig. 7.20b). An alternative anterior recon struction uses single clamps and one ro (Fig. 7.20c). This should only be used to supplemen posterior fixation. The single clamp may be adde to the double clamp construct if purchase on th bone graft is felt necessary (Fig. 7.21).

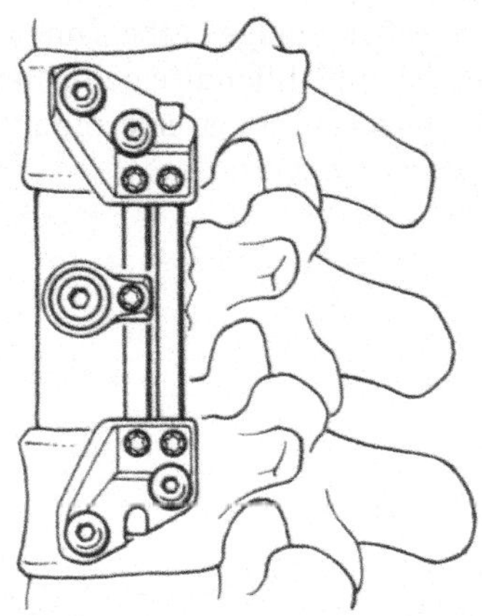

Fig. 7.21 Double-rod clamp system with additional single clamp

7.2 Posterior Techniques

7.2.1 Translaminar Screw Fixation

Stabilization of a posterior fusion over one or two motion segments is achieved by transfixing the facet joints.

Indications
- Pure dislocations or subluxations from T12 – L1 to the lumbosacral junction (minor articular process fractures can be ignored.)
- Supplementary internal fixation of degenerative spinal segments treated by an interbody fusion.
- Posterior alar-transverse or intertransverse fusion in degenerative disease of the spine.

Advantages
- Short segment fixation.
- Relatively easy technique.
- No major inherent risk.
- The stability achieved is superior to that with other facet joint screw fixations (e.g., Boucher's) or with posterior wiring techniques.

Disadvantages
- Not recommended in severe osteoporosis.
- Not applicable when the lamina is fractured.

Surgical Techniques (Figs. 7.22, 7.23)

Posterior Midline Approach. The first step is exposure of the posterior vertebral elements including the bases of the transverse processes of the lower vertebra. Using an *oscillating drill*, the screw canals are prepared with a special long 3.2-mm drill. The 3.2-mm drill with drill guide is directed so that the drill passes through the base of the spinous process, into the lamina, transverses the facet joint and exits near the base of the transverse process (Fig. 7.22a). To avoid a long incision or forced soft tissue retraction, the drill and guide which helps to direct the drill precisely can be placed through a small hole in the soft tissue.

At the L5 – S1 level, the screws are inserted into the base of the spinous processes and exit into the alar of the sacrum. The length of each screw canal is mea-

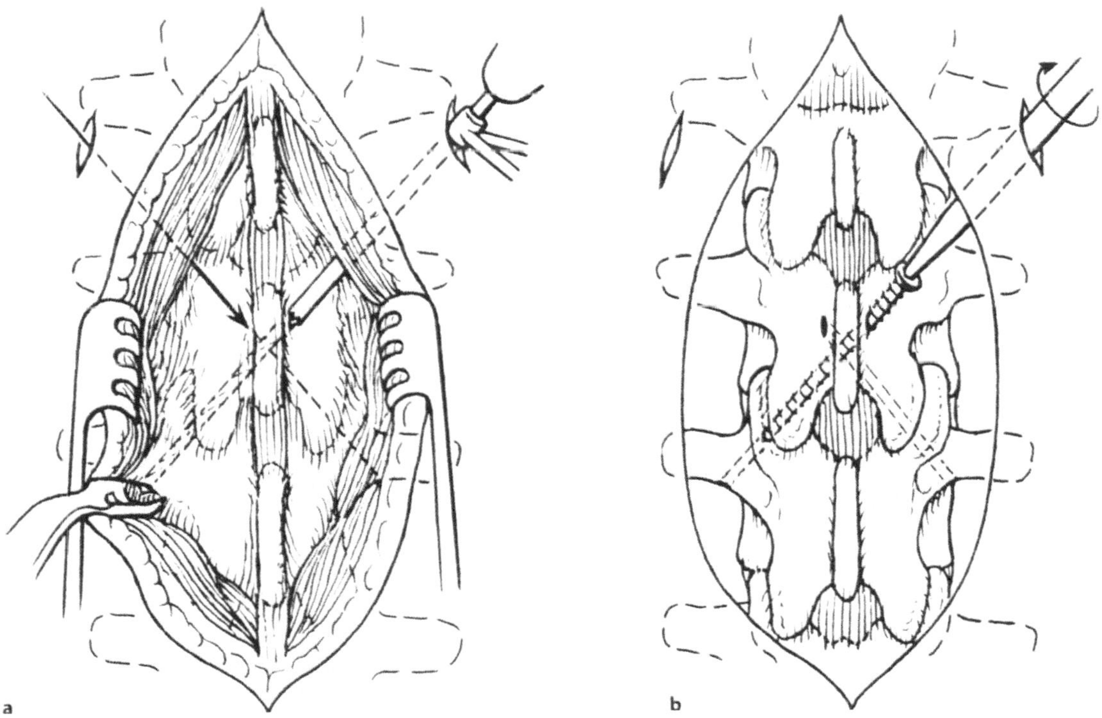

a b

Fig. 7.22 Translaminar screw fixation
a Positioning and direction of the special long 3.2-mm drill, protected with a drill sleeve – an oscillatory drill is used – through a slab wound of the skin
b Insertion of the appropriate-length 4.5-mm cortical screw

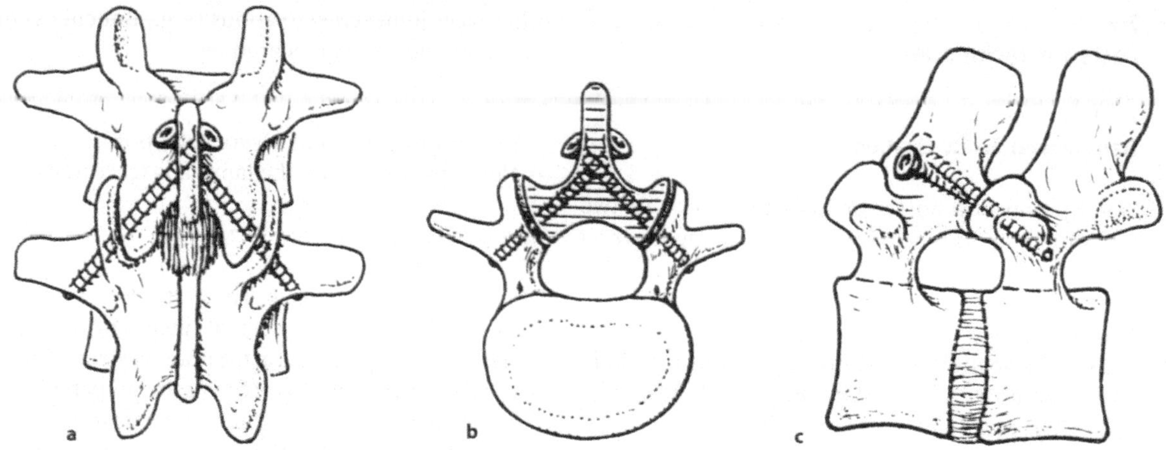

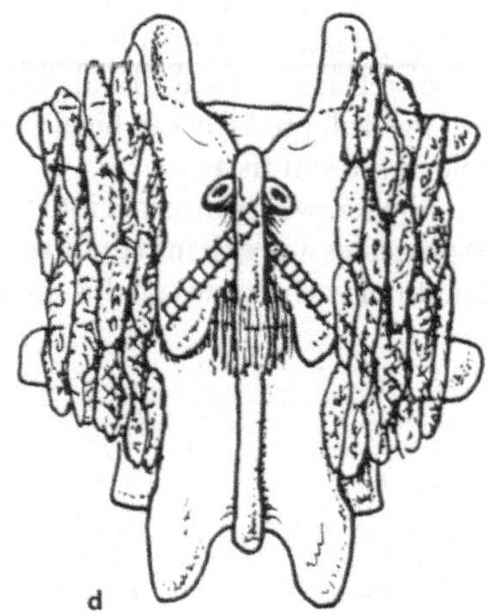

Fig. 7.23 Position of the translaminar screws
a Positioning of the translaminar screws seen from posterior
b Screws seen in the horizontal plane
c Screws seen from the side
d Posterior vertebral elements, including the posterior half of the joints, are carefully decorticated and cancellous bone graft is applied

sured, and the beginning of the screw canals is tapped with the 4.5-mm tap. The tap needs only to cross the facet joints if the joints are very sclerotic. The appropriate-length 4.5-mm cortex screw is then inserted (Fig. 7.22b).

When preparing the first screw canal on the spinous processes, it is important to appreciate that two screws are to be inserted; therefore, the first one should enter the spinous process and lamina slightly out of the ideal position either cranially or caudally in order to leave enough space for the second screw (Fig. 7.23a). Given their diverging direction, the screws cannot be lagged. Translaminar screws function as threaded bolts which prevent motion in the respective segment but do not exert compression in the facet joints (Fig. 7.23b, c).

After insertion of the screws, the posterior vertebral elements including the posterior half of the joints are carefully decorticated and cancellous bone graft is applied (Fig. 7.23d).

Postoperative Care
The patient is mobilized when comfortable and wears a hyperextension brace for 10–12 weeks. The brace may be removed for daily care and during bed rest.

7.2.2 Pedicle Fixation

Determining the Position of the Transpedicular Screws
Exact evaluation of the pedicles is an essential prerequisite for posterior plating and the application of fixator systems. The pedicles are short conical tubes with an oval cross-section. The objective is to insert the screws through the center of the pedicles, approximately parallel to the upper end plates or angled downward. The screws should converge toward the midline to an end plate or be angled downward. The screws should converge toward the midline to a

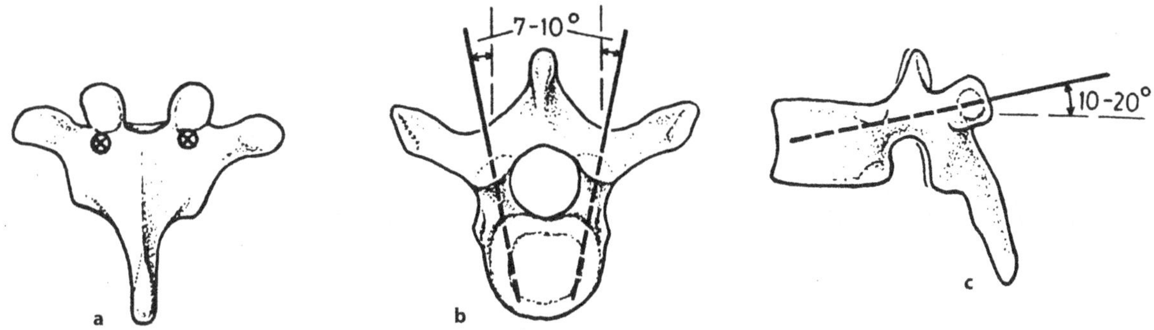

Fig. 7.24 Determining the position of the transpedicular screw: thoracic spine
a The point of entry is just below the rim of the upper facet joint
b, c The screw should be angled 7–10° towards the midline and 10–20° caudally

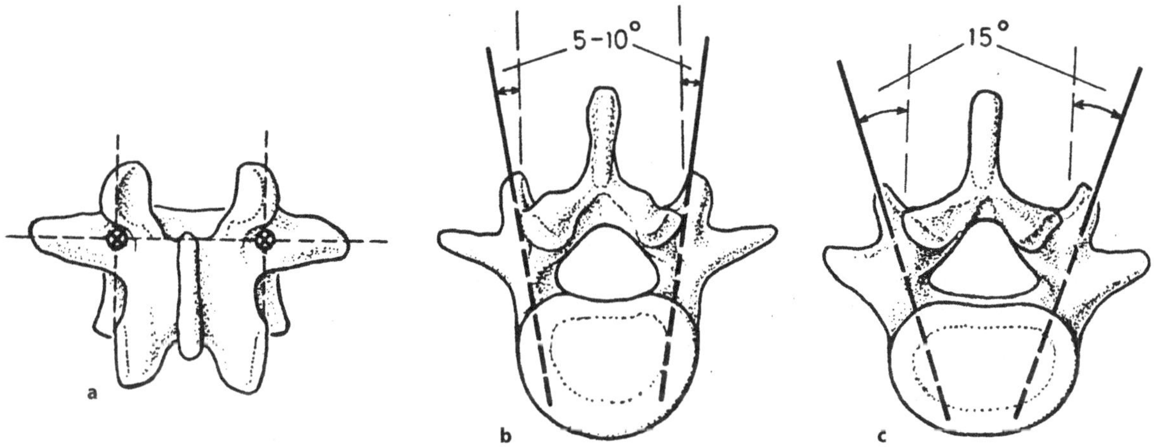

Fig. 7.25 Determining the position of the transpedicular screw: lumbar spine
a The entry point for the pedicle is at the intersection of a vertical line tangential to the lateral border of the superior articular process and a horizontal line bisecting the transverse process
b The screws should converge by 5° at the thoracolumbar junction
c The screws should converge by 10° at L2, increasing to 15° at L5

certain extent – up to 20 % depending on the spinal level – in order to ensure that they do not penetrate the lateral wall of the vertebral body. The long axis of the pedicle can be identified either by direct exposure or by image intensification. Although each method is reliable by itself, it is best to use a combination of the two. In addition, there are other aids for deciding screw position which are useful particularly when the anatomic landmarks are difficult to define due to distorted anatomic relationships.

Thoracic Spine. The point of entry is just below the rim of the upper facet joint (Fig. 7.24a), 3 mm lateral to the center of the joint near the base of the transverse process. This screw should be angled 7–10° towards the midline (Fig. 7.24b) and 10–20° caudally (Fig. 7.24c).

Lumbar Spine. At practically all levels, the long axis of the pedicle pierces the lamina at the intersection of two lines: a vertical line tangential to the lateral border of the superior articular process, and a horizontal line bisecting the transverse process (Fig. 7.25a). Their point of intersection lies in the angle between the superior articular process and the base of the transverse process. The screws should converge by 5° at the thoracolumbar junction (Fig. 7.25b) and by 10–15° as one progresses from L2 to L5 (Fig. 7.25c).

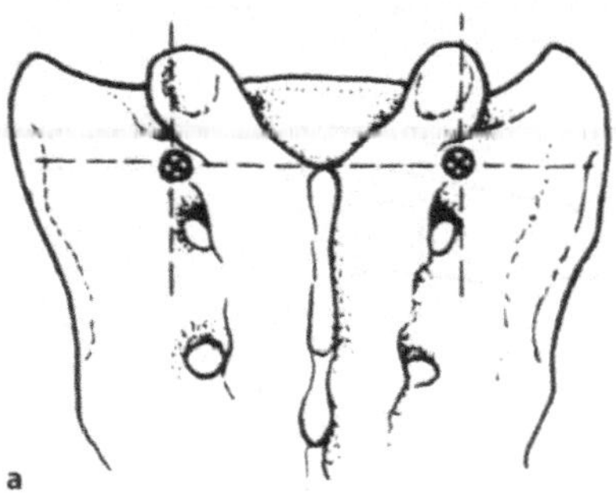

a

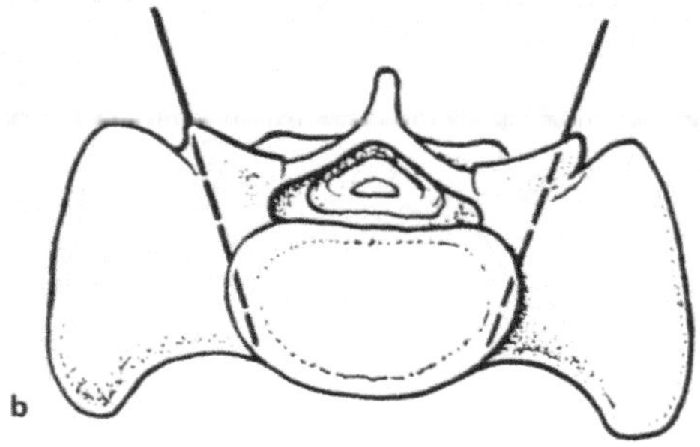

b

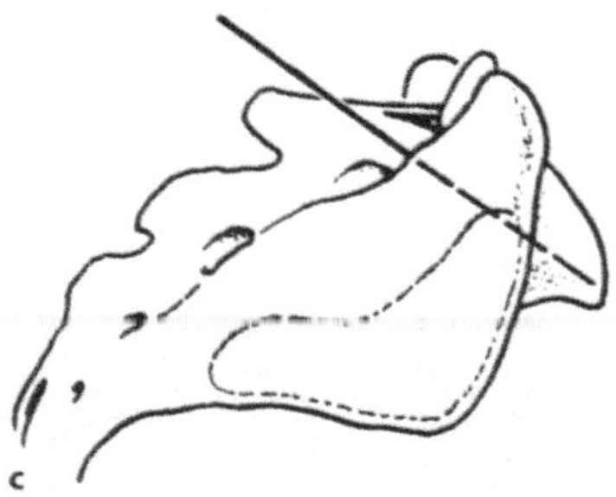

c

Fig. 7.26 Determining the position of the transpedicular screw: sacrum
a The entry point for the S1 pedicle is located at the intersection of a vertical line tangential to the lateral border of the S1 facet and a horizontal line tangential to its inferior border
b The screws converge toward the midline
c The screws aim toward the anterior corner of the promontorium

Sacrum. Proper placement of screws in the sacrum is difficult because of its variable anatomy. The screws may be introduced at different points and in different directions, depending upon the instrumentation and the quality of the bone. In general, the entry point is located at the intersection of two lines: a vertical line tangential to the lateral border of the S1 facet, and a horizontal line tangential to the inferior border of this facet (Fig. 7.26a). In most cases, the screws converge towards the midline (Fig. 7.26b) and aim towards the anterior corner of the promontorium (Fig. 7.26c). An alternative possibility is to insert the screws more sagittally or parallel to the surface of the sacroiliac joint. The entry point shifts slightly medially as the screw direction diverges. Screws inserted parallel to the sacroiliac joint aim towards the anterior superior angle of the lateral mass of the sacrum. When positioning screws in the sacrum so as to achieve optimal purchase, it is necessary to note the density of the bone – the subchondral bone is the strongest, whereas the lateral mass of the sacrum is often very osteoporotic, sometimes even hollow.

Radiographic control of Screw Position
In any case, anteroposterior (AP) and lateral preoperative X-rays are indispensable. If there is any suggestion of anatomic variations, then CT scans are essential. They give information about pedicle diameter and direction; intraoperatively, the use of image intensification is indispensable, too. It confirms the location and direction of the screws. In every difficult case, intraoperative myelography with image intensification helps to identify the medial border in relationship to the nerve root.

Direct Visualization of the Pedicle
At the lumbar spine, the inferior and inferior lateral aspect of the pedicle can be exposed by dissecting subperiosteally from the base of the transverse process anteriorly. The soft tissues together with the spinal nerve and blood vessels are carefully retracted with a curved dissector. A small curved dissector is used to probe the lateral wall of the pedicle. If necessary, the inferior part of the medial wall may also be probed. In addition, osteotomy of the base of the transverse process can help to identify the pedicle. Alternatively, the spinal canal can be opened and the medial wall of the pedicle identified. The latter two techniques are usually not necessary in routine procedures. At the sacral level, it is very helpful to expose the S1 nerve root, which allows visualization of the lateral wall of the S1 canal.

Preparation of the Screw Canal
After identification of the entry point and the direction of the pedicle, the posterior cortex is perforated for approximately 5 mm using a 3.5-mm drill, preferably with the oscillating attachment. Continued drilling of the pedicle can be dangerous. A safer

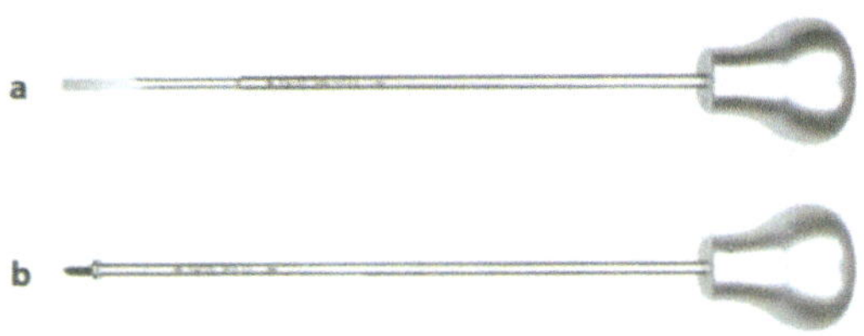

Fig. 7.27 Instruments for the preparation of the screw canal
a USS pedicle probe 3.8 mm diameter
b USS pedicle awl

technique is to prepare the entry points with the pedicle awl (Fig. 7.27a) and to open the pedicle with a pedicle feeler (Fig. 7.27b). This preparation is performed to the junction between the pedicle and vertebral body. The circumference of the canal is checked with the tip of the AO depth gauge, which has an angled tip to ensure that perforation of the bone has not occurred, particularly medially. Image intensification with the gauge or a Kirschner wire in place confirms the proper position. The depth gauge may be inserted into the cancellous bone of the vertebral body and the anterior cortex is not perforated. If there is doubt regarding the depth, take a lateral radiograph and ensure that the depth gauge does not penetrate more than 80 % of the AP body diameter, then the anterior cortex will not be perforated.

7.2.2.1 *Notched Thoracolumbar Plates* (Fig. 7.28)

Principle

The plate functions as a splint when the vertebral body is not able to support axial load. If the anterior column is intact, the plate functions as a posterior tension band.

Indications

- Fracture dislocations from T6 to S1.
- Supplementary stabilization to anterior interbody fusions.

Advantage

- Relatively easy to use.

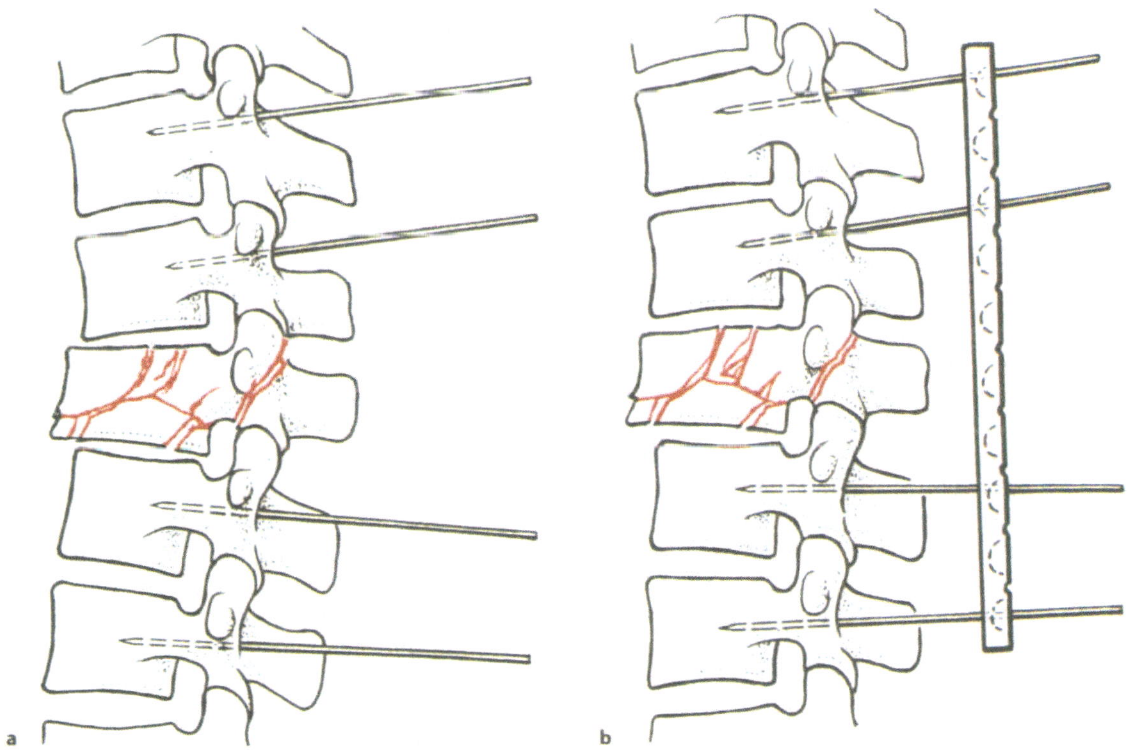

Fig. 7.28 Notched plates for the thoracolumbar spine: surgical technique
a The upper and lower screw canals are prepared; the pedicles are entered in the usual manner and Kirschner wires are inserted into each hole
b The two plates are fitted into position over the Kirschner wires

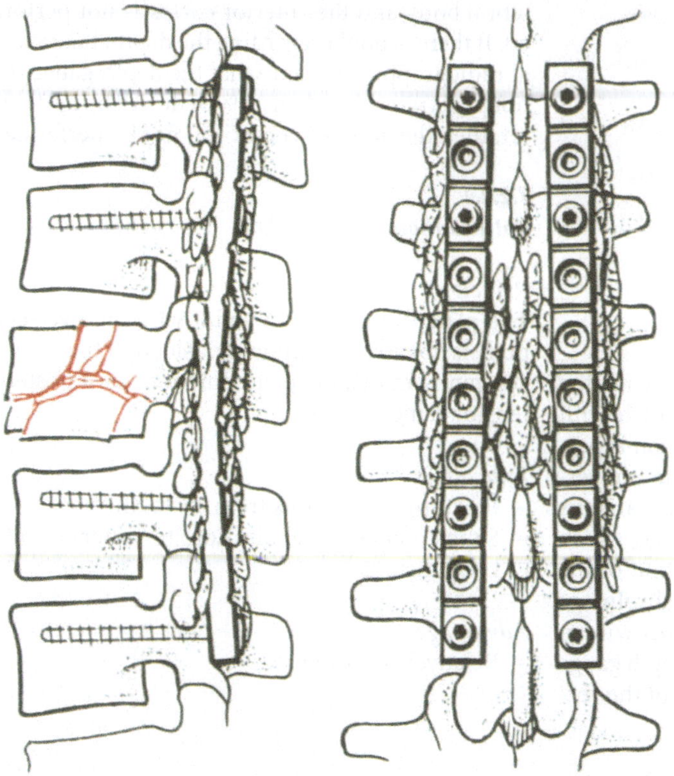
c

(Fig. 7.28)
c A cancellous bone graft is placed over the decorticated lamina and transverse processes of the injured and the two adjacent vertebrae

Disadvantages
- A minimum of five vertebrae are bridged.
- In most cases, reduction of the fracture needs to be undertaken before application of the plate.

Surgical Technique
The fracture may be reduced with the aid of an image intensifier prior to surgery on the operating table. Through a midline incision, the spinous processes, laminae, facet joints and transverse processes are exposed. If reduction of the spinal fracture has not been fully achieved, further manipulation to apply distraction can be undertaken using the Harrington outrigger inserted one level above and below the intended plated levels. A plate of appropriate length is placed over the posterior aspect of the spine and transverse processes and, if necessary, a bed is made to allow the plate to lie snugly on the bone. Initially the upper and lower screw canals are prepared. The pedicles of two vertebrae above and below are entered in the usual manner and Kirschner wires are inserted into each hole (Fig. 7.28a).

The two plates are fitted into position over the Kirschner wires (Fig. 7.28). The appropriate-length 4.5-mm cortex screws are inserted. The screws are tightened alternatively, allowing the spine to adapt to the plate. Where possible, the remaining holes in the plates are then prepared and the screws inserted. A cancellous bone graft is placed over the decorticated laminae and transverse processes (Fig. 7.28c).

Correction of Kyphosis (Fig. 7.29)
If a kyphosis is present, the plates may be used for correction. They are not fully bent to match the deformity of the spine but are contoured to attain a normal curve. Both plates are screwed to the two vertebrae below the fracture. The prominent upper portions of the plates are then manually approximated to the spine and the remaining screws inserted (Fig. 7.29a). An alternative method of reduction is to contour the plate into the normal curve and then prepare the screw holes. Each screw is loosely inserted; then alternate ones are tightened from the apex of the deformity outwards so that the fracture is slowly reduced (Fig. 7.29b).

Postoperative Care
Early mobilization is allowed without external support.

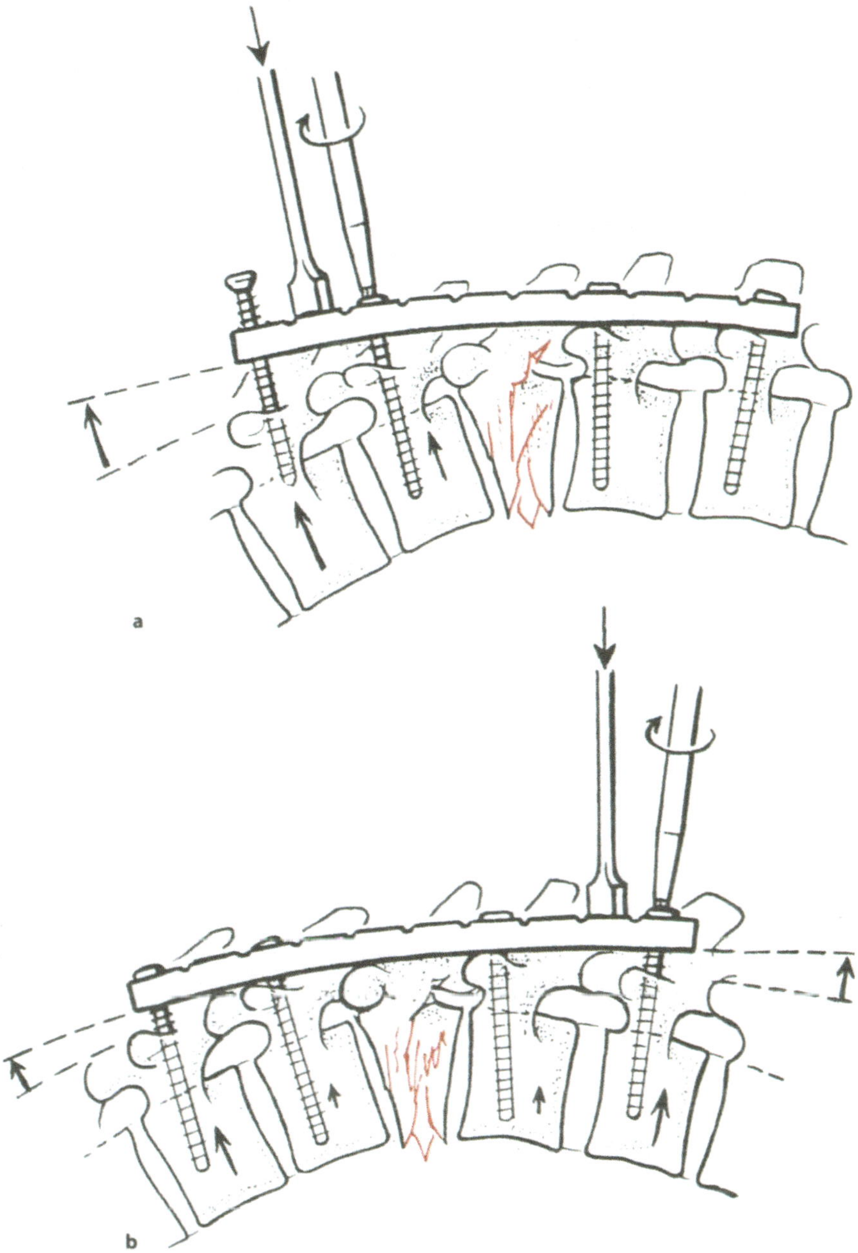

Fig. 7.29 Correction of kyphosis
a The prominent upper portions of the plates are manually approximated to the spine using a pusher and the remaining screws inserted
b Each screw is loosely inserted, then alternate ones are tightened from the apex of the deformity outwards so that the fracture is slowly reduced

7.2.2.2
Fracture Module of the USS (See also Chap. 9)

Introduction

The fracture module is a modification of the AO internal fixator, incorporated into the USS from an early stage. The clamp with the posterior opening nut of the internal fixator is modified for attachment to the 6-mm hard rod.

Principle

The internal fixator is a device which allows stabilization and reduction of the spine. Long Schanz screws are inserted in the pedicles of the vertebral bodies and are connected to the 6-mm hard rod by fully adjustable posterior opening clamps. The implant acts as a tension band, a buttress or neutralization system; it allows distraction, compression as well as fixation in a neutral position. Kyphosis or lordosis can be created in the construct.

Indications
- Lower thoracic and lumbar spine fractures.
- Stabilization and correction of spinal segments in nontraumatic disorders of the spine (degenerative disease, tumors, deformities, infections, etc.)

Advantages
- A simple versatile system.
- Its use is independent of the fracture type.
- Short segment fixation.
- Schanz screws allow easy reduction.

Disadvantages
- It should not be used in the upper thoracic spine (above T6) because the pedicles are too small.
- In the treatment of certain A-type fractures, an additional anterior reconstruction may be necessary either by anterior surgery or by transpedicular bone grafting.

Implants and Instruments
Implants and instruments are shown in Fig. 7.30.
Surgical Technique

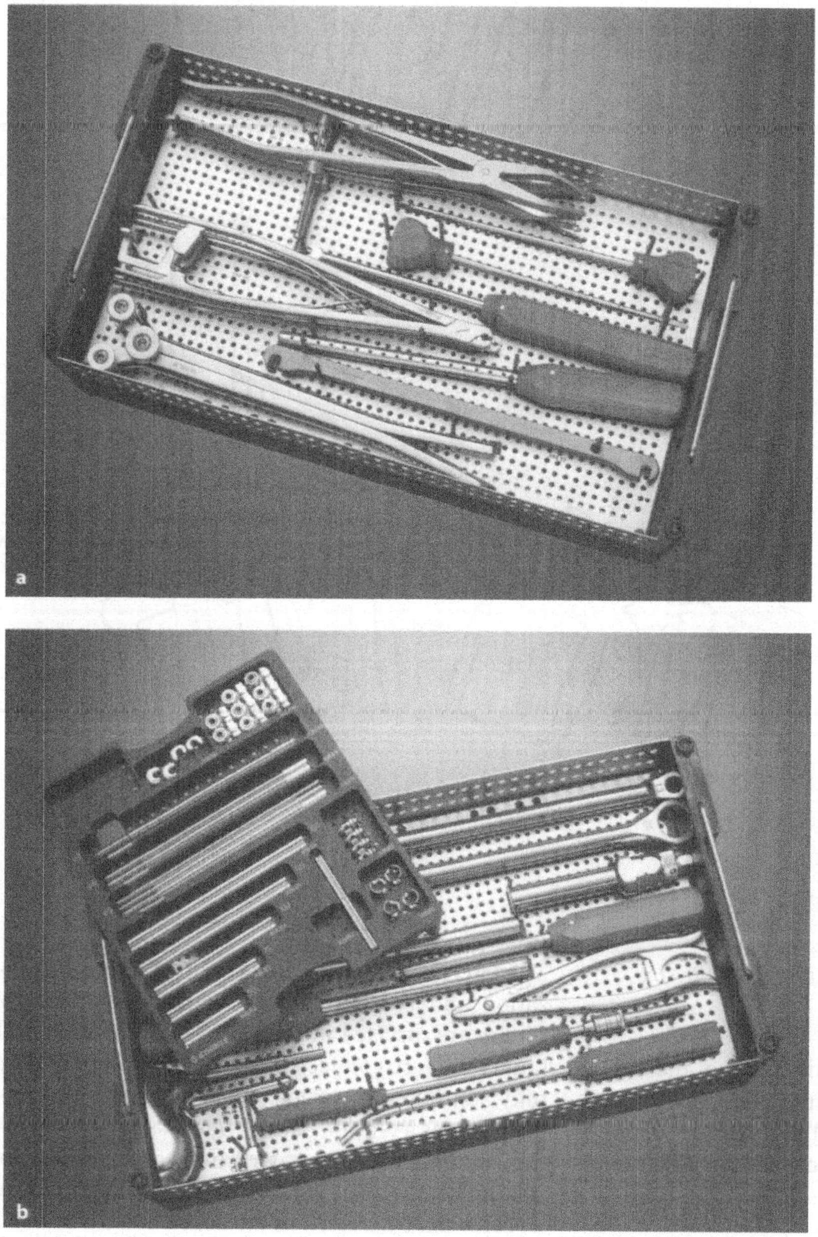

Fig. 7.30 Implants, and Instruments for fracture treatment
a VARIO case for USS general instruments
b VARIO case for USS Schanz screws
c Schanz screws 5, 6 and 7 mm diameter
d USS clamp with posterior nut for USS rods
e USS rod 6.0 mm diameter, hard
f USS rod 3.5 mm diameter for USS cross-link system
g USS cross-link clamp for USS rods 6.0 mm diameter
h USS pedicle probe 3.8 mm diameter
i USS pedicle awl
j Universal chuck with T-handle
k Simple handle
l USS socket wrench 6 mm
m USS socket wrench 11 mm
n Screwdriver, hexagonal, small with groove
o USS holding sleeve
p Bolt cutter head 5.0 mm diameter, long
q Handle for bolt cutter 13 mm
r Handle for bolt cutter 24 mm
s USS half-ring
t USS spreader forceps
u USS compression forceps

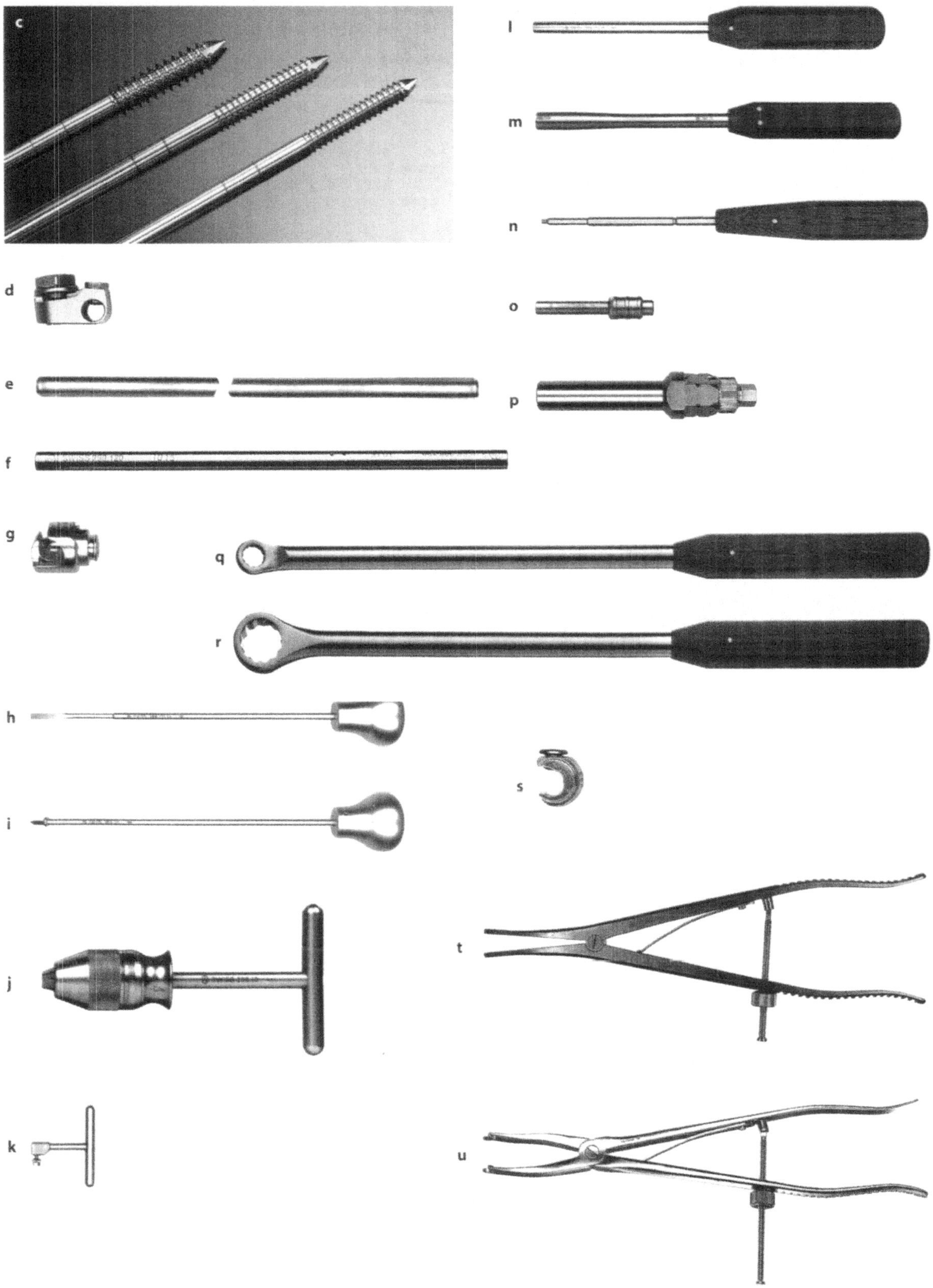
c
d
e
f
g
h
i
j
k
l
m
n
o
p
q
r
s
t
u

v

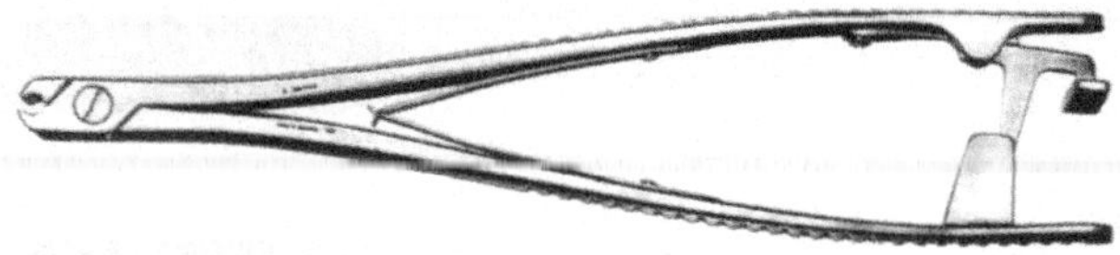

w

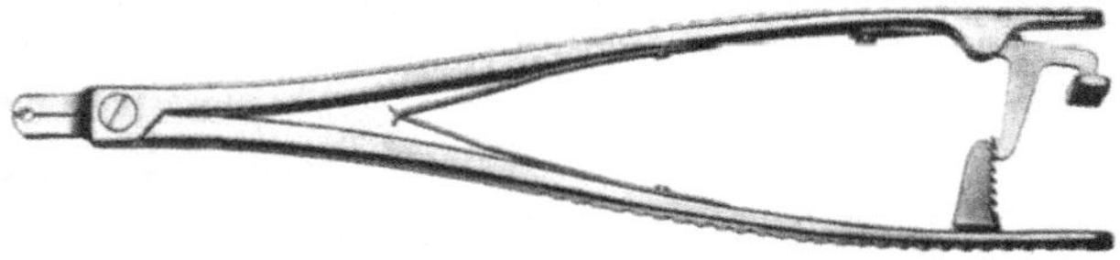

x

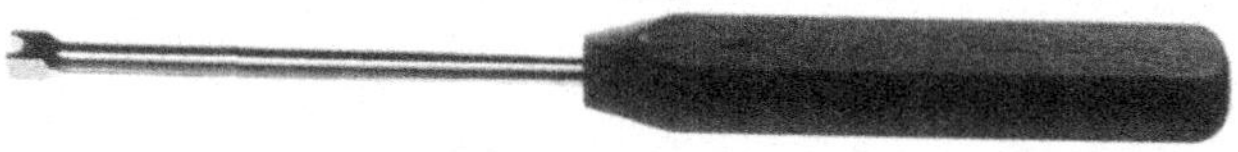

y

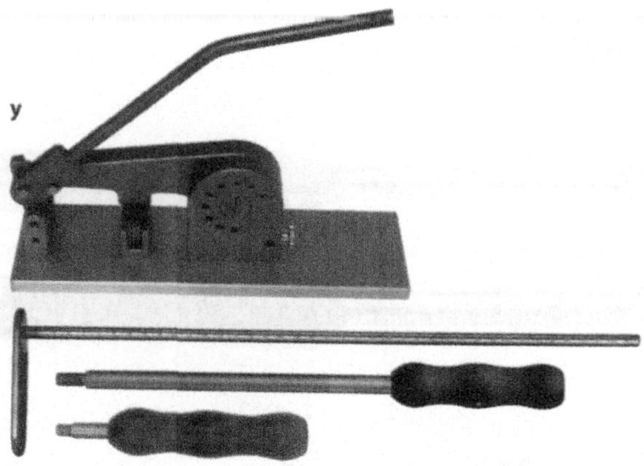

z

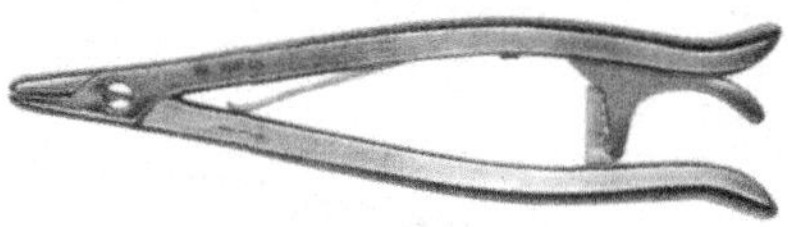

a′

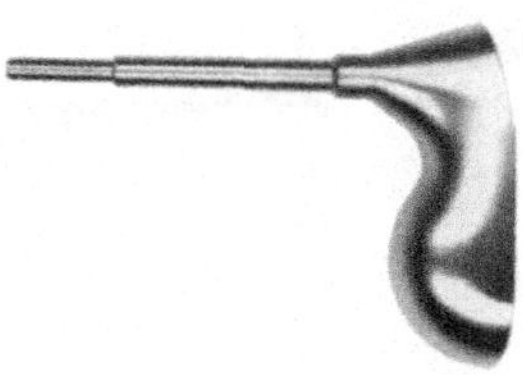

b′

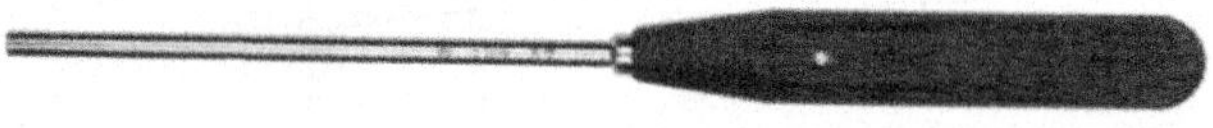

c′

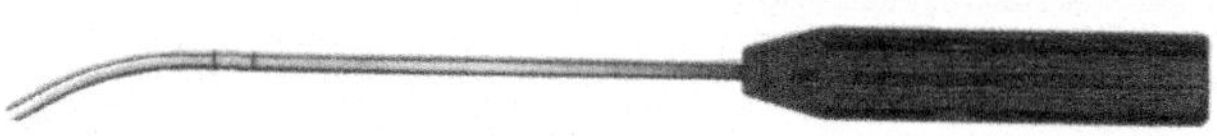

(Fig. 7.30)
v USS holding forceps for USS rods 6.0 mm diameter
w USS holding forceps for USS rods 3.5 and 4.5 mm diameter
x USS rod pusher for USS rods 6.0 mm diameter
y USS rod cutting and bending device
z Forceps for screw removal
a′ Bone graft funnel
b′ Cancellous bone impactor, straight
c′ Cancellous bone impactor, curved

Posterior Midline Approach. Subperiosteal dissection of the laminae laterally to the intervertebral joints is performed. The entry points for the Schanz screws are determined carefully as described above. The entry point for the Schanz screw is started with the pedicle awl (Fig. 7.31a); the entry point is deepened by 3 cm with the pedicle probe (Fig. 7.31b). A K-wire is then inserted into the opened pedicle using the image intensifier to check the orientation of the pedicle hole (Fig. 7.31c). In the lateral projection, the level and the direction of the wires in relation to the end plate are determined. In the AP projection, the tips of the K-wires should converge but not cross. The image intensifier in the AP direction is repositioned for each K-wire exactly parallel to the axis of the wire: thus, the wire will be seen as a point, and its position in relation to the oval of the pedicle can be determined unequivocally.

When the K-wires are correctly sited (Fig. 7.31d), the hole is enlarged with the pedicle probe and a depth gauge is used as a probe to ensure that the hole is surrounded by bone and penetration through the side of the pedicle wall has not occurred (Fig. 7.31e). The 5-, 6- or 7 mm self-cutting Schanz screw is easily inserted with the simple handle to a depth of two-thirds of the depth of the vertebral body (Fig. 7.31f). Lateral fluoroscopic control ensures that the anterior vertebral cortex is not perforated (Fig. 7.31g).

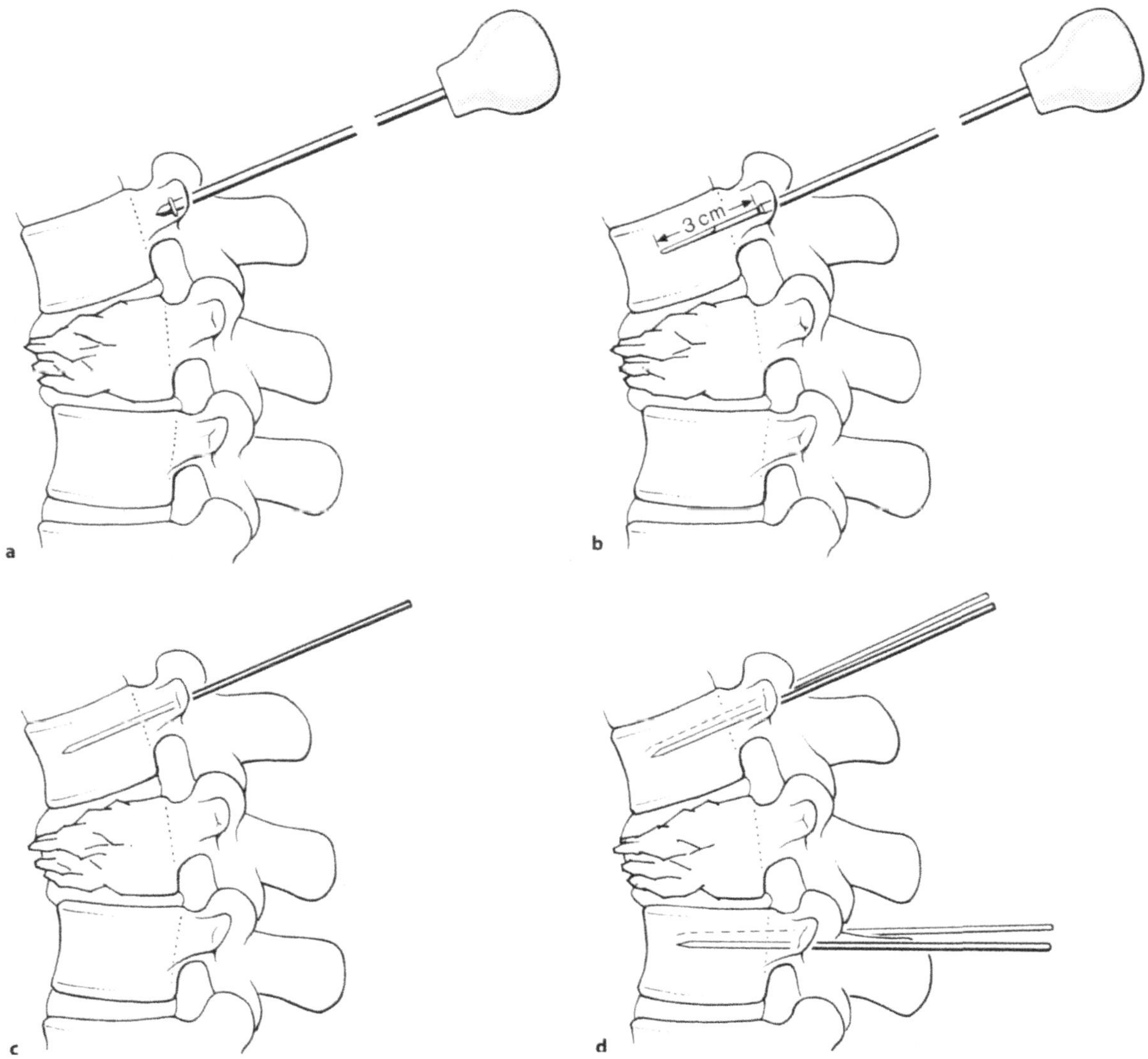

Fig. 7.31 Surgical technique for the USS internal fixator
a The entry points for the Schanz screws are started with the pedicle awl
b The entry point is deepened by 3 cm with the pedicle probe
c K-wires are inserted in the opened pedicles for checking with an image intensifie
d All the K-wires are correctly sited

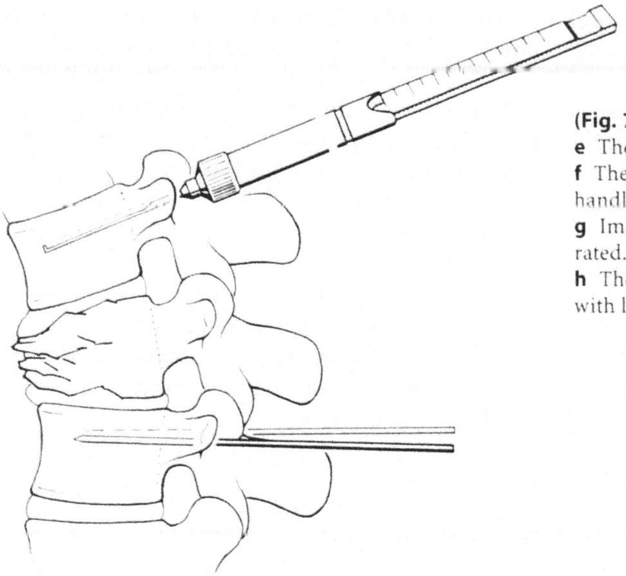

e

(Fig. 7.31)
e The depth gauge is used as a probe
f The self-cutting Schanz screw is inserted with the simple T-handle
g Image intensifier checking that anterior cortex is not perforated.
h The two 6-mm rods are applied to the four Schanz screws with loose clamps

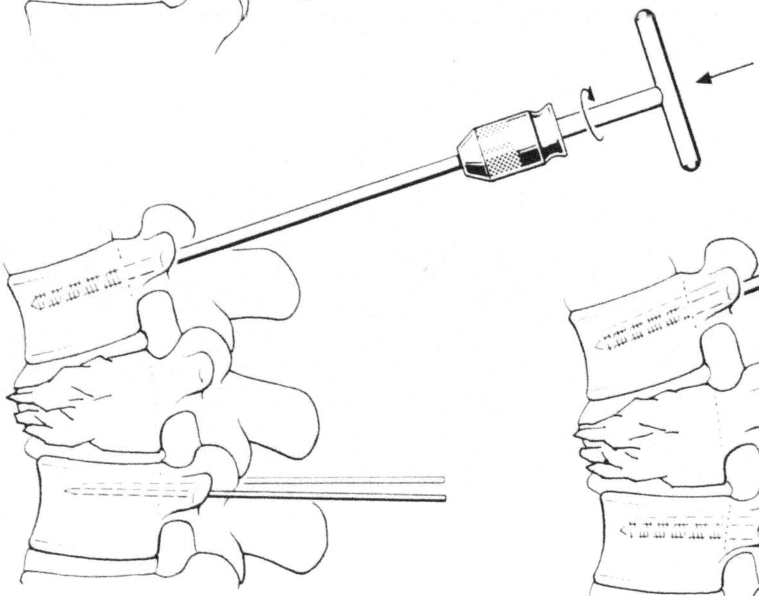

f

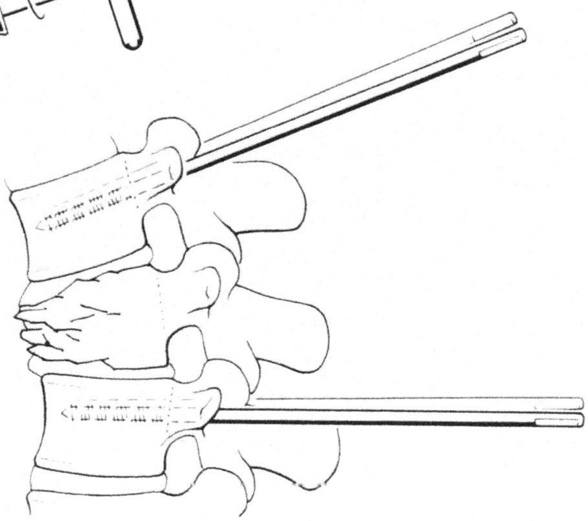

g

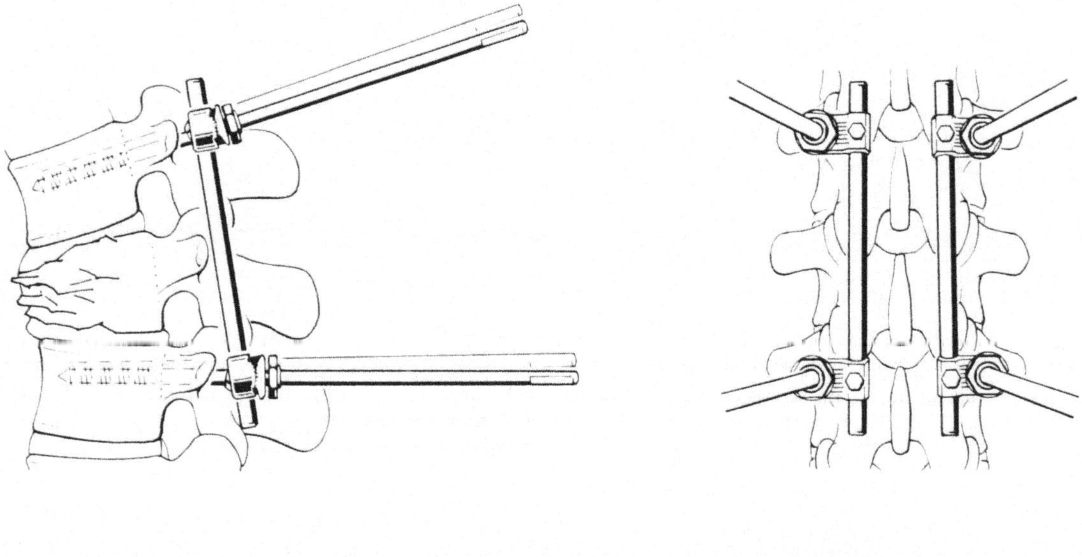

h

When all four Schanz screws are in place, the rods of the internal fixator with loose clamps and clamp elements are applied, the rods lying medially to the screws (Fig. 7.31h). The reduction technique depends on the type of fracture.

7.2.2.2.1
Anterior Vertebral Body Fracture with Intact Posterior Wall (Type A-1 and A-2) (Fig. 7.32a)

Principle

The dorsal ends of the Schanz screws are manually approximated until the desired correction of the kyphosis has been attained (Fig. 7.32b). The set screws on the clamps must remain loose so that the clamps are allowed to slide freely towards each other during the maneuver. The center of rotation then lies at the posterior edge of the vertebral body. By creating the lordosis, the vertebral body anteriorly will be distracted and the vertebral disk space and height will be restored by ligamentotaxis (tightening of the anterior longitudinal ligament and annulus of the disk).

Technique

Place two cannulated socket wrenches over the caudal Schanz screws and tilt the wrenches cranially to lordose the spine (Fig. 7.32c). The posterior nuts are locked. A similar procedure is performed on the cranial Schanz screws in order to reestablish the correct sagittal plane (Fig. 7.32d). The appropriate posterior nuts are tightened to fix the angle between the Schanz screws and the rods (Fig. 7.32c and d). At this stage, it is necessary to distract the Schanz screws to reestablish the normal height of the injured segment (disk). A half-ring is placed in the center of each 6-mm rod between the clamps and locked (Fig. 7.32e). Apply distraction with the spreader forceps checking the procedure with the image intensifier (Fig. 7.32f). The set screws are tightened when the desired distraction has been obtained (Fig. 7.32n). The half-rings are removed. Alternatively, the 6-mm rod holders can be used instead of the half-rings (Fig. 7.32g). This distraction force reconstitutes the height of the anterior portion of the vertebral body and relieves the pressure from the intervertebral disk and completes the vertebral body reduction.

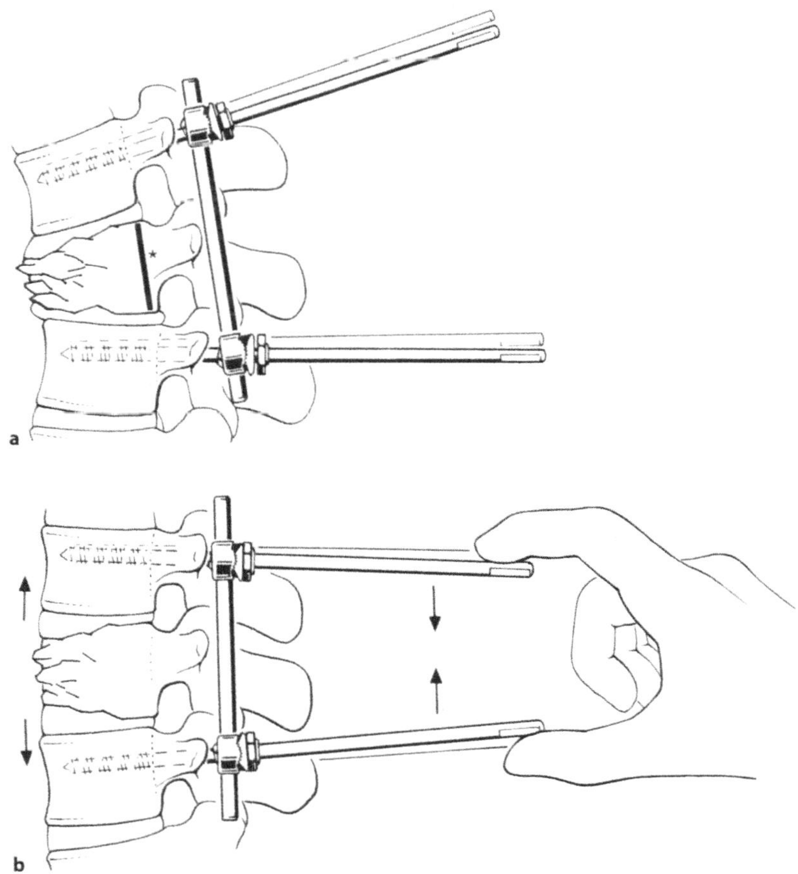

Fig. 7.32 Correction of anterior vertebral body fracture with intact posterior wall (type A)
a Posterior vertebral body wall intact (*)
b Correction of kyphosis by manually approximating the dorsal ends of the Schanz screws

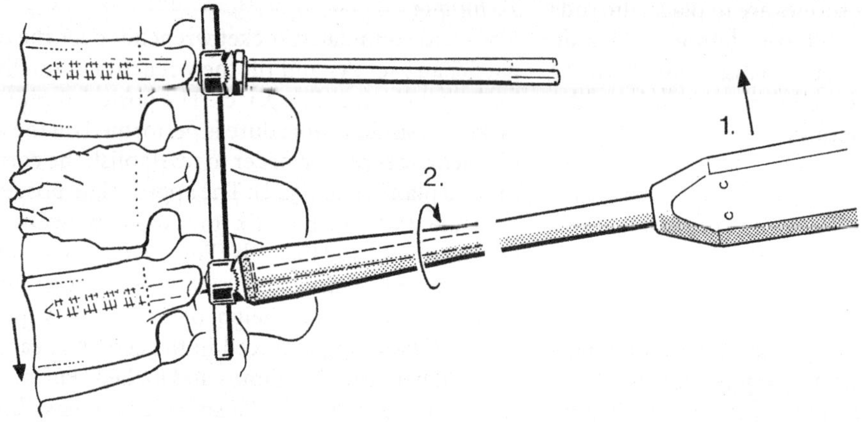

c

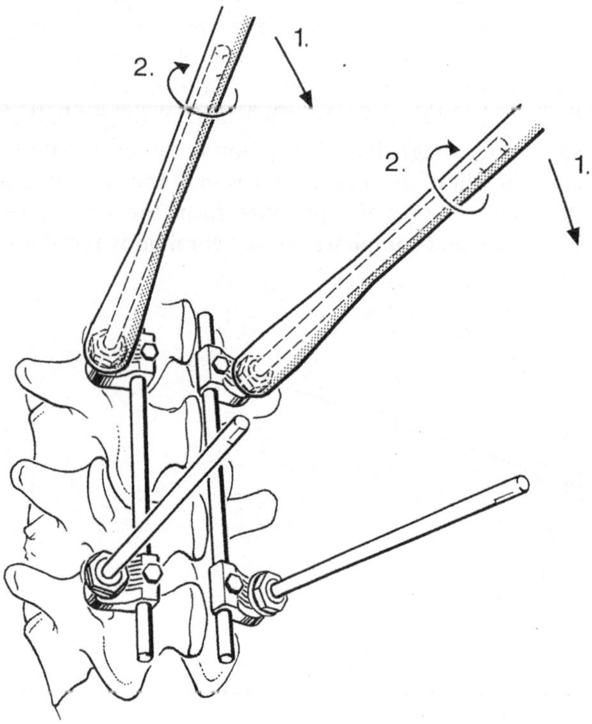

d

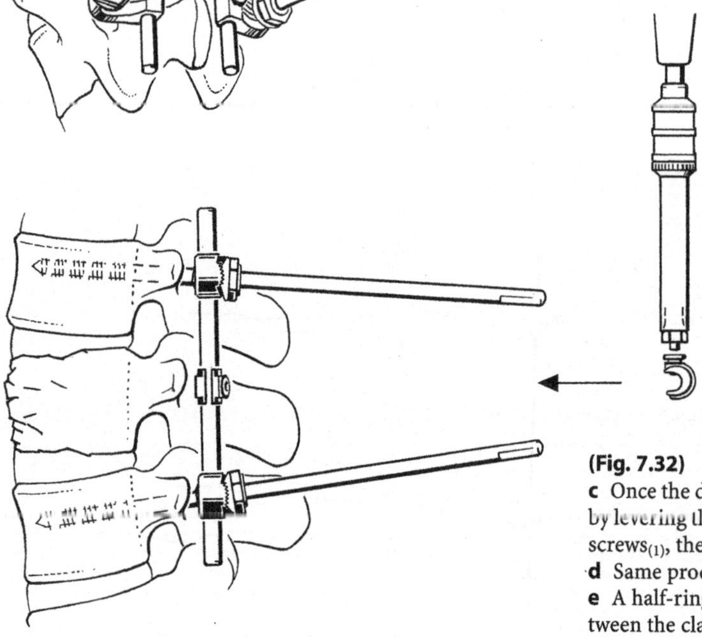

e

(Fig. 7.32)
c Once the distal Schanz screws are in the desired position by levering the cannulated socket wrenches with the Schanz screws$_{(1)}$, the nuts are locked in the final position$_{(2)}$
d Same procedure on the cranial Schanz screws
e A half-ring is placed in the center of each 6-mm rod between the clamps and locked

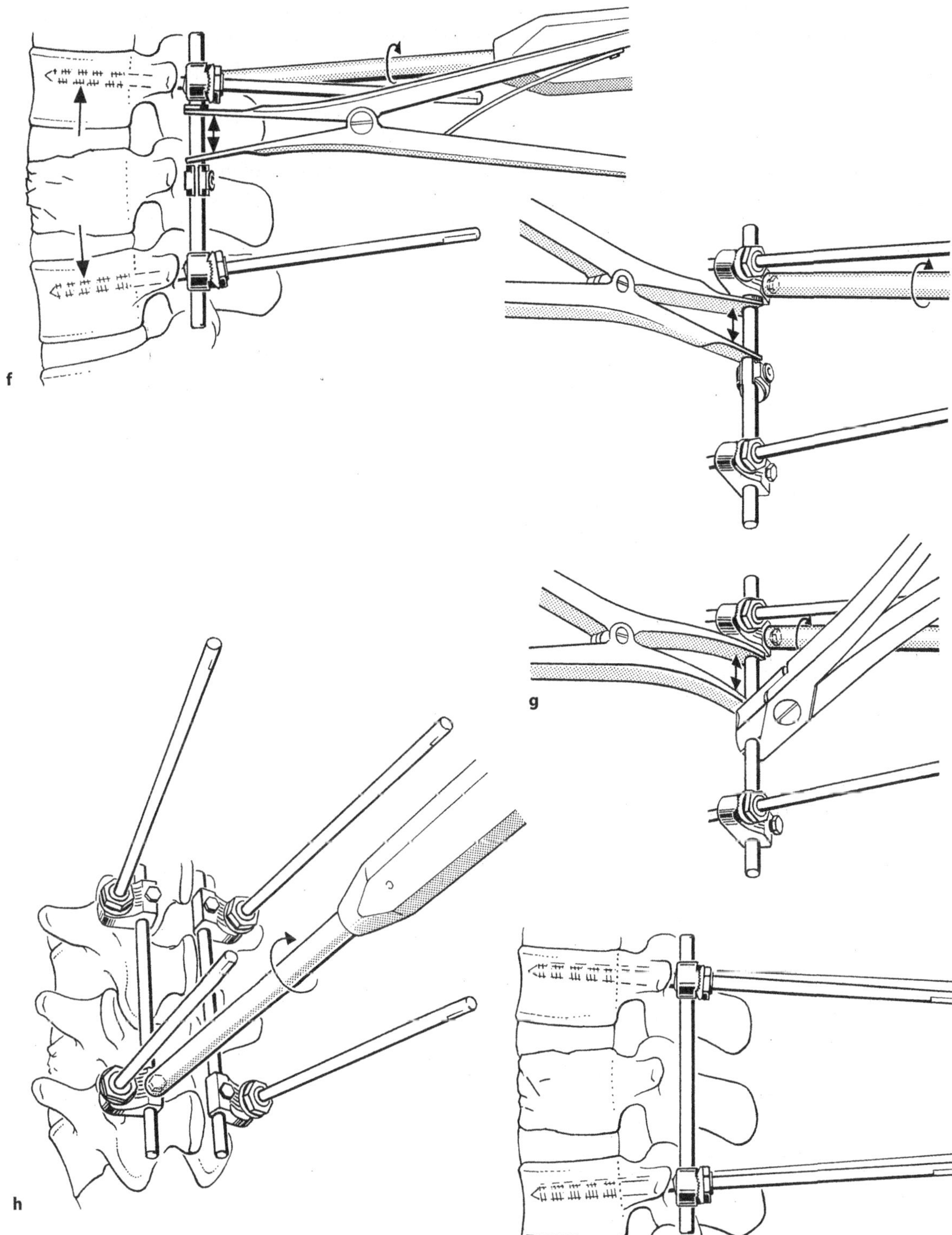

(Fig. 7.32)
f Application of distraction with the spreader forceps. (Check with image intensifier)
g Alternatively, the 6-mm rod holder can be used instead of the half-rings
h Completed vertebral body reduction with resolved height of the body and the discs. The set screws are tightened

7.2.2.2.2
Anterior Vertebral Body Fracture with Fractured Posterior Wall (Type A-3) (Fig. 7.33a)

Principle

In this type of fracture, there is a theoretical danger that posterior wall fragments might displace posteriorly into the canal during correction of the kyphosis by compressing together the posterior opening clamps of the Schanz screws. The posterior wall must be protected against compression. Distraction is used to reconstitute the height of the vertebral body.

Technique

Posterior wall decompression can be achieved by the following technique. Two 5-mm half-rings are placed on each of the 6-mm rods prior to the reduction with the Schanz screws; a distance of 5 mm between the half-rings/rod holder and the clamp is allowed for every 10° of attempted kyphosis correction (Fig. 7.33b). When approximating the ends of the Schanz screws, the clamps will soon touch the half-rings and the center of rotation is transferred posteriorly to the level of the rods. The force now required to correct the kyphosis is much greater. The lordosis is checked on the lateral image of the intensifier. The posterior opening nuts are tightened to secure correction and the set screws on the clamps are tightened (Fig. 7.33c). The same procedure is repeated for the other Schanz screws (Fig. 7.33d). The half-rings are removed. Distraction as described in the previous section is now exerted to restore the original height of the vertebra (Fig. 7.33e, f).

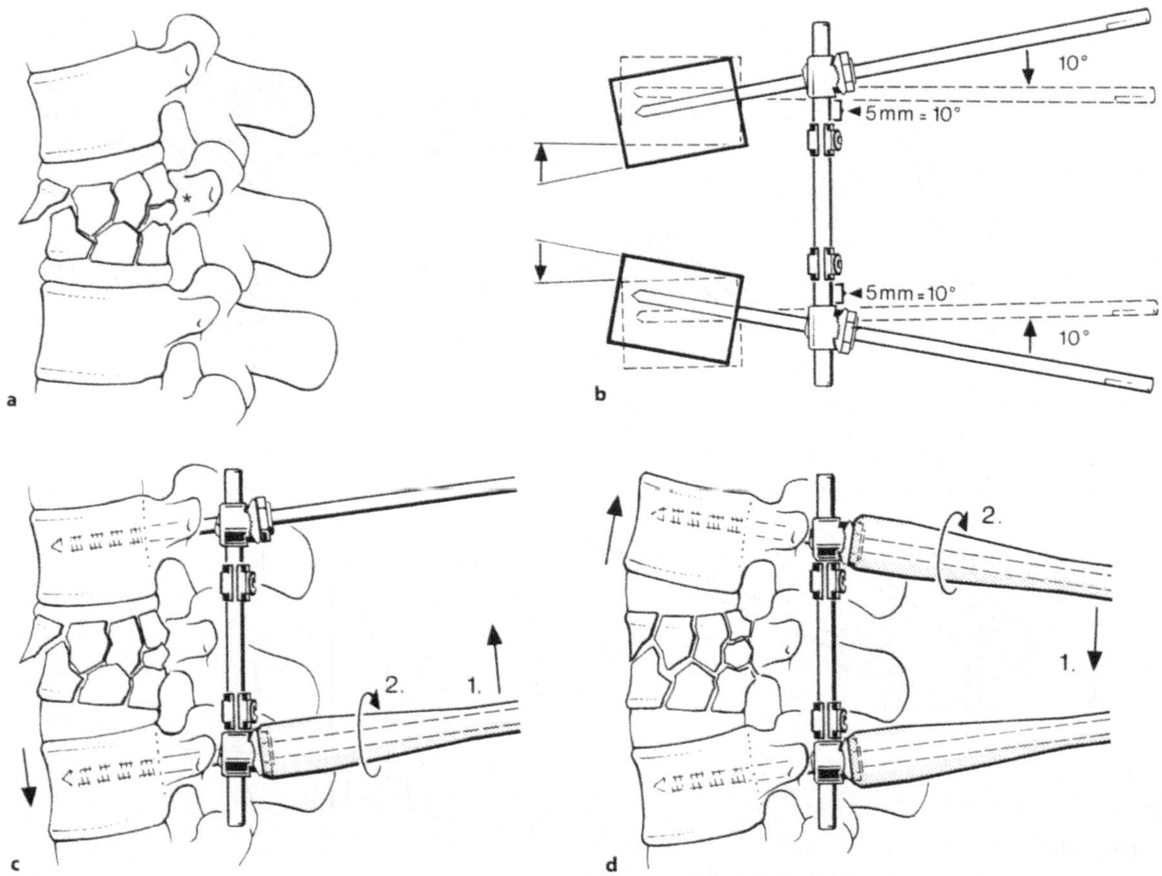

Fig. 7.33 Anterior vertebral body fracture with fractured posterior wall
a Burst fracture (*)
b 5 mm distance for the clamp on the rod allows for 10° kyphosis correction
c Tightening of the nuts of the clamps to secure correction. The posterior vertebral body wall is maintained by the preset distance of the C-rings
d Same procedure for the cranial Schanz screws and tightening of the set screws on the clamp

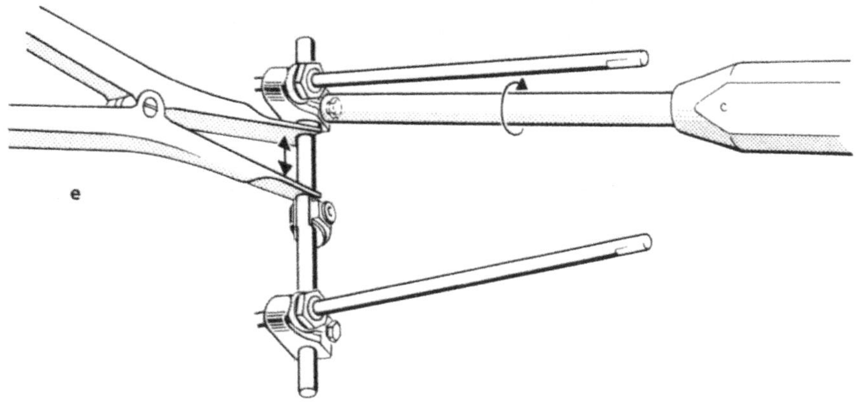

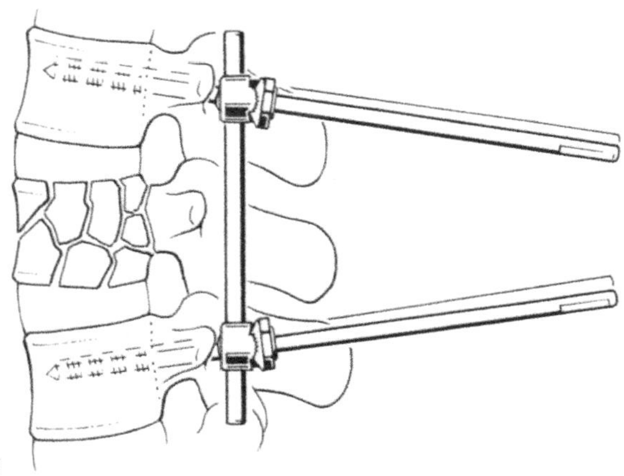

(Fig. 7.33)
e Distraction applied by spreader forceps
f Final correction

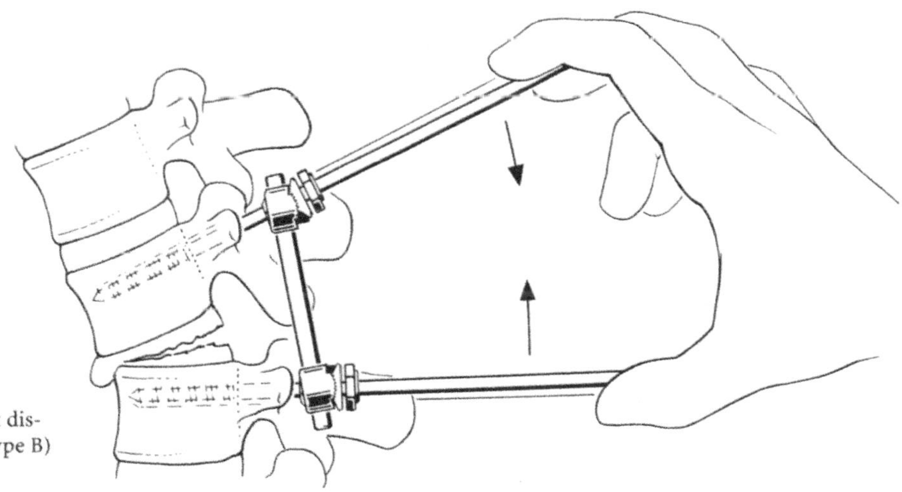

Fig 7.34 Posterior element disruption with distraction (type B)
a Reduction maneuver

7.2.2.2.3
Posterior Element Fractures or Disruption with Distraction (Type B) (Fig. 7.34)

The implant acts as a pure tension band. Therefore, after reduction in the above-described manner with the clamp elements sliding freely, no distraction is carried out but slight compression is applied (Fig. 7.34a–c). To achieve compression, the half-rings or 6-mm rod holders are placed between the posterior opening clamps and the compression forceps applied across the posterior clamps and half-rings/6-mm rod holders (Fig. 7.34d). The set screws on the clamps are tightened. The protruding ends of the Schanz' screws are cut with the bolt cutter (Fig. 7.35a, b).

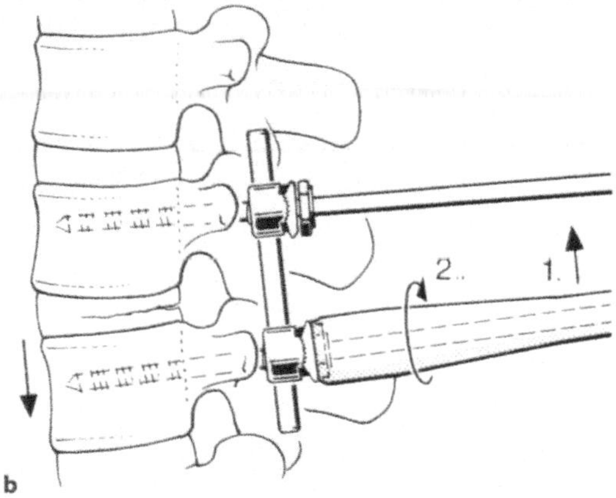

b

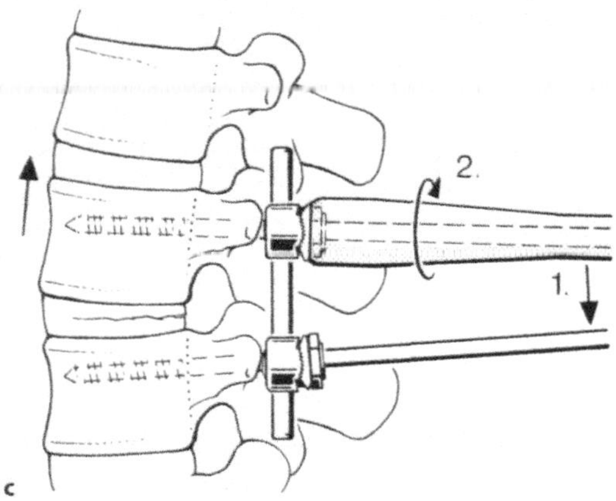

c

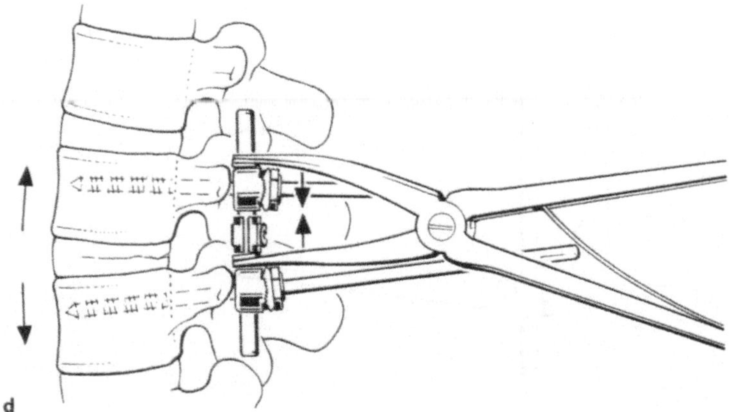

d

(Fig 7.34)
b Tightening the distal nuts with cannulated socket wrench
c Tightening the proximal nuts after maximal lordosis has been achieved
d Compression forceps are used to achieve optimal tension banding fixation

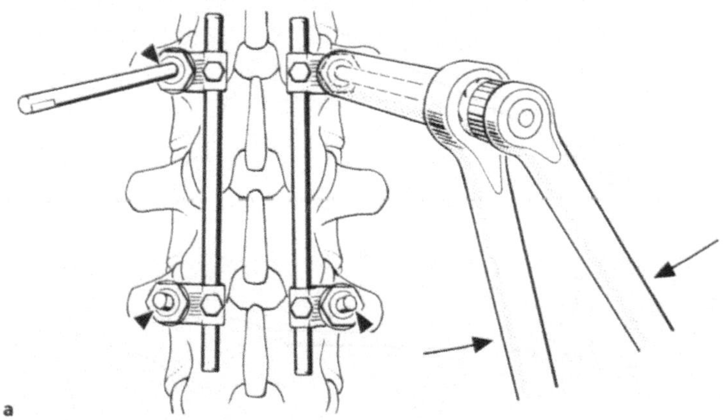

a

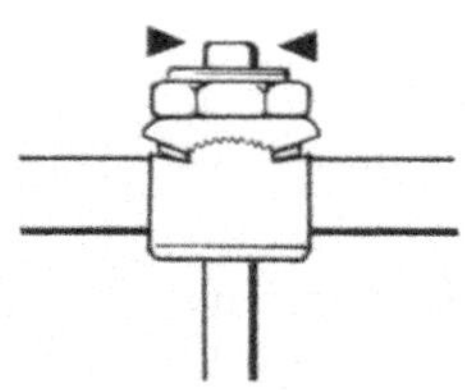

b

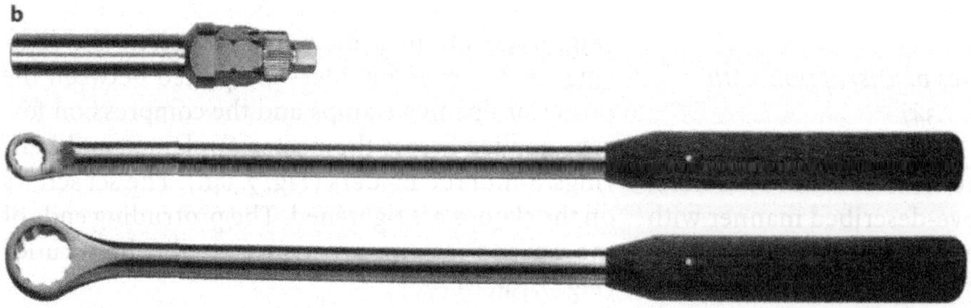

Fig. 7.35 Cut off the protruding ends of the Schanz screws
a Protruding ends cut off
b Bolt cutter with handles

7.2.2.2.4
Complete Disruption of the Anterior and Posterior Elements with Rotation (Type C)

The internal fixator acts as a neutralization device. The reduction technique is similar to that described for No. 3 above. If there is any doubt regarding stability of the fracture particularly in rotation or shear (type C fracture), then it is essential to cross-link the two 6-mm rods (Fig. 7.36). (See Chap. 8.2.1, Fig. 8.6a,b). Take care to hold the handles steadily. The hexagonal screwdriver with holding sleeve is attached to the cross-link clamp (Fig. 7.36a); the special sleeve with the two notches on the top is placed on the holder (Fig. 7.36b), and the clamp is placed on the 6-mm rod and the sleeve positioned over the rod and cross-link clamp. The 3-mm rod is cut to the appropriate length in order to link the two 6-mm rods and then placed in the side opening of the cross-link clamp (Fig. 7.36c); the hexagonal screwdriver and holding sleeve are removed, leaving the set screw loose. Another cross-link clamp is placed on the opposite rod and the 3-mm rod pushed through the clamp (Fig. 7.36d). Both set screws on the cross-link clamps are tightened (Fig. 7.36e), the second one only after applying distraction along the 3-mm rod with the USS spreader, thus loading the vertical rods and the pedicle screw heads (Fig. 7.36f). The excessive length of the 3-mm rod is finally cut on the lateral side of the clamp (Fig. 7.36g) in order to create the final construct (Fig. 7.36h).

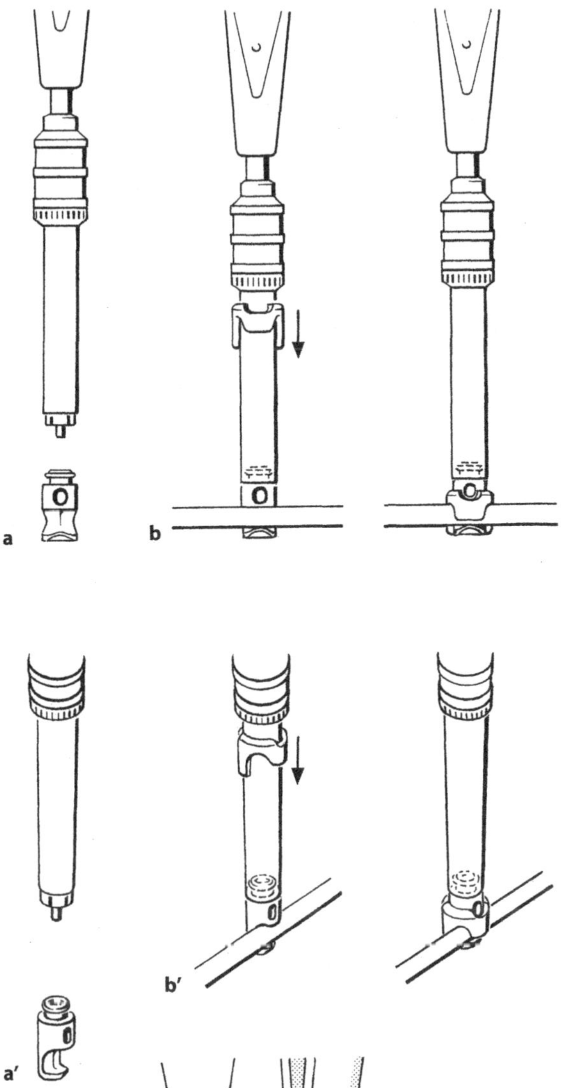

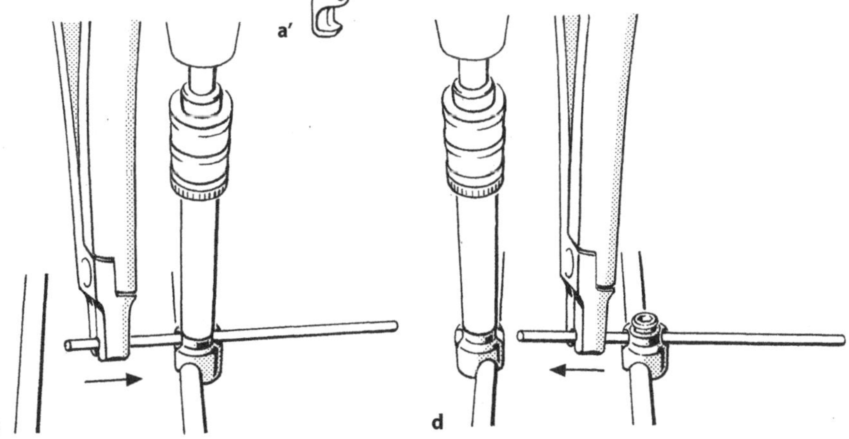

Fig. 7.36 Application of a cross-link (indicated in some B and C fractures)

a/a′ Cross-link clamp is attached to the hexagonal screwdriver with holding sleeve
b/b′ The special sleeve is placed on the holder and the cross-link clamp is brought to the 6-mm rod
c 3-mm rod is placed in the side-opening of the cross-link clamp
d The 3-mm rod is pushed through the clamp on the opposite rod

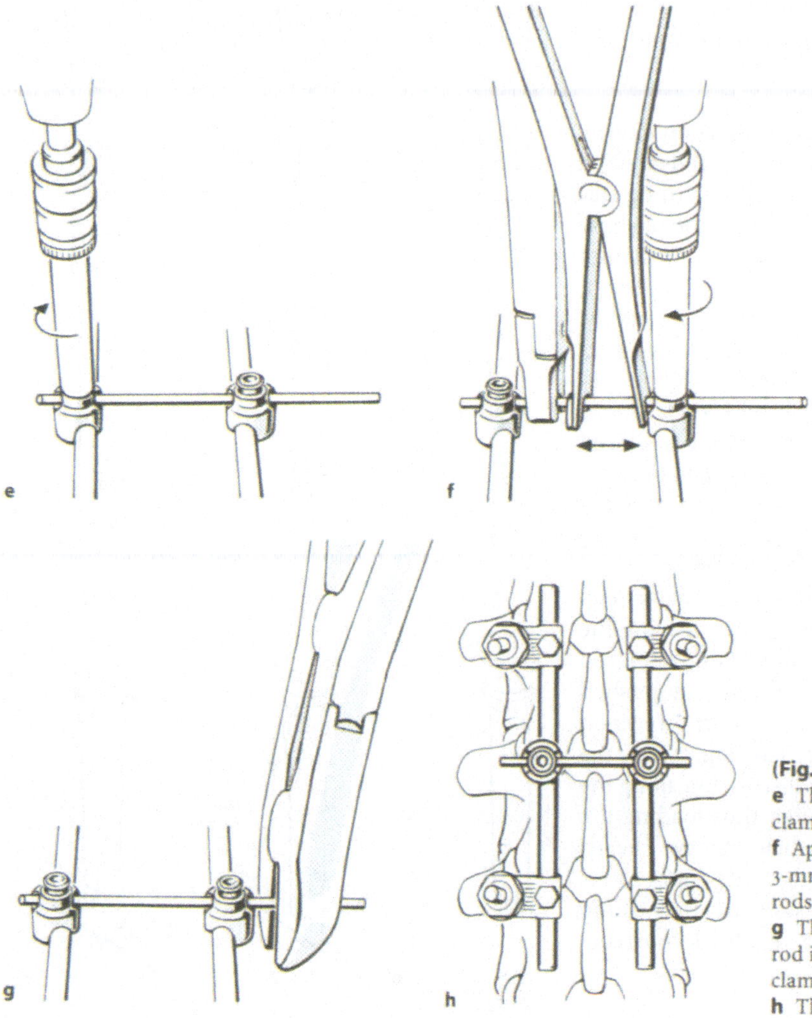

(Fig. 7.36)
e The set screws on the cross-link clamps are tightened
f Application of distraction along the 3-mm rod in order to load the 6-mm rods and the connected pedicle screws
g The excessive length of the 3-mm rod is cut on the lateral side of the clamp
h The final construct

Additional Measures

1. In the majority of cases, reduction results in a large defect of bone stock in the vertebral body. It is an integral part of the fixator instrumentation to fill the anterior defects with autologous bone grafts. This is possible using the same posterior approach by the transpedicular bone-grafting procedure described by Daniaux (1986): a channel of 6 mm diameter is made into the pedicle of the fractured vertebra, and the pedicle entered as previously described. The hole is made initially with the pedicle probe and the position is controlled by the image intensifier (Fig. 7.37a). A depth gauge is placed down the pedicle to ensure bone surrounds the hole, which is then enlarged to 6 mm with the use of an *oscillating* drill, the drill being directed slightly cranially towards the defect (Fig. 7.37b). In order not only to fill the fractured vertebral body with cancellous bone but to enhance an anterior fusion between the vertebral body above and the fractured vertebra, disk material can be removed through the 6-mm pedicular channel with a pituitary rongeur, and the lower end plate of the vertebra above can even be freshened up (Fig. 7.37c). As the entry point lies in line with the already inserted Schanz screws, it is situated lateral to the longitudinal rod and can be reached without impairment. The special long funnel is then inserted into the drill hole (Fig. 7.37d) until the stop touches the posterior cortex of the lamina: the tip then automatically reaches into the center of the vertebral body and *protects the vertebral canal from unintended intrusion of bone graft particles through a fracture gap in the pedicle.* The transplanted bone is pushed anteriorly into the defect zone (Fig. 7.37e).

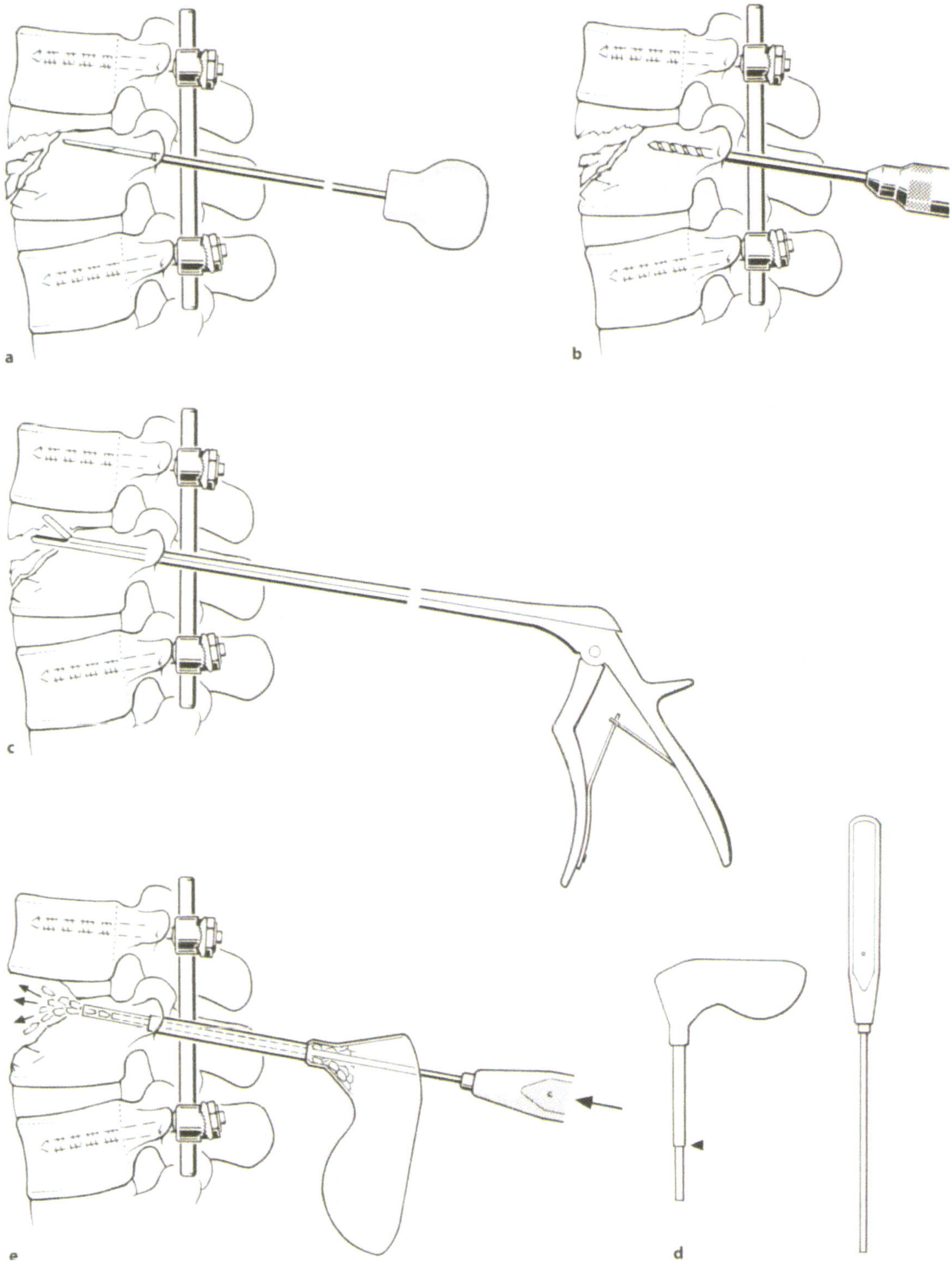

Fig. 7.37 Transpedicular bone grafting
a The initial hole is made with the pedicle probe
b The pedicle opening is enlarged with a 6-mm oscillating drill, directed slightly cranially
c Disk material can be removed and the lower end plates freshened up with a pituitary rongeur through the pedicle
d Special long funnel with a stop rim and the bone pusher
e The bone graft is pushed anteriorly into the defect zone

2. If the patency of the spinal canal has not been restored and posterior wall fragments continue to protrude, hemilaminectomy and resection of one pedicle of the fractured vertebra is performed to reduce by impaction, or to extract, the posterior wall fragments: an alternative would be anterior decompression through a second approach.
3. Posterolateral fusion is recommended.
4. Anterior bone grafting is necessary in the case of significant defect with mechanical impairment of the anterior column, since the incidence of fatigue fractures of the Schanz screws will, otherwise, increase.

Postoperative Care

Early mobilization is allowed with a three-point fixation bracc (Jcwctt bracc) to prevent excessive flexion or extension for 6 – 12 weeks postoperatively.

CHAPTER 8

Modular Stabilization System: The Universal Spine System

8.1 Basic Concepts

The Universal Spine System (USS) involves four basic concepts:

- Independent anchorage of hooks and/or screws to the spine and independent rod positioning.
- Easy connection between the anchorage and the rod.
- Standardization and simplification of implants, *which can all be handled from the top.* No lateral nuts are used.
- Segmental correction and stabilization.

These four basic concepts are essential and are necessary to allow a completely free choice of the anchorage of the screws or hooks to the spine, using the best possible anatomic location. This immediately implies that the connection device between the rod and screws/hooks must be adjustable with a variable distance between the anchorage site (hook or screw) and the vertical bar (rod). In addition, the vertical bar must be adjustable to the desired curvature of the spine; therefore, it must be able to be bent. It is clear that such a system cannot consist of a plate and screws, but rather a rod system which is anchored to the bone with either screws or hooks.

The anatomy of the deformed or degenerated spine does not allow the placement of all the screws or hooks in a straight line. These hooks/screws should be placed in the best-defined anatomic position, with no regard for the fit with the longitudinal bar. However, it is essential to limit the number of implants and to simplify their use; therefore, a concept was developed which allows a simple connection between the rods and variable positions of the anchorage (hooks and/or screws).

In addition, the connection between the rod and the hook/screw should be designed in a way that this concept can be used with the hook-based or screw-based system. The system should also be used as an anterior system. To meet these requirements, a uniformity must be achieved with the designed implants in terms of the underlying concept, to simplify its use as much as possible and also to simplify the instrumentation which is necessary to handle these implants. The screw and the hook head must either accept the rod in different positions, or the connection system. The connection system must provide the freedom to adapt the variable positions of the anchorage to the vertical bar.

Furthermore, experience with the internal fixator for the spine has taught us that a connection device which needs to be tightened from laterally is too 'fiddly' and needs considerable dexterity and should be replaced by a clamp which can be *completely handled from the posterior or above.* This concept has already been adopted in the second generation of the internal fixator and was to be applied in any new development.

Experience with the CD (Cotrel Dubousset) Instrumentation has shown that the concept of derotation in scoliotic spines through the rotation of the rod does not, in reality, always involve significant derotation, or when it does, it may be associated with an important unbalancing of the spine above and/or below the spinal area included in the fixation. The principle is based on the assumption that by adapting the rod to the curve in the frontal plane and attaching it along the concavity of the curve, the scoliosis in the thoracic spine, which is in reality a lordosis, can be transformed into a kyphosis by rotating the bent rod from the frontal plane into the sagittal plane. The spinal area which is fixed with the instrumentation is pulled along with the rotated rod into the desired kyphotic form. *This global rotation has a significant torque effect on the rest of the spine.*

Derotation should be based on individual vertebrae. Clinical experience in scoliosis with the internal fixator allowed us to design the concept of a 'frame technique', where the frame is constructed by the anchorage of screws or hooks in the end vertebrae, cranially as well as caudally, which are attached to the two vertical rods. Therefore, all vertebrae within this frame, or relative to the frame, can then be 'derotated' and/or 'translated' into the frame by individual manipulation of each vertebra. It is clear that the strongest lever arm for the manipulation of a vertebra is a pedicle screw with a long handle (Schanz screw). Therefore, instrumentation was designed which could convert the hook or screw into a Schanz screw temporarily for the derotation manoeuver. It is important that the anchorage in the vertebra is very strong and provides a stable fixation angle. This can be achieved with a pedicular screw, or with the completely newly designed specialized pedicle hook, which allows a stable fixation to the pedicle. This concept necessitates a whole new set of implants as well as instruments to perform these complex manipulations.

8.2 The System

In order to obtain a universal spine system, it was built on a modular concept. The three major areas of spinal surgery, (1) traumatic fracture and pathological spinal treatment, (2) deformity treatment, and (3) degenerative spine disease treatment, demand individual techniques which require specific instrumentation solutions. These three areas have in common a basic instrumentation set and a modular section which addresses each of the individual problems specifically.

8.2.1 Instruments and Implants

The first common implant is the rod. The rods are smooth with a 6 mm diameter and are available in different lengths from 50 to 500 mm. There are *hard* rods for fractures or tumors as well as for deformity surgery, and *soft* rods for low back surgery (Fig. 8.1). There are different instruments to bend the rods: a rod holder (Fig. 8.2) and rod-bending irons, with straight or angled notches, for in situ lordosing or kyphosing of the rod (Fig. 8.3a).

A USS tubular rod bender (Fig. 8.3b), USS bending pliers (Fig. 8.3c) and a USS 6-mm bending template are available (Fig. 8.3d). Different devices have been designed to extend the versatility of the rods: an extension connector (Fig. 8.4a), which allows the direct connection of two 6-mm rods, a parallel connector (Fig. 8.4b), which allows parallel connection of two 6-mm rods, and the half-ring, which is used as an aid for distraction or compression (Fig. 8.4c). All three devices have set screws which accept the small fragment-set hexagonal screwdriver. To perform appropriate distraction and compression, spreader as well as compression forceps have been developed (Fig. 8.5a, b). This is a clear departure from the original threaded rod in the internal fixa-

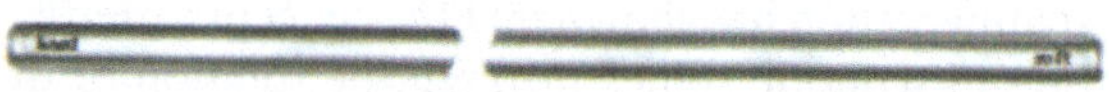

Fig. 8.1 Hard and soft rods

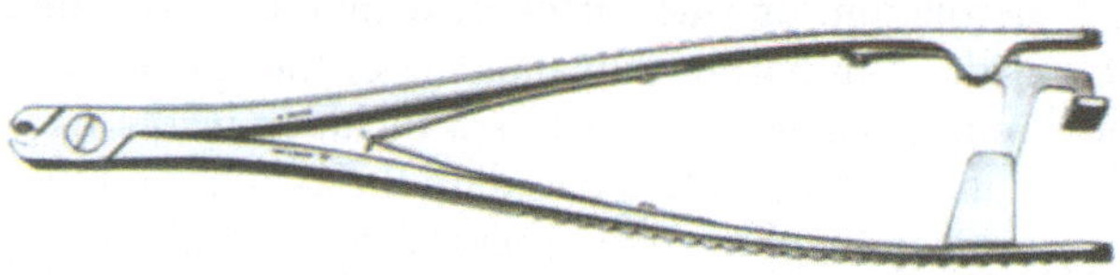

Fig. 8.2 Rod-holding forceps

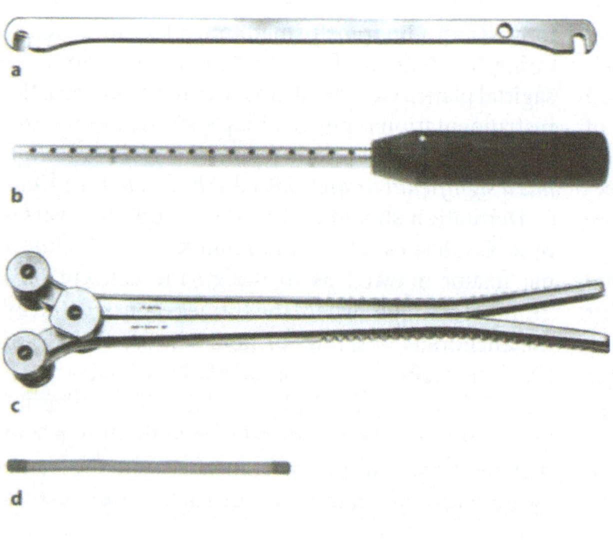

Fig. 8.3
a Rod-bending irons, with straight and angled notches
b USS tubular rod bender
c USS bending pliers
d USS 6-mm template for USS rods

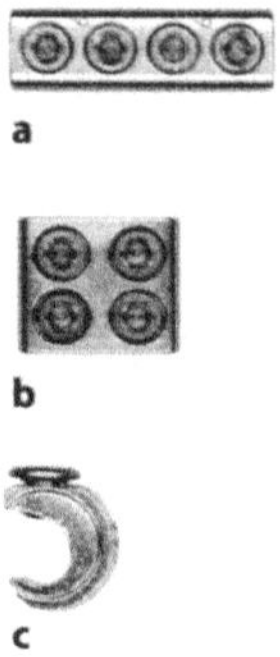

Fig. 8.4
a USS extension connector for rods of 6.0 mm diameter
b USS parallel connector for rods of 6.0 mm diameter
c USS half ring

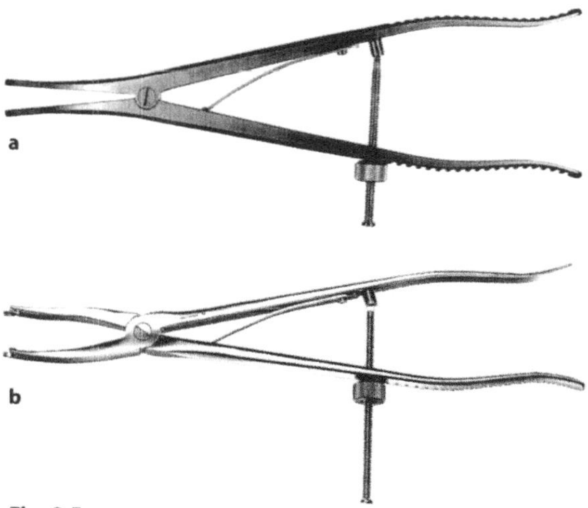

Fig. 8.5
a USS spreader forceps
b USS compression forceps

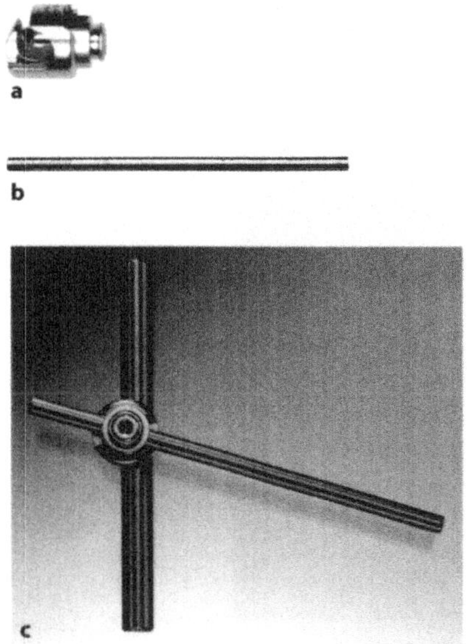

Fig. 8.6
a USS cross-link clamp for USS rods 6.0 mm diameter
b USS rod 3.5 mm diameter for USS cross-link system
c Angulation of cross-link system +/-20 °

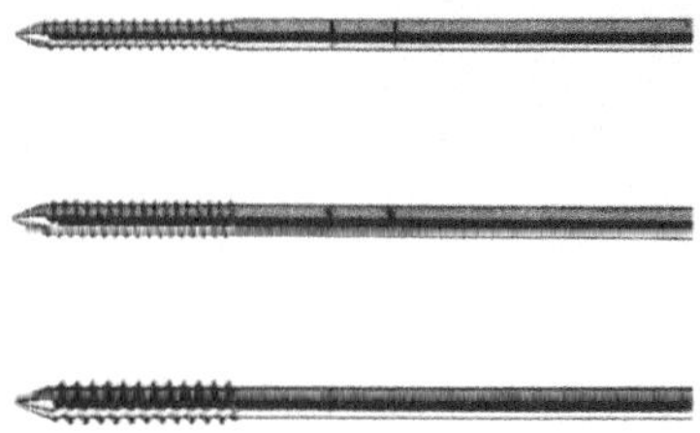

Fig. 8.7 Schanz screws. 7 mm, 6 mm and 5 mm. The shaft of all three screw types is the same (5 mm)

tor which allowed a continuous distraction or compression by tightening the nuts on the threaded rod.

To link the longitudinal bars together cross-links were created. The cross-link includes two cross-linkage clamps and a connecting rod (Fig. 8.6a, b). The clamp may be swiveled to allow various angles of connection between the two rods, each clamp allowing up to 20 ° in either direction (Fig. 8.6c). Two cross-links are available and their use is dictated by the distance between the implants on the 6-mm rods.

8.2.1.1 Fracture Module

For the fracture set, specific implants with very similar instrumentation to the basic set are used. The main component of this instrumentation has been adapted for use with transpedicular Schanz screws of 5, 6 or 7 mm diameter (Fig. 8.7). The Schanz screw allows a significant lever arm for reduction of the fracture. A second-generation internal fixator clamp with posterior nuts – a further development of the original, laterally tightened clamp, which can now be adjusted completely from above – has been adapted to the USS to connect the rod with the Schanz screws (Fig. 8.8a). The clamp has an adjustability range of 36 ° in the sagittal plane (Fig. 8.8b). A single set screw tightens the clamp onto the rod (Fig. 8.8c). If a much higher range of adjustability is required, the rod is bent to increase the amount of lordosis.

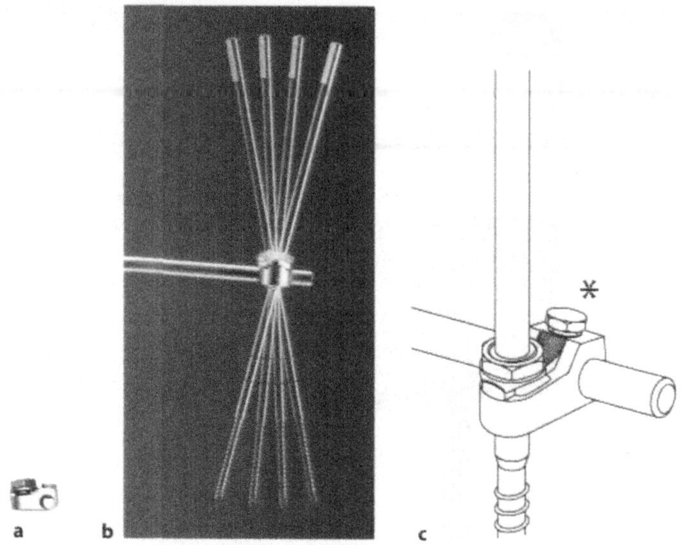

Fig. 8.8
a USS clamp with posterior nut for USS rods
b Schanz screw with clamp, angled. Range of motion +/- 18° in the sagittal plane
c single set screw (*) tightening the clamp onto the rod

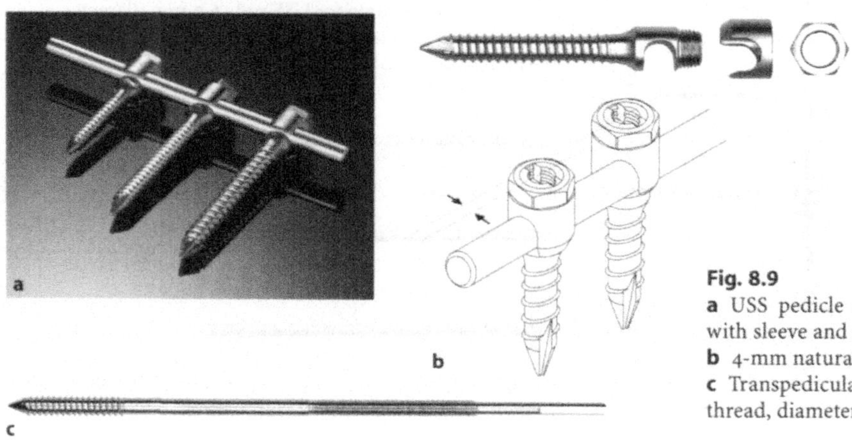

Fig. 8.9
a USS pedicle screw,side-opening complete with sleeve and nut, diameter 5,6,7 mm
b 4-mm natural offset (see also Fig. 8.39)
c Transpedicular Schanz screw with double thread, diameter 6 mm

8.2.1.2 Low Back Surgery Module

For the low back surgery set, different screws with side-openings for the rod (Fig. 8.9a)and Schanz screws with a double thread (Fig. 8.9c) have been developed for treating the different clinical pathology of the lumbar spine, in the context of degenerative lumbar spine disease such as scoliotic and kyphotic deformity, spinal stenosis, degenerative spondylolisthesis, degenerative segmental instability and osteoporotic weakening of the bone.

The side-opening screws have exactly the same head as the hooks (Figs. 8.9a, 8.11, 8.13 and 8.14). The side-opening allows the screws to be inserted retrospectively (once a rod is in place). They are, therefore, easier to replace without removing the complete construct, if a revision is necessary. The side-opening screws are often used in conjunction with the hooks for the treatment of deformities. The natural 4-mm offset of the opening in the screws allows the rod to be more easily accommodated with various positions of the screws, rather than having to bend the rod (Fig. 8.9b). For even more versatility, rod connectors allow the complete adjustment of an independently inserted pedicle screw to the rod, which may be completely offset relative to the screw and also allows free angulation (Fig. 8.10a). The rod connector allows indirect connection of the side-opening screw to the rod (Fig. 8.10b). In addition, the same connectors can be used with the frontal-opening hook (Fig. 8.10c). The open rod connectors can be connected to the rod retrospectively, after adjacent implants and the rod have already been

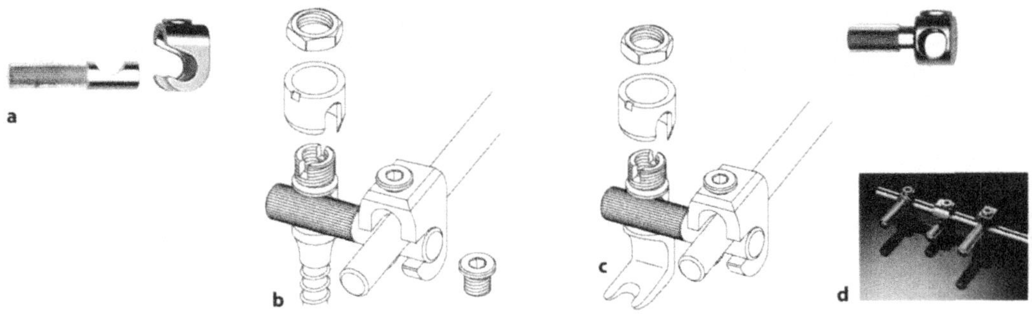

Fig. 8.10
a USS rod connector, open, length 15, 20, 25 mm
b Rod connector attached to pedicle screw
c USS rod connector attached to frontally open hook
d USS rod connector, closed, length 15, 20, 26 mm

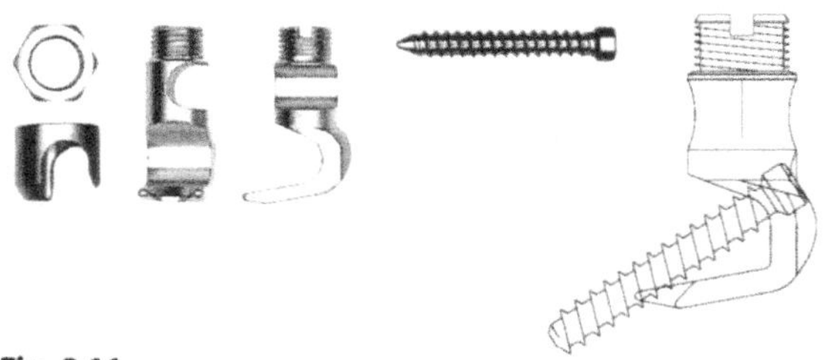

Fig. 8.11
USS pedicle hook, side-opening with USS screws 3.2 mm for USS pedicle hooks.

placed. Closed rod connectors can be used at the end of a construct where they can be added at the end of a procedure. They are smaller than the open rod connectors (Fig. 8.10d).

Soft rods are used in low back construction because they are more easily contoured.

8.2.1.3
Scoliosis and Deformity Module

The scoliosis instrumentation is the most interesting because the system is built on an innovative concept of scoliosis treatment. The USS offers the possibility of segmental correction and realignment of the spine to the sagittally placed rod.

In order to achieve reduction of the spine to the rod, special instruments have been developed and innovative hooks designed. A segmental derotation and translation can only be achieved when the implants are firmly anchored to the spine. The ideal fixation to the spine is a pedicle screw. A specialized pedicle hook has been designed to allow fixation to the vertebra, a 3.2-mm self-cutting screw passing through the pedicle into the end plate of the vertebra (Fig. 8.11). These special hooks allow, for the first time, translation and pulling forces to be applied without the hooks loosening or jumping out and *do not require distraction* to keep them in place. The locking mechanism of the hooks to the rod is exactly the same as for screws. The hooks and screws are inserted and manipulated with the screw holders,

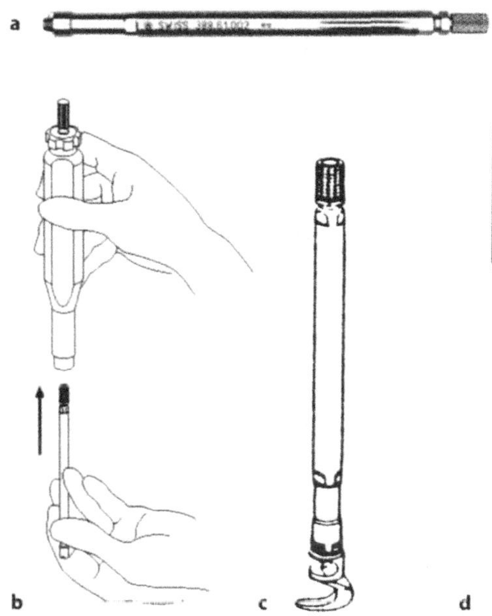

Fig. 8.12
a USS hook and USS screw holder
b USS hook and USS screw holder assembled with universal handle
c USS hook and USS screw holder attached to hook
d USS hook and USS screw holder attached to screw assembled with universal handle

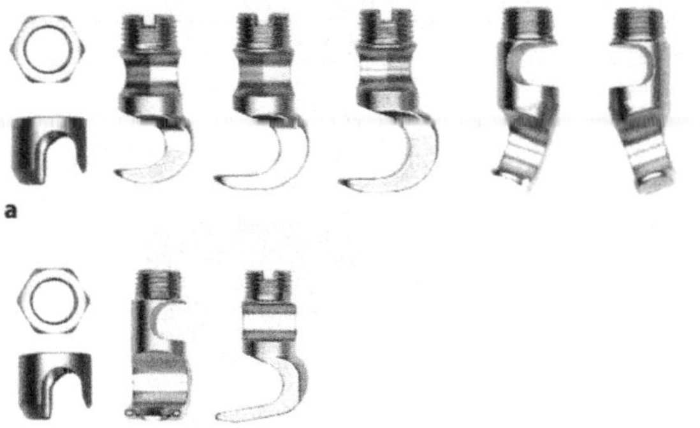

Fig. 8.13 Types of hooks
a USS lamina hook (large, medium, small, angled, side-opening)
b USS pedicle hook

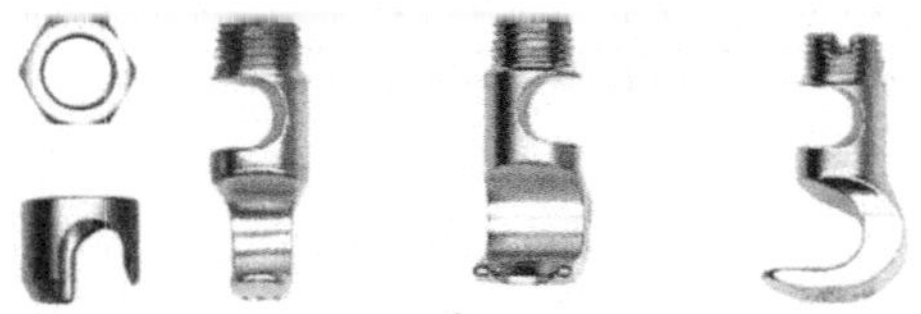

Fig. 8.14
a USS lamina hook, left open
b USS pedicle hook, right opening
c USS lamina hook, frontal opening

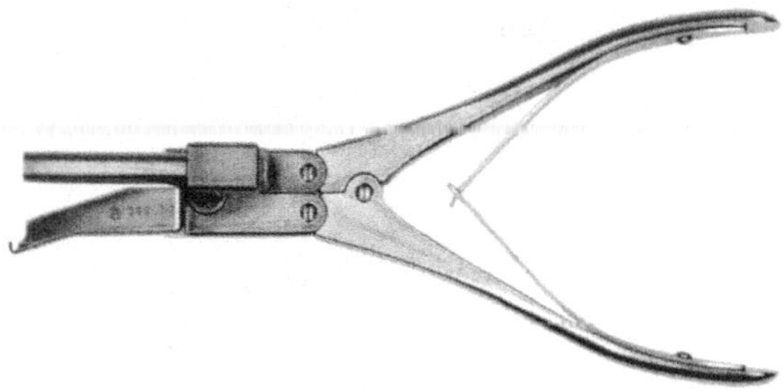

Fig. 8.15 USS complex reduction forceps ("persuader")

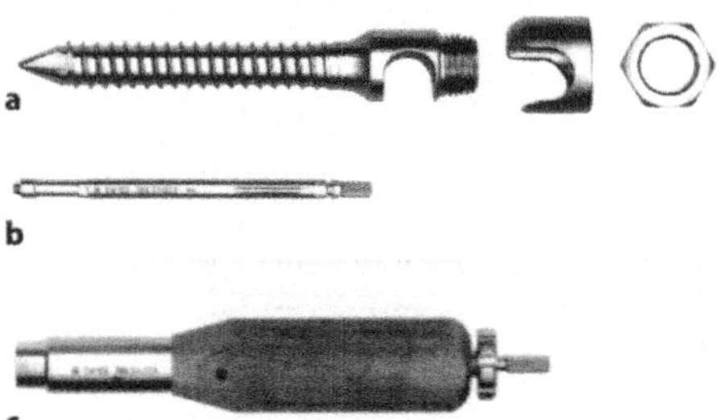

Fig. 8.16 Implants/instruments
a USS pedicle screw, side opening, complete with nut and sleeve
b USS screw and hook holder (stick)
c USS universal handle

which are often called extension sticks and which are fixed within the hook or screw head, imitating a Schanz screw (Fig. 8.12a–d). Since all the hooks are either laterally or frontally open, it should be appreciated that at any time during the insertion of implants at the end of the construct, further additional hooks or screws can be added where necessary. There are five types of hooks (Fig. 8.13a, b): laminar hooks – large, medium, small, angled – and pedicle hooks. Each type of hook has either a left, right or frontal opening (Fig. 8.14a–c)

The side-openings in the hooks or screws are especially useful in the treatment of kyphosis, where progressive fixation of the kyphosis from cranially to caudally is extremely helpful, and does not really require insertion of all hooks at the same time.

The USS open implants simplify pre- and intraoperative planning, allowing easy connection to the 6-mm rods. They can easily be added or removed from a construct without removing the entire implant system.

In order to manipulate the vertebrae, a set of specific instruments is available. The key instrument for the segmental derotation maneuver is the complex reduction forceps, the 'persuader', which allows lifting and translation at the same time, in order to bring the hook or the screw over the rod (Fig. 8.15). *This underlines the concept of a modular system with a high degree of versatility.*

8.2.1.4 Specific Implants and Instruments

8.2.1.4.1 USS Side-Opening Pedicle Screws

Implant and Instruments (Fig. 8.16)

Insertion Technique

The screws are inserted with the use of the screw holder (extension stick) attached to the universal handle (Fig. 8.16b, c). Initially the screw holder is connected to the universal handle (Fig. 8.17a, b). The screw holder is connected to the screw by rotating the cog wheel, which allows the thread of the screw holder to engage to the top of the screw (Fig. 8.18); alternatively, the screw holder can be tightened to the screw by hand (Fig. 8.19). The screw

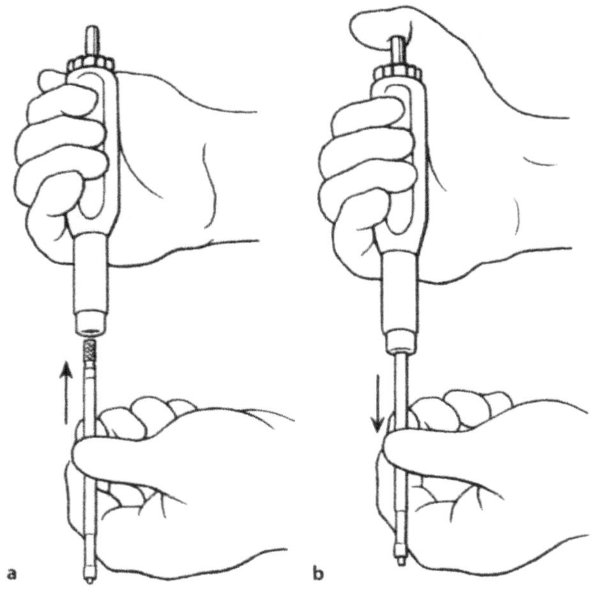

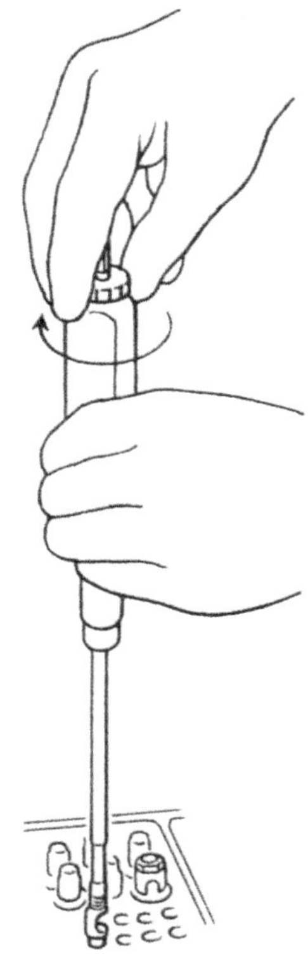

Fig. 8.18

Fig. 8.17
a Attachment of universal handle to the screw holder (extension stick)
b Release of universal handle from the screw holder (extension stick)

Fig. 8.18 Connection of screw holder to screw by rotating the cog-wheel

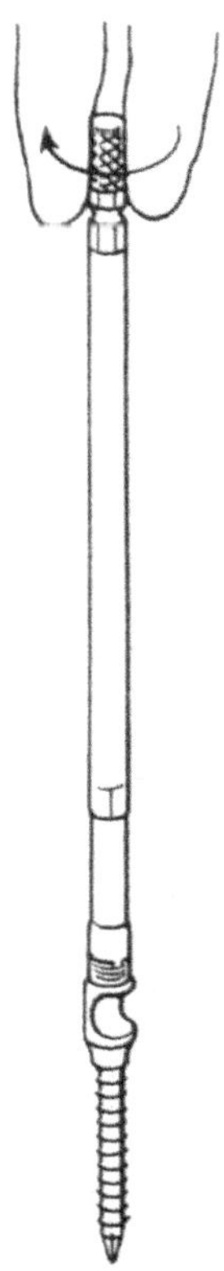

Fig. 8.19

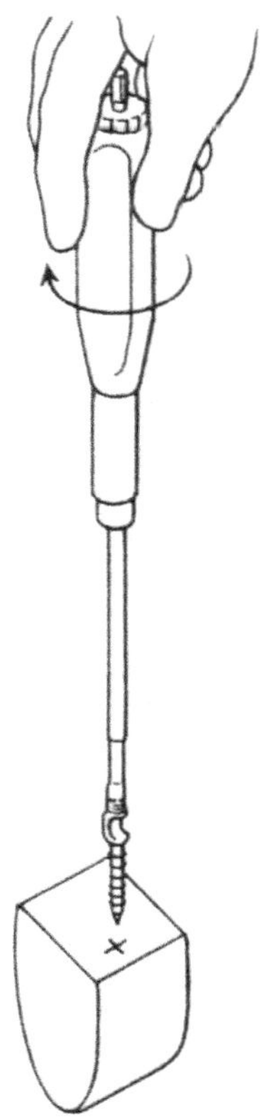

Fig. 8.20

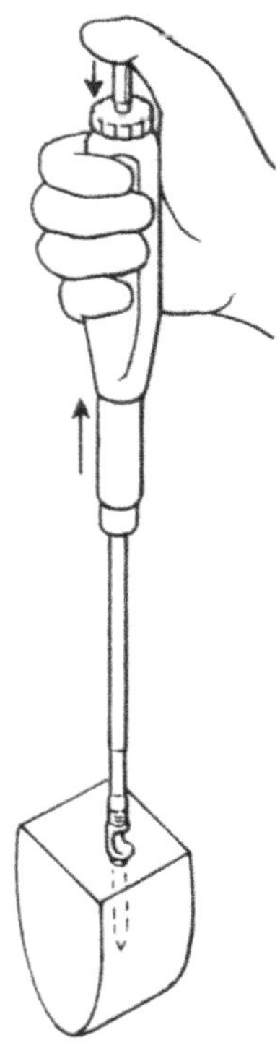

Fig. 8.21

Fig. 8.19 Tightening of screw holder to screw by hand

Fig. 8.20 Insertion of the screw

Fig. 8.21 Release of the screw holder from the universal handle, when screw inserted

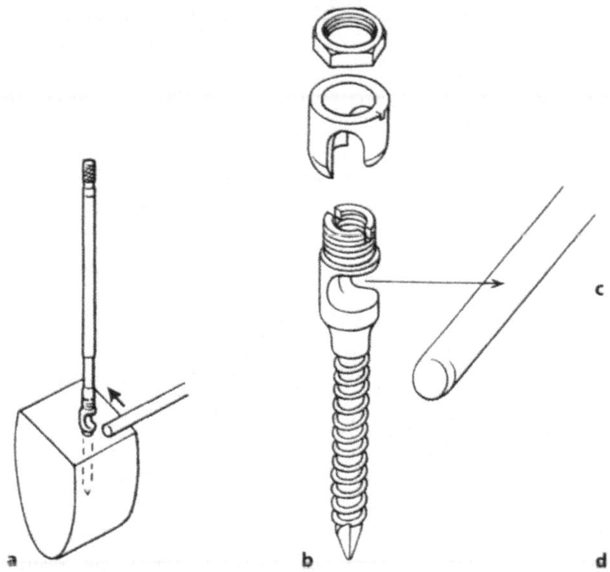

Fig. 8.22 a–e Steps of the insertion of the rod

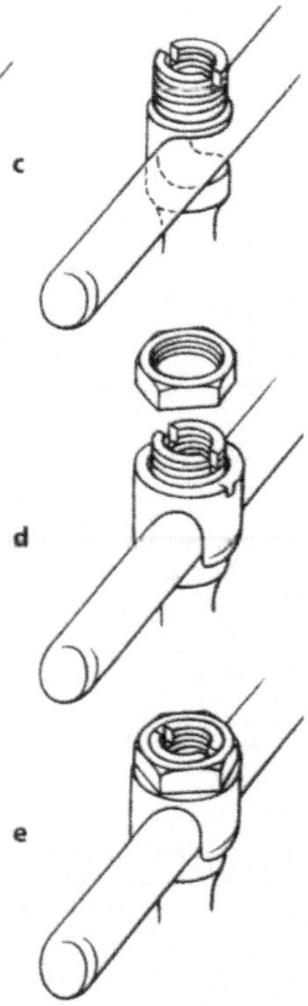

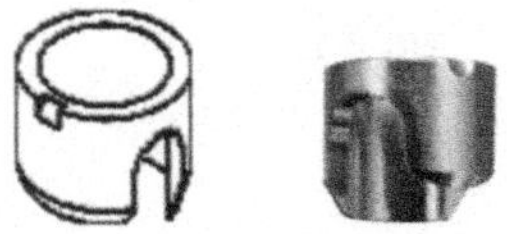

Fig. 8.23 Sleeve with short and long legs, small mark on the top of short leg.

can now be inserted into the bone (Fig. 8.20). The screw holder is disconnected from the handle by pressing the top of the handle (Fig. 8.21). A 6-mm rod can now be inserted into the screw (Fig. 8.22a). The 6-mm rod is held in place with a sleeve and nut (Fig. 8.22b-e).

The sleeve has a long and short leg – the latter slides over the open side of the implant and has a small mark on the top of the short leg for identification (Fig. 8.23). The nut and sleeve can be inserted into the universal handle (Fig. 8.24a). The universal handle is attached to the screw holder and the top of the universal handle is depressed causing the sleeve and nut to be released (Fig. 8.24b). The nut is tightened by the use of the 11-mm L-handed socket wrench and the USS 6.0-mm socket wrench (Fig. 8.24c). The 6-mm socket wrench is held firmly to control the screw to prevent torque of the implant when the nut is tightened (Fig. 8.24d).

8.2.1.4.2
USS Hooks: Laminar Hooks

Implants and Instrument (Fig. 8.25)

Insertion Technique
The lamina hook can be placed around either the superior or inferior portion of the lamina. The ligamentum flavum is carefully removed with a rongeur; to ensure the hook fits snugly onto the lamina, a small portion of the lamina is removed with a bone rongeur (Fig. 8.26a, b). The lamina feeler is carefully put around the lamina to ensure a close fit for the hook (Fig. 8.26c). The appropriate-size hook is mounted onto a stick with handle (Fig. 8.27a). The lamina hook is gently eased into place around the lamina (Fig. 8.27b, b'). *Ensure the foot of the hook does not lie too deep and press upon the spinal cord.* The inferior part of the hook must fit close to the lamina (Fig. 8.27c). The hook is attached to the screw holder in the same manner as the screw. The

Fig. 8.24
a Insertion of sleeve and nut onto the universal handle
b Release of sleeve and nut
c Tightening of nut with 11-mm L-handed socket wrench and 6.0-mm socket wrench
d The 6-mm socket wrench controls the rotation of the implant through the screw holder as the 11-mm L-handed socket wrench tightens the nut

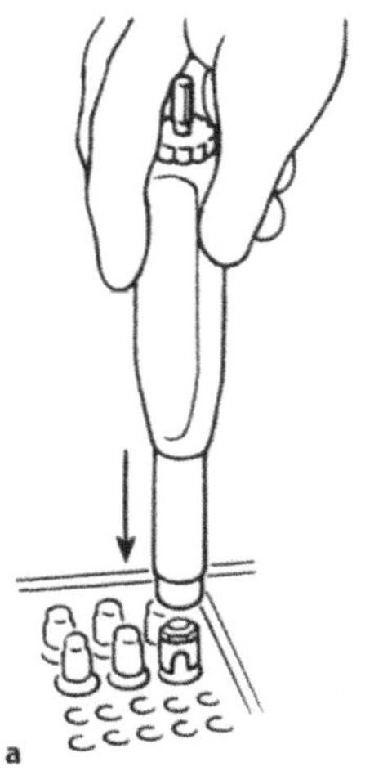

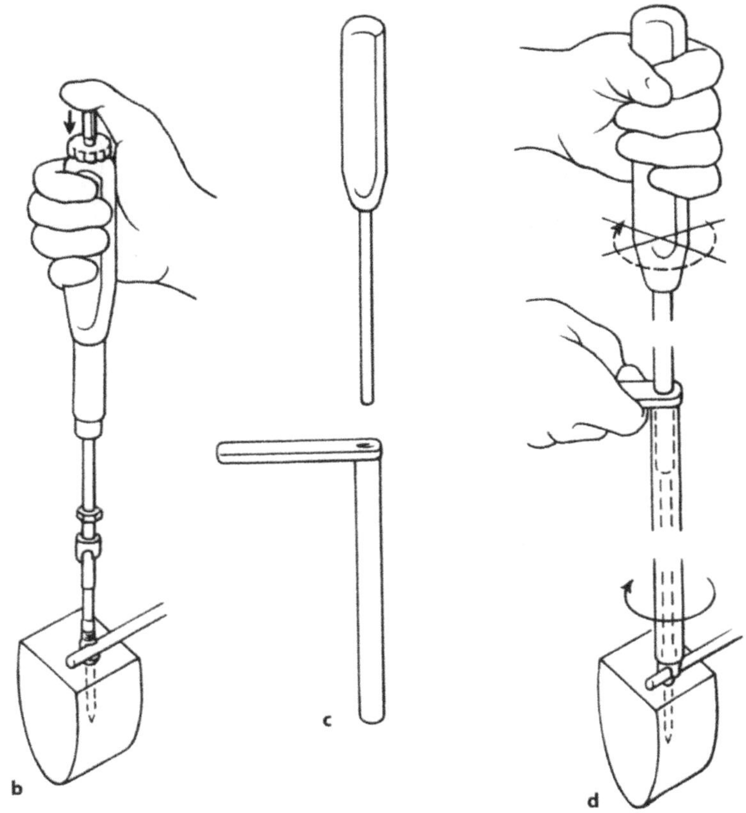

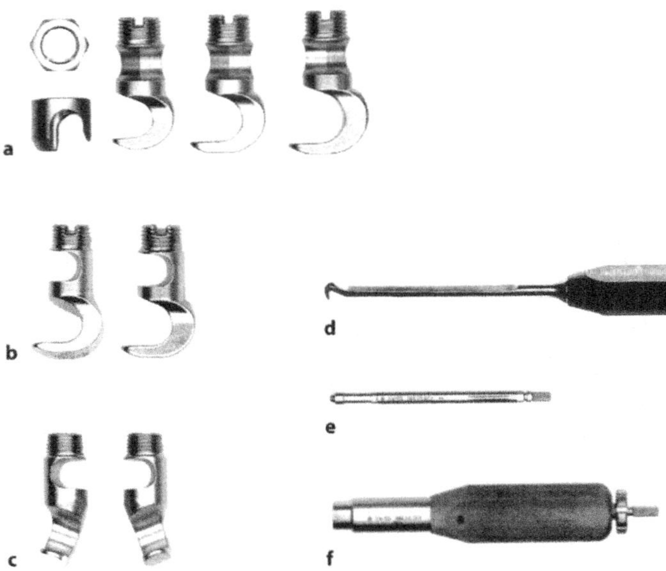

Fig. 8.25 Implants and Instrument
a USS laminar hook, side-opening small, medium, large
b USS laminar hook, front opening
c USS laminar hook, side-opening, angled
d USS lamina feeler
e USS hook and screw holder
f USS universal handle

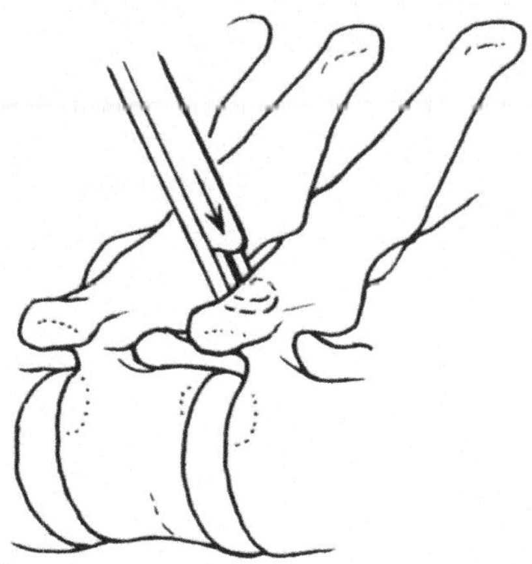
a

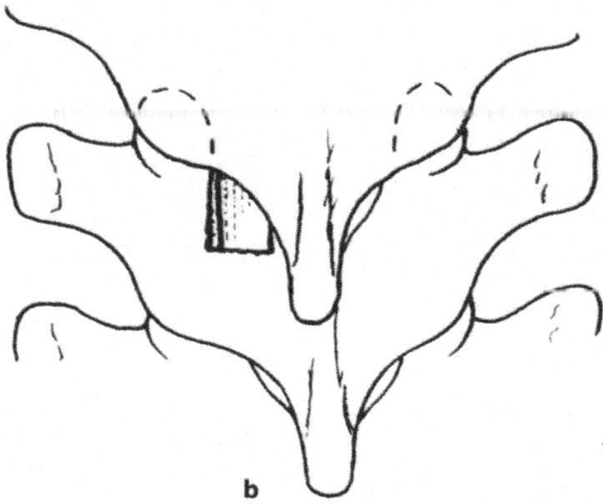
b

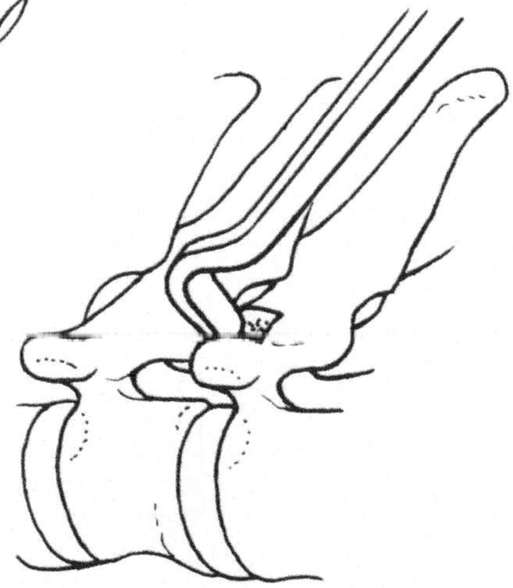
c

Fig. 8.26
a For laminar hook positioning, a small portion of the lamina is removed
b Prepared cranial position of the lamina, ready to seat a hook
c Lamina feeler is put carefully around the lamina

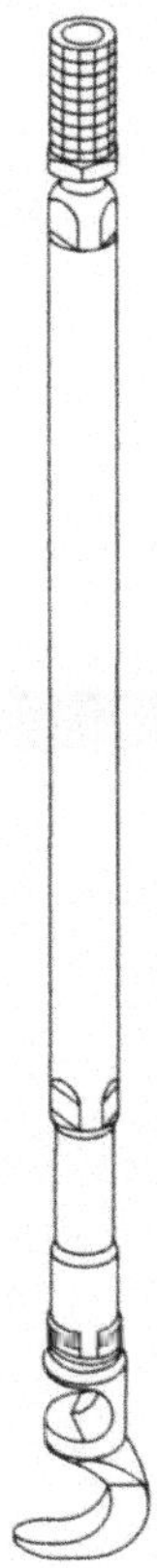
a

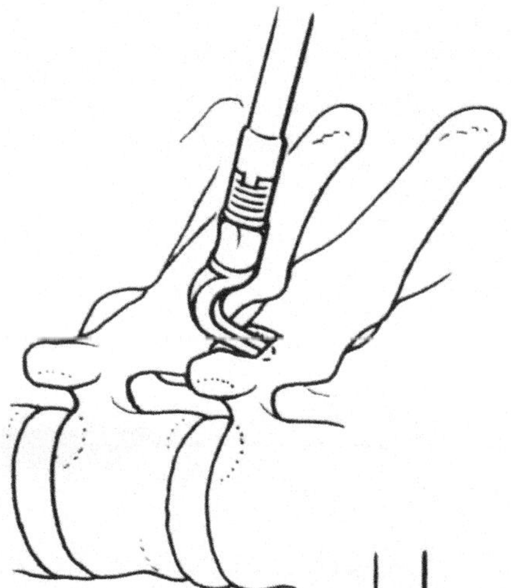
b

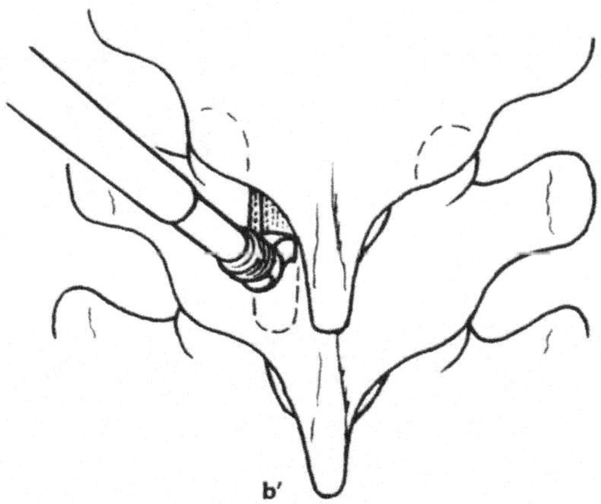
b′

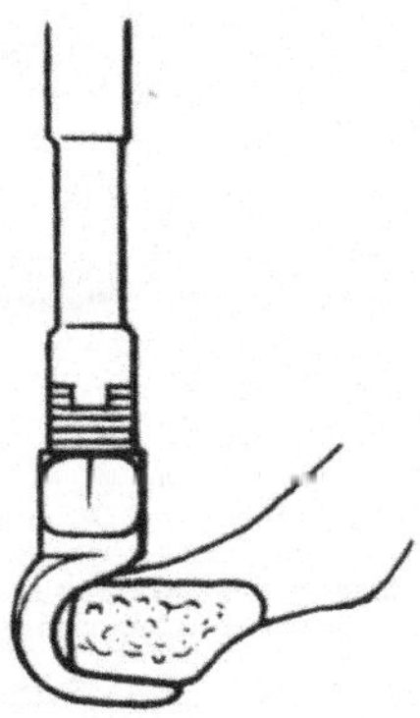
c

Fig. 8.27 The hook is controlled with the USS hook holder
a Attachment of the hook to the hook holder (extension stick)
b, b′ Lamina hook gently eased into place around the lamina
c The inferior part of the hook must fit close to the lamina

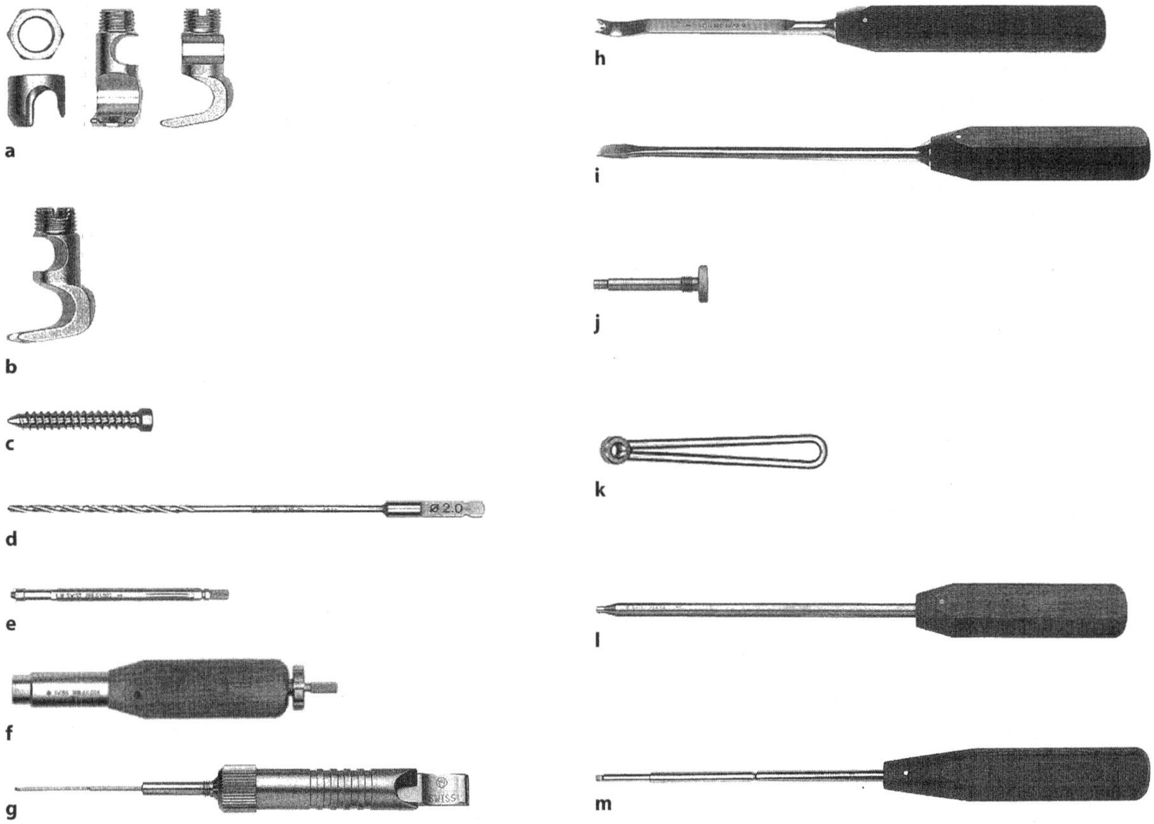

Fig. 8.28 Specialized pedicle hook
a USS pedicle hook, side-opening
b USS pedicle hook, front opening
c USS screws for USS pedicle hooks, 3.2 mm diameter
d 3-flute drill bit for quick coupling, 2.0 mm diameter
e USS hook and screw holder
f USS universal handle
g Depth gauge
h USS pedicle feeler
i USS chisel 9 mm
j USS drill guide 2.0
k Handle for drill guide
l USS hook positioner
m Screwdriver, hexagonal, small, self-holding

various hooks are attached to the 6-mm rod using the same technique as the screw.

8.2.1.4.3
USS Hooks: Specialized Pedicle Hook

Instruments and Implants (Fig. 8.28)

Technique
The special pedicle hook is attached to the screw holder and universal handle.

Bone Preparation
The level in the thoracic spine for the insertion of the specialized pedicle hook is identified. The pedicle feeler is placed between the inferior and superior facet joints. The feeler must go into the articular joint and not into bone of the inferior facet (Fig. 8.29). To facilitate insertion of the pedicle feeler, a small portion of the inferior facet may be removed with an osteotome – *aim the osteotome laterally* (Fig. 8.30a–c). Ensure the pedicle feeler is around the pedicle by exertion axial loading and also ease the feeler laterally – *N.B. Do not push medially* (Fig. 8.31). Once the feeler is around the pedicle, it may be necessary to remove further bone from the inferior facet to allow the pedicle hook to sit around the pedicle. The pedicle feeler has six lines on the blade; when the last line is reached, sufficient bone has been removed to accommodate the hook around the pedicle (Fig. 8.30c).

Insertion
The specialized pedicle hook with extension stick and introducing handle are now inserted into the prepared site. The hook positioner is placed into the small hole in the back of the pedicle (Fig. 8.32a, b). The hook is now eased around the inferior aspect of

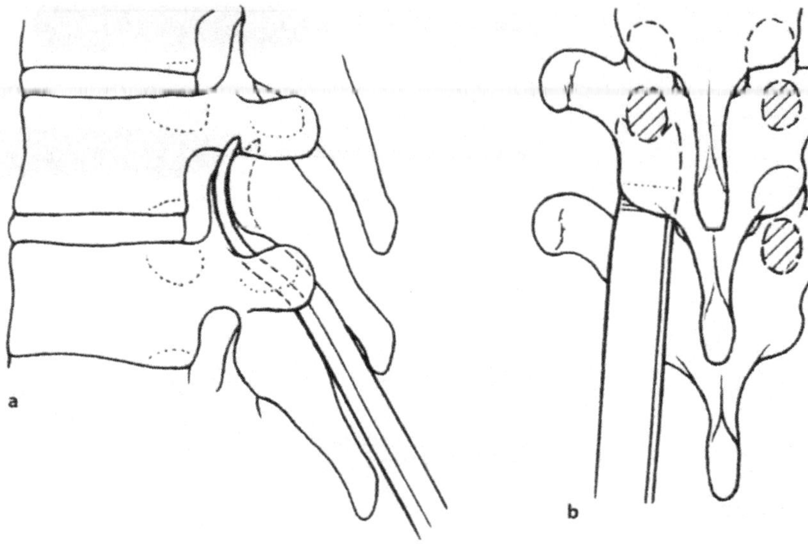

Fig. 8.29 Pedicle feeler inserted around pedicle
a Lateral view
b Frontal view

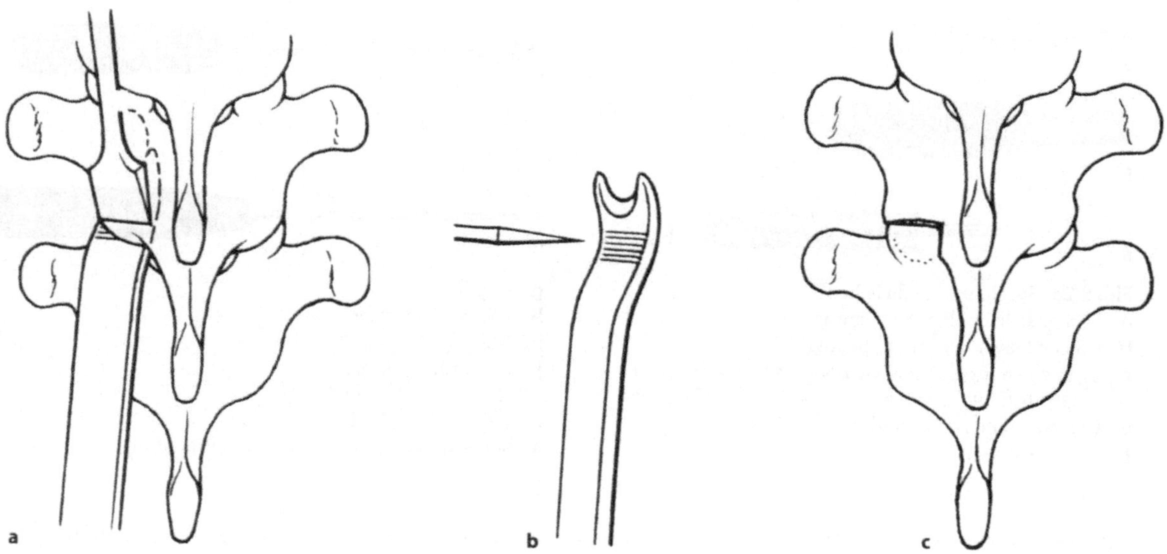

Fig. 8.30 Removal of bone from the inferior facet until the sixth line on the pedicle feeler is exposed
a Osteotomy
b Pedicle feeler with marker
c Osteotomy executed

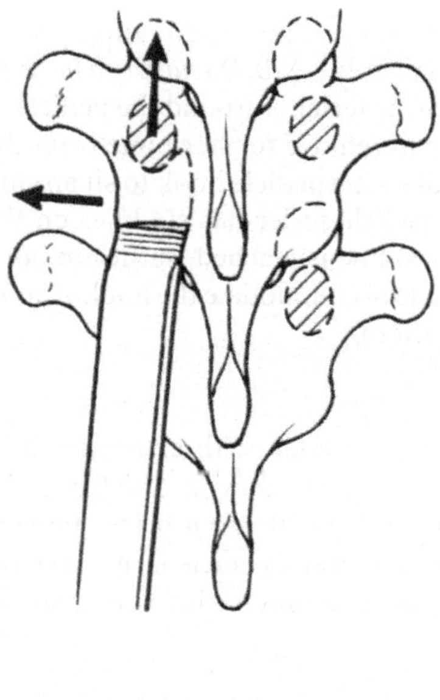

Fig. 8.31 Ensure the pedicle feeler is in the correct position by axial loading and lateral motion

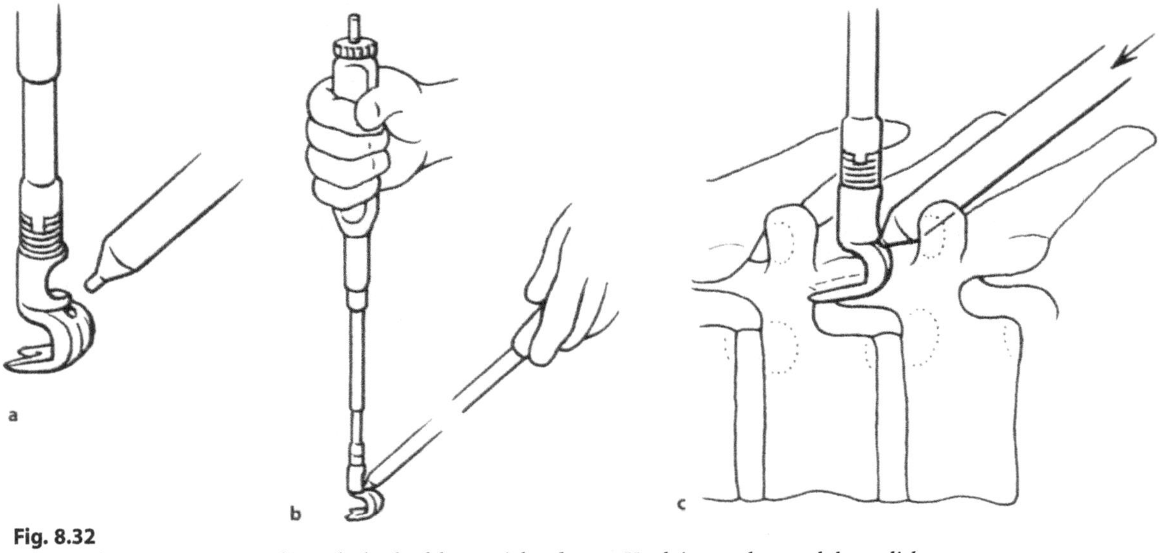

Fig. 8.32
a, b Hook positioner inserted into the back of the special pedicle hook **c** Hook inserted around the pedicle

the pedicle (Fig. 8.32c). Once in place, check if it is snug around the pedicle by axial loading of the hook positioner and also by pushing laterally. If it does not move, then the pedicle hook is around the pedicle. The hook positioner is gently tapped with a hammer to site the hook. The pedicle hook drill-guide is inserted into the hole in the back of the pedicle hook (Fig. 8.33a). A three-fluted 2.0-mm drill is placed into the drill-guide and, using the oscillating drill, the tip is advanced until it passes through the end plate (Fig. 8.33b). *Do not start the power drill if the drill does not hit bone after passing through the drill-guide.* The drill-guide is removed and the depth to the end plate is measured with the small-fragment AO depth gauge (this is approximately 25–30 mm) (Fig. 8.33c). The self-cutting 3.2-mm cortical screw is inserted (Fig. 8.33d). The specialized pedicle hook is now firmly fixed to the pedicle and end plate.

8.2.1.4.4
USS Hooks: Transverse Process Hook

Instruments and Implants (see Fig. 8.34)
The chosen transverse process is cleared of soft tissue. The lamina feeler is placed around the transverse process elevating the soft tissue attachments from the anterior portion of the transverse process (Fig. 8.35a). An appropriate-size lamina hook is mounted onto an extension stick with handle, as the hook is eased around the transverse process using the hook positioner (Fig. 8.35b).

8.2.1.4.5
USS Rod Introduction into Side-Opening Implants

Instrument (Fig. 8.36)

Technique
The 6-mm rod can be eased, if necessary, onto the side-opening implants with the rod-crimping pliers (Fig. 8.37). The sleeve and rod are then released and dropped over the construct (Fig. 8.38). The screw/hook side-openings are offset by 4 mm when the implants are aligned. If the implants are not in perfect alignment, rotating the screw by 90° or changing the hook will allow the rod to be more easily inserted (Fig. 8.39).

8.2.1.4.6
Complex Reduction Forceps – the 'Persuader' (Fig. 8.40)

Principle
At times, it is not possible to ease the hook screw into the rod as a result of the distance between the rod and anchorage. The anchorage can be lifted and translated to the rod with the complex reduction forceps (CRF) – the 'persuader' (Fig. 8.40).

Technique
The sleeve is placed onto the cylinder of the persuader so that the short leg of the sleeve faces in the direction of the 6-mm bar (Fig. 8.41a). The sleeve clips onto the top of the cylinder (Fig. 8.41b). The cylinder of the persuader is slid over the extension

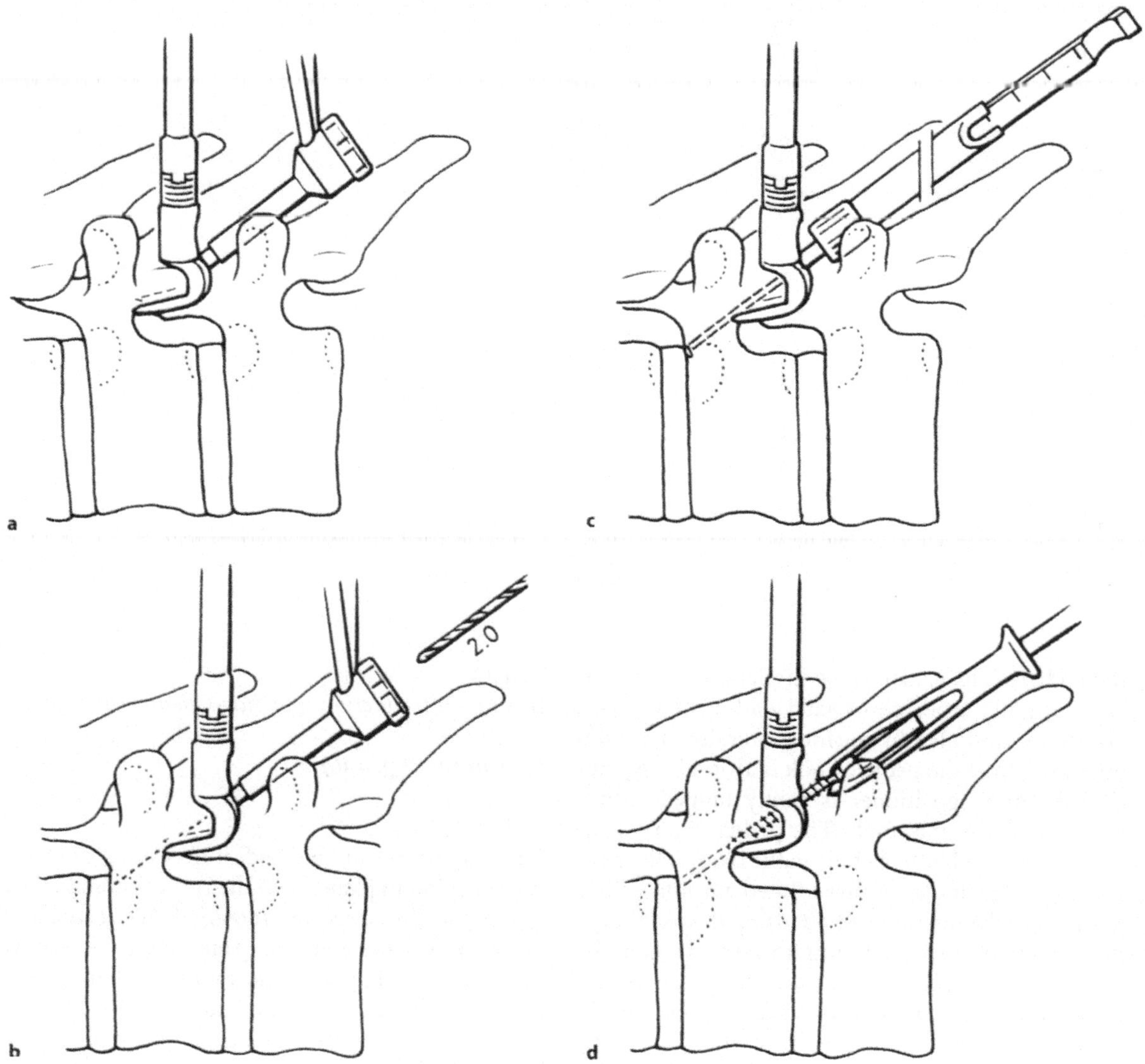

Fig. 8.33
a Pedicle hook drill-guide is inserted into the hole at the back of the pedicle hook
b Fluted 2.0 mm drill is drilled through the pedicle to the end plate
c Measurement of depth with a small-fragment depth gauge
d The 3.2-mm self-tapping cortical screw is inserted

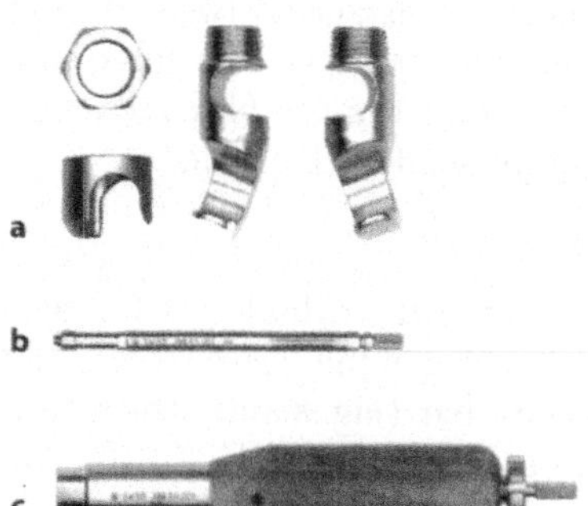

Fig. 8.34
a USS lamina hook, angled, side-opening
b USS hook and screw holder
c USS universal handle

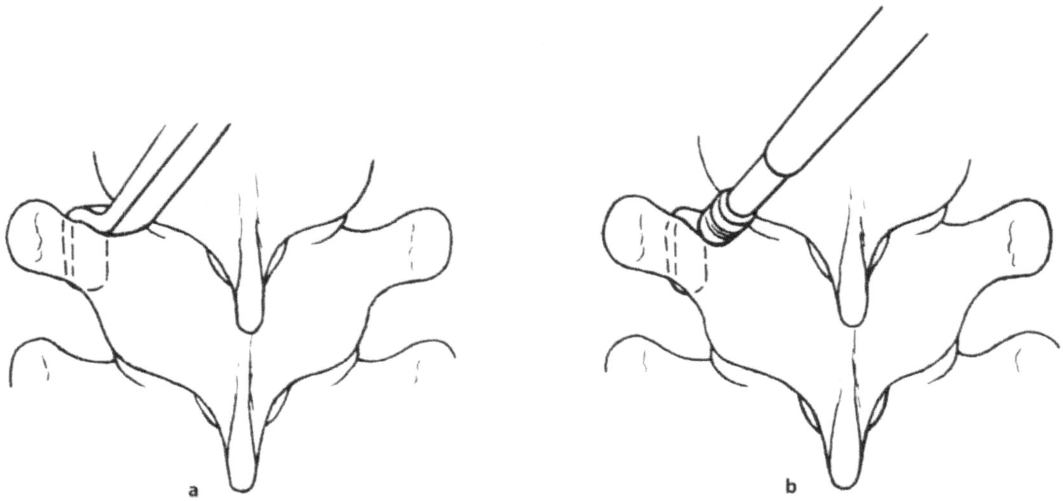

Fig. 8.35
a Laminar feeler placed around the transverse process **b** Hook placed around the transverse process

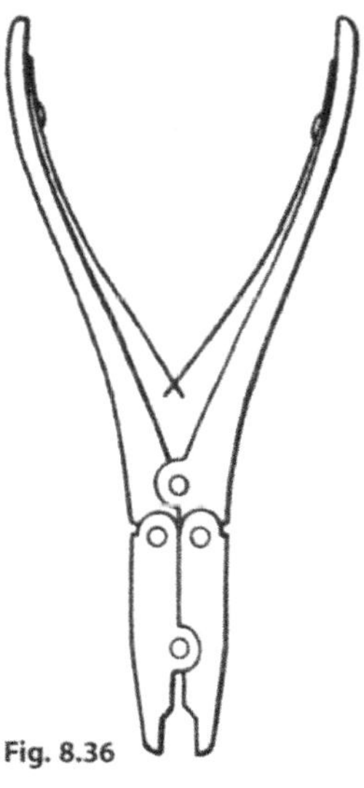

Fig. 8.36

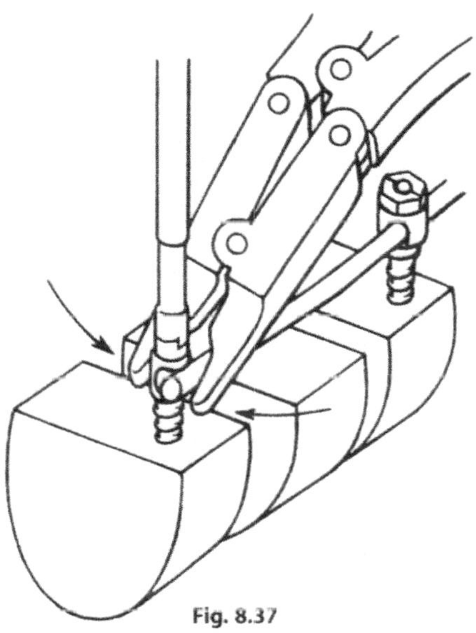

Fig. 8.37

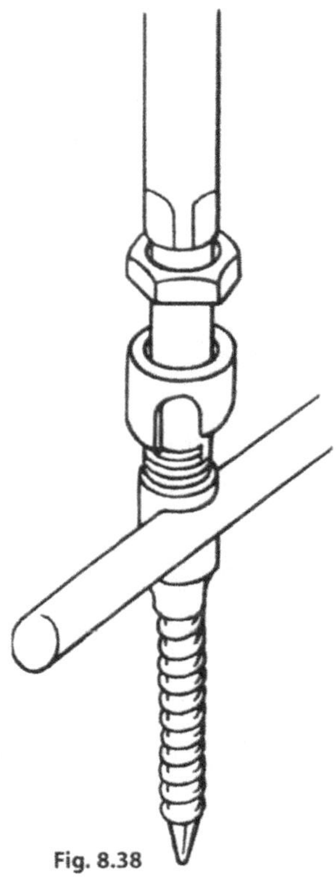

Fig. 8.38

Fig. 8.36 Instrument: the USS rod-crimping pliers

Fig. 8.37 Insertion of 6-mm rod into the side-opening implant with the rod-crimping pliers

Fig. 8.38 Release of sleeve and nut onto rod/anchorage

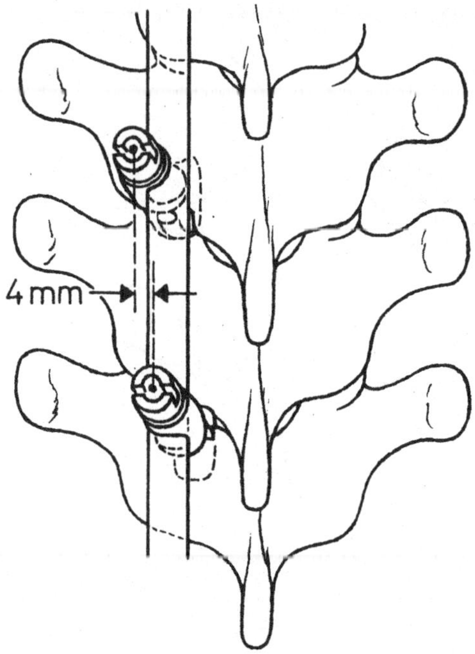

Fig. 8.39 The hook/screw offset

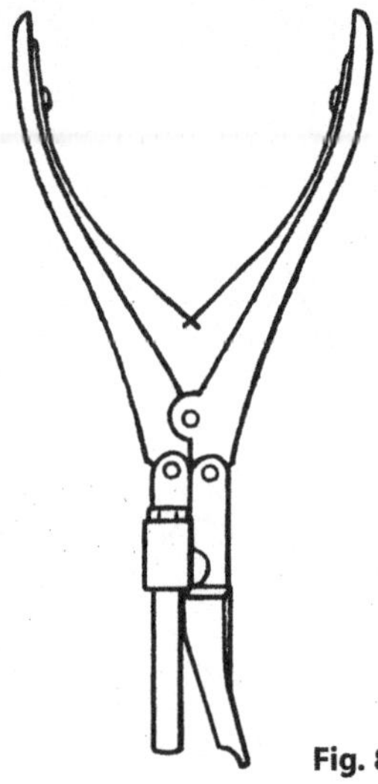

Fig. 8.40 USS complex reduction forcep

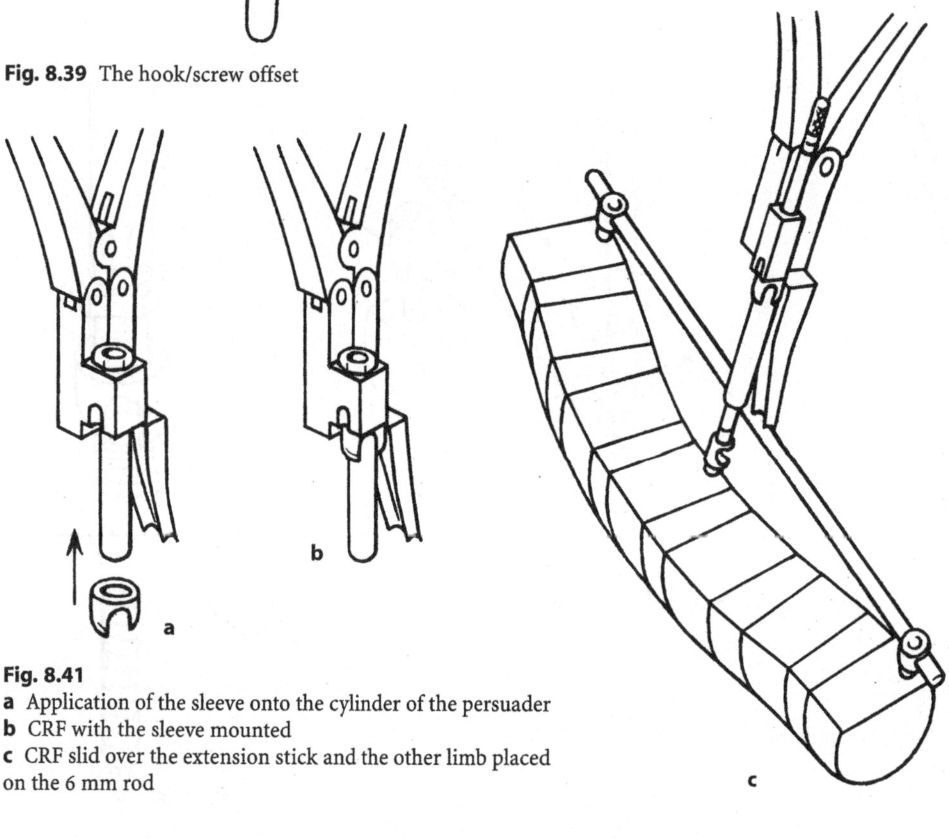

Fig. 8.41
a Application of the sleeve onto the cylinder of the persuader
b CRF with the sleeve mounted
c CRF slid over the extension stick and the other limb placed on the 6 mm rod

stick of the screw/hook, and the limb of the forceps is placed on the bar (Fig. 8.41c). The 6-mm rod holder or extension stick clamp is placed on the protruding extension stick (Fig. 8.42a, b). Controlling the rod holder or extension stick clamp will prevent rotation of the hook or screw.

The forceps are now gently closed bringing the anchorage towards the rod (Fig. 8.43a); *do not completely close the forceps. Beware. This is a most powerful instrument.* Controlling the forceps and ensuring the limb of the forceps remains on the rod, a spreader is placed between the clamp and the cylinder. The spreader is slowly opened bringing the hook upwards towards the rod (Fig. 8.43b); when the side-opening is opposite the rod, the persuader is closed allowing the anchorage to engage onto the rod (Fig. 8.43c). The sleeve is pushed down the cylinder and placed over the rod and anchorage. If the sleeve will not ease onto the anchorage, place the rod pusher onto the sleeve and gently tap the sleeve into place (Fig. 8.43d). The 6-mm rod holder or clamp is removed, the persuader is removed and a nut dropped over the extension stick and loosely attached to the hook or screw (Fig. 8.43e).

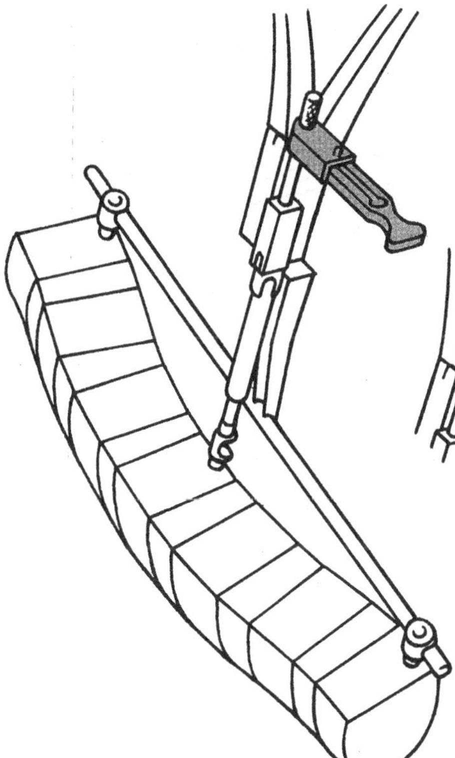

a

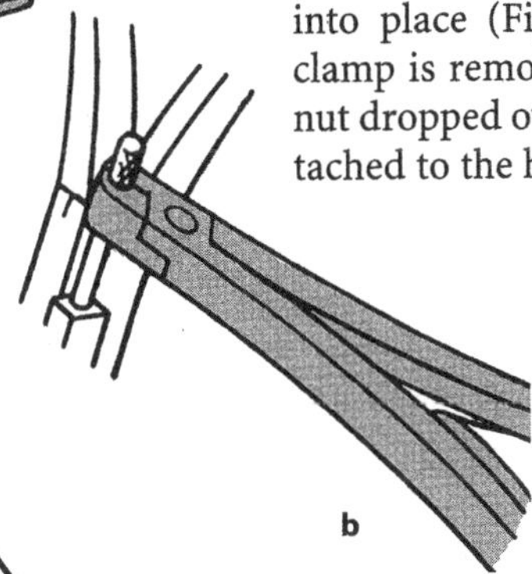

b

Fig. 8.42
a A special clamp for the top of the screw holder (extension stick)
b 6-mm rod holder attached to screw holder (alternative)

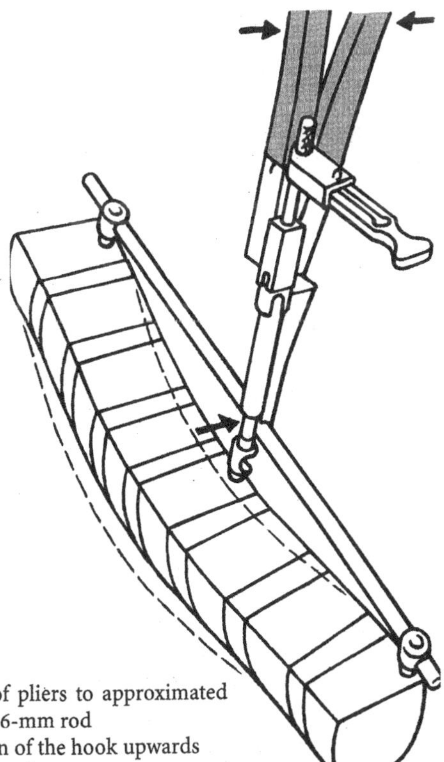

a

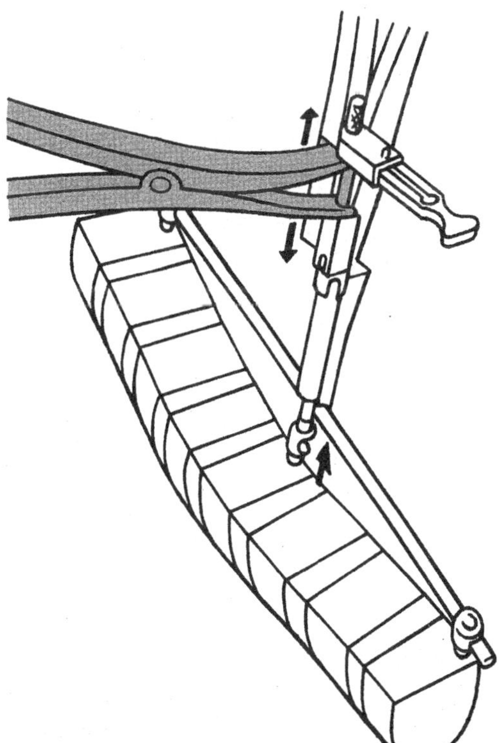

b

Fig. 8.43
a Closure of pliers to approximated hook to the 6-mm rod
b Reduction of the hook upwards towards the rod

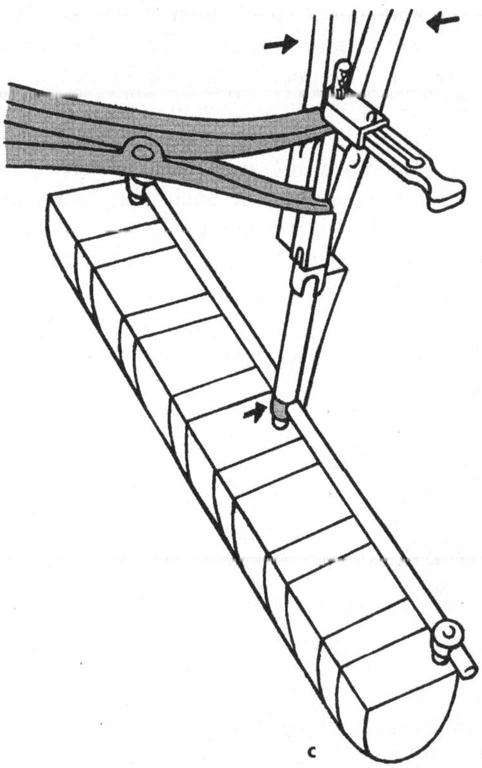

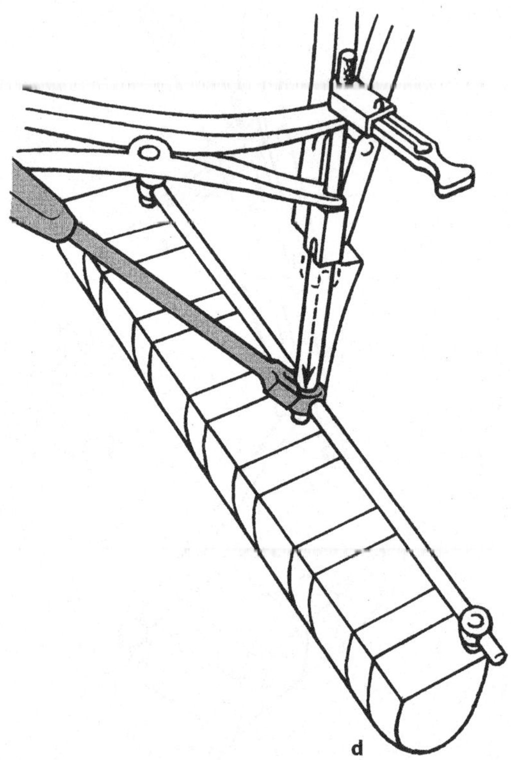

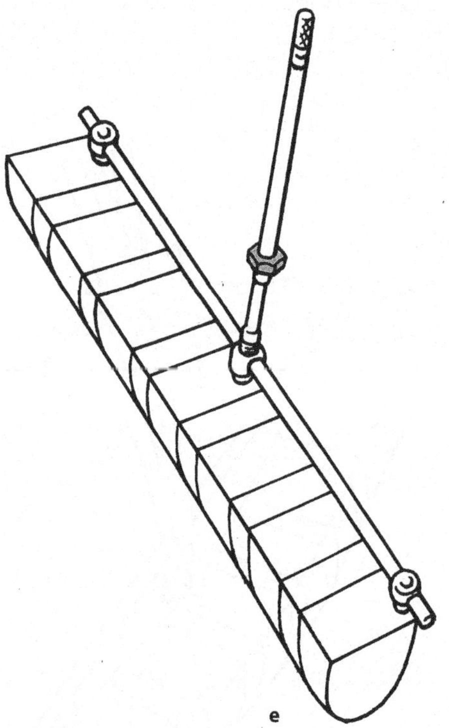

(Fig. 8.43)
c Closure of pliers to attach side-opening implant to the rod
d Rod pusher used to tap sleeve into place if slightly tight (ensure sleeve legs are correctly positioned)
e Nut dropped on stick and attached to hook/screw

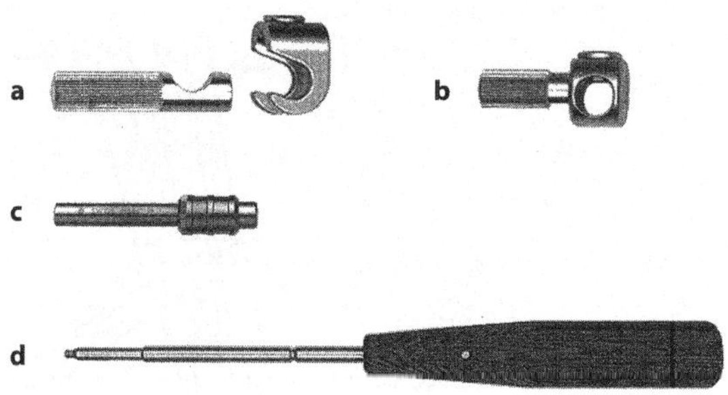

Fig. 8.44 Instruments and implants
a USS rod connector, open
b USS rod connector, closed
c USS holding sleeve
d Screwdriver, hexagonal, small

8.2.1.4.7
Rod Connectors

Implants and Instruments (Fig. 8.44)

Principle
There are times when the anchorage will not reach the rod. Experience will dictate whether the persuader will bring the anchorage to the rod. *If too much force is exerted on the anchorage, it will tear out of the bone.* When the anchorage does not reach

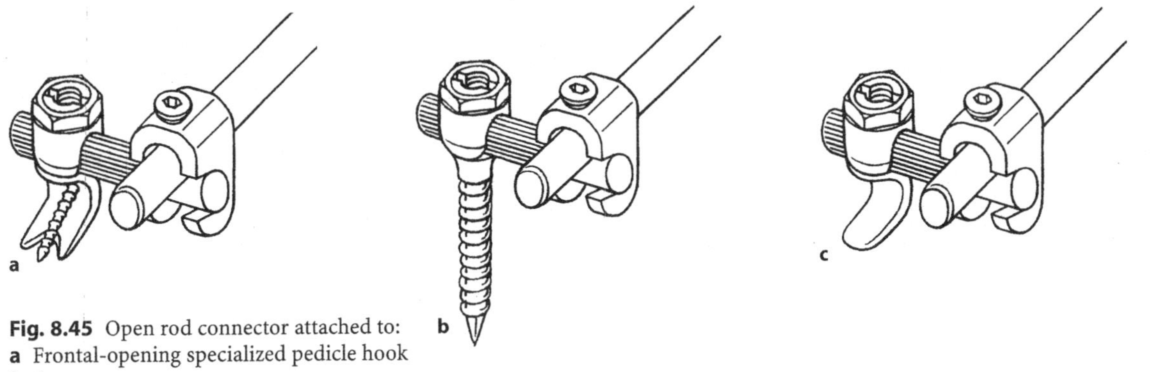

Fig. 8.45 Open rod connector attached to:
a Frontal-opening specialized pedicle hook
b Screw
c Lamina hook

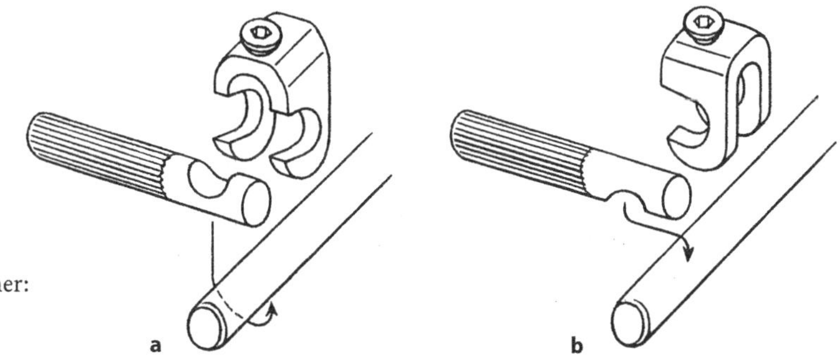

Fig. 8.46 Open rod connector placed either:
a Beneath or
b On top of the 6-mm rod

the rod, then it is necessary to use the rod connectors. When using the rod connector, the *frontal opening hooks* must be used or the screw turned 90° to become the front opening. The rod connector fits into the hook or screw at a right angle (Fig. 8.45a–c).

Technique
The appropriate-length rod connector is placed either beneath or on top of the 6-mm rod (Fig. 8.46a, b). The position of the rod and anchorage dictate this position. The small hexagonal screwdriver and holding sleeve is placed onto the connector clamp (Fig. 8.47a). *Ensure the screw is not protruding inside the connector clamp.* The connector clamp is clipped onto the bar and rod connector and tightened (Fig. 8.47b). The rod connector is now placed into the front open hook or screw; the sleeve and nut are dropped onto the anchorage (Fig. 8.47c). The anchorage can be approximated to the rod with the compression forceps (Fig. 8.48). The nut is finally tightened on the hook, with the L-handed socket wrench. The hook/screw rotation is controlled with the small 6-mm socket wrench. At this stage, the vertebra can be rotated by loosening the screw on the open rod connector; the extension stick on the anchorage is tilted to derotate the vertebra and, finally, the screw on the open rod connector is tightened (Fig. 8.49). At either end of the construct, a closed rod connector can be used – it has a lower profile (Fig. 8.50a, b).

8.2.1.4.8
USS Cross-link System

There are two cross-links: a standard cross-link and a specialized cross-link, which are only used if there is insufficient space between the implants to allow application of the standard cross-link.

Instruments and Implants (Fig. 8.51)

Standard Cross-link
The cross-link system connects the two 6-mm rods, and the use of the cross-link significantly increases the stiffness of the construction. For fracture construct, it is *absolutely essential* if there is rotational instability. To increase the stiffness, the clamps can be compressed toward each other. *N.B. The sleeve for the cross-link system is different from the standard sleeve.* The sleeve has a section cut away at the top on each side. This allows the rod to be angled up to 20° in each direction (Fig. 8.52).

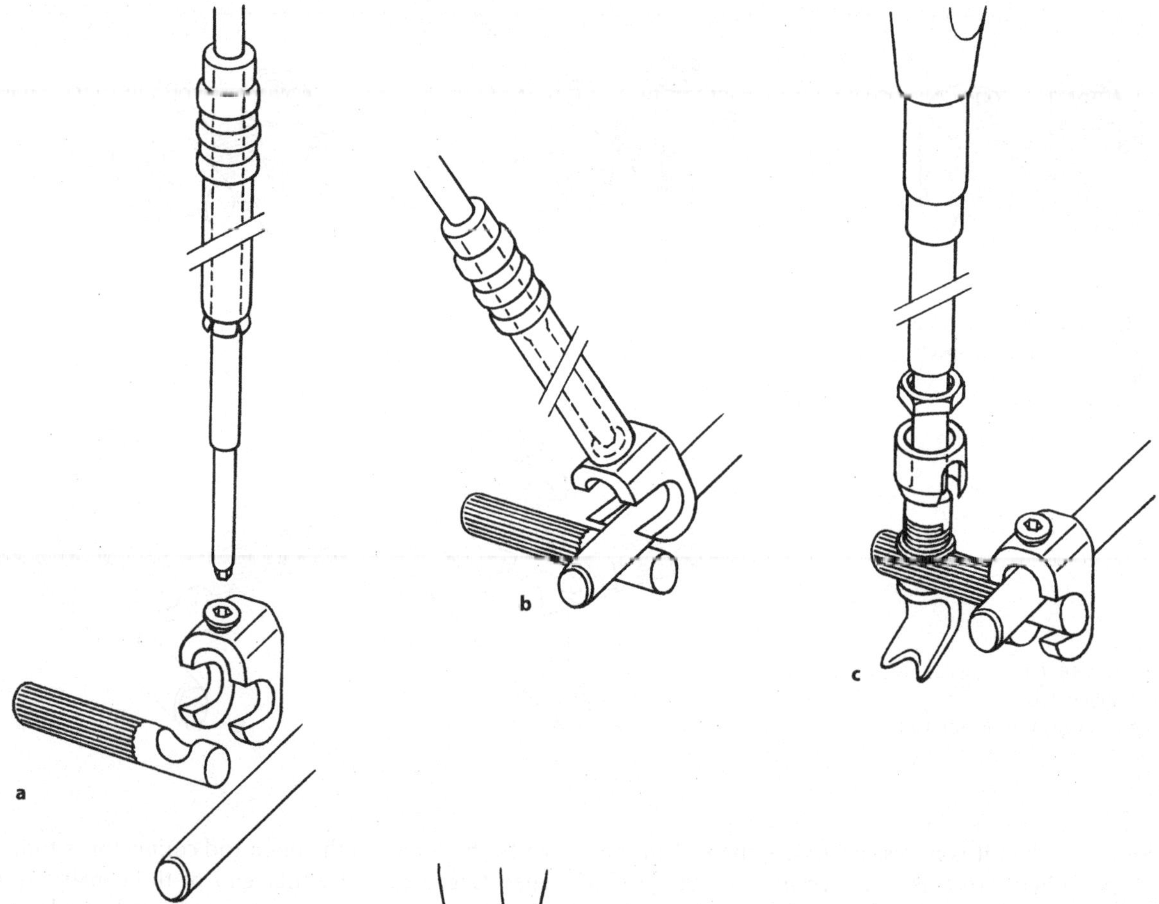

Fig. 8.47
a Small hexagonal screwdriver and holding sleeve being connected to the connector clamp (N.B. ensure thread is not protruding inside clamp)
b Connection clamp is clipped onto the bar and rod connector and tightened
c Rod connector attached to the frontal-opening pedicle hook/screw and the nut dropped onto the anchorage

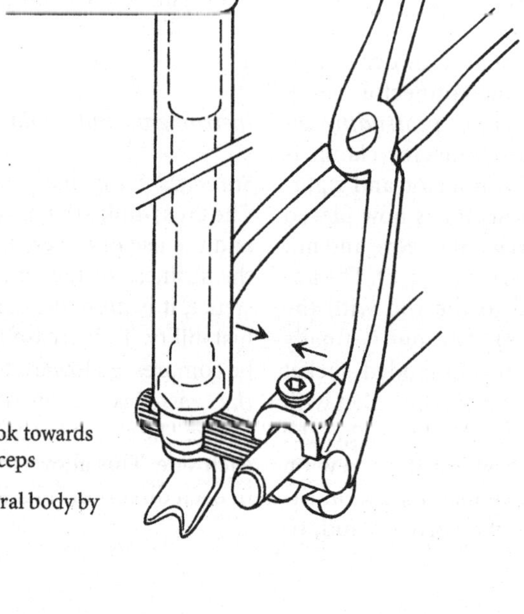

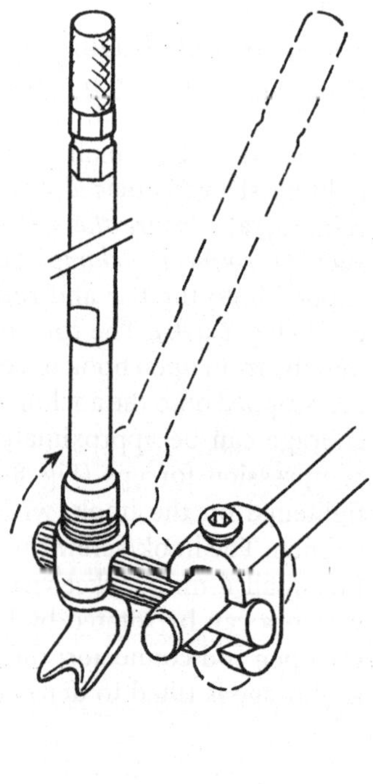

Fig. 8.48 Approximation of hook towards the clamp with compression forceps

Fig. 8.49 Rotation of the vertebral body by manipulating the hook

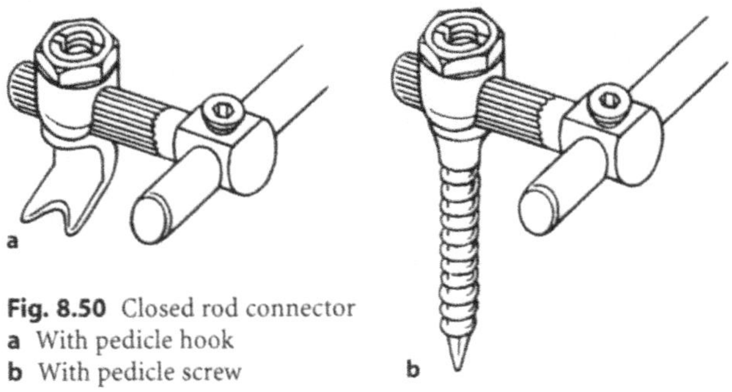

Fig. 8.50 Closed rod connector
a With pedicle hook
b With pedicle screw

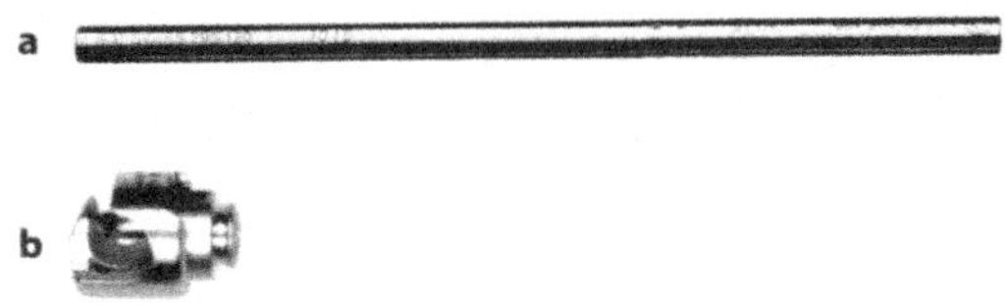

Fig. 8.51 Implants and instruments
a USS rod 3.5 mm diameter
b USS cross-link clamp

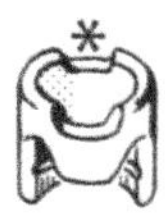

Fig. 8.52 Cross-link sleeve with a section cut away* allowing a range of angulation of the cross-link rod (see Fig. 8.6)

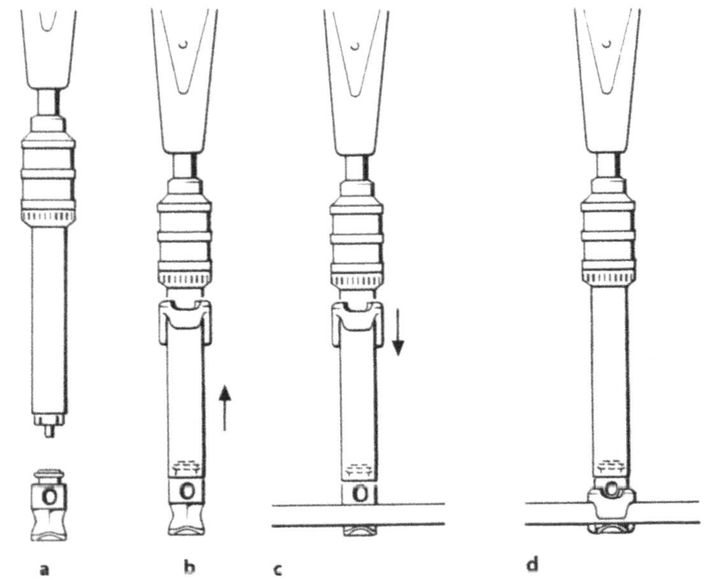

Fig. 8.53a Small hexagonal screwdriver with groove with the holding sleeve being attached to the clamp
b The special cross-link sleeve is attached to the cylinder of the holding sleeve
c The clamp is attached to the 6-mm rod
d The sleeve is dropped into place

Technique. The small hexagonal screwdriver with groove and with the holding sleeve is connected to the USS cross-link clamp (Fig. 8.52). The special cross-link sleeve (Fig. 8.53b) is now placed upon the cylinder of the holding sleeve (Fig. 8.53b). The clamp is placed on the 6-mm rod (Fig. 8.53c), the sleeve is dropped into place (Fig. 8.53d) and the 3.5-mm rod can be inserted into the clamp (Fig. 8.54). The nut is then tightened after removal of the holding sleeve.

Assembly of Cross-linkage to Two Parallel 6-mm Rods. The first clamp and sleeve is applied to the 6-mm rod. The 3.5-mm rod is then held with the 3.5-mm rod holder and threaded through the first clamp (Fig. 8.54). The second clamp and sleeve are attached to the second 6-mm rod and then the 3.5-mm rod is pushed through the clamp (Fig. 8.56). When the rod is applied 0.5 cm beyond the clamp, the hexagonal nut is tightened (Fig. 8.57). The 3.5-mm rod holder is reattached to the center of the bar and, using the USS spreader, the clamp and rod are distracted and the clamp tightened (Fig. 8.58). The rod is cut (Fig. 8.59) and the final position of the cross-link is noted (Fig. 8.60).

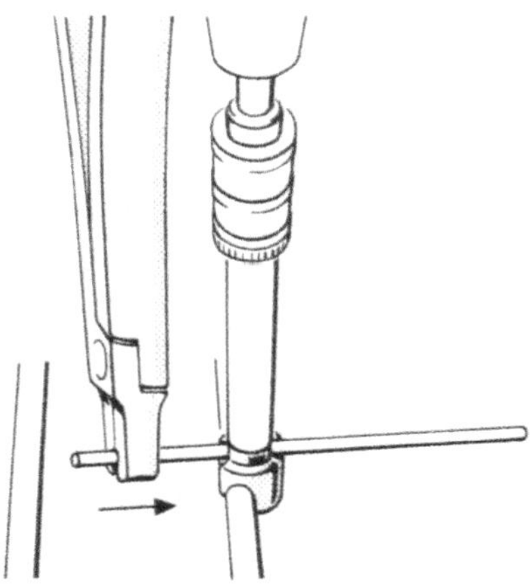

Fig. 8.54 Insertion of 3.5-mm cross-link rod onto the clamp.

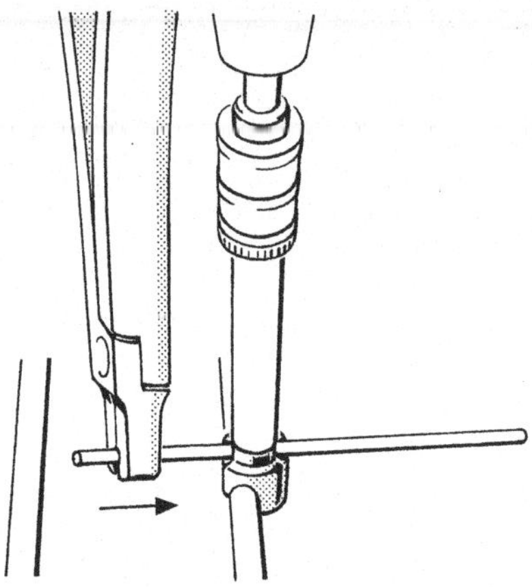

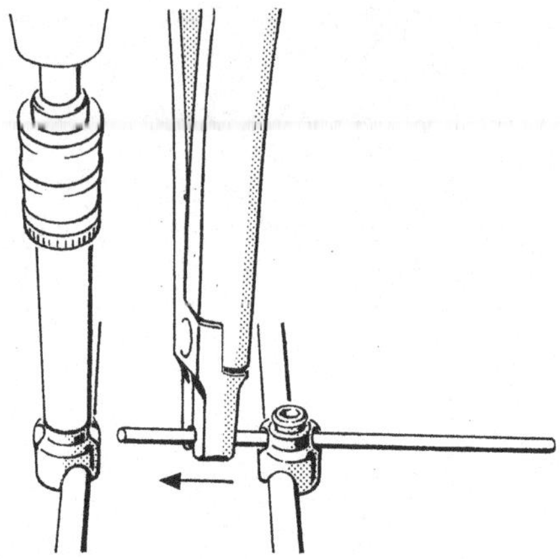

Fig. 8.55 The clamp applied and the 3.5-mm cross-link rod connected with the aid of the 3.5-mm rod holder

Fig. 8.56 The second clamp and sleeve is applied to the 6-mm rod and the 3.5-mm cross-link rod is pushed through

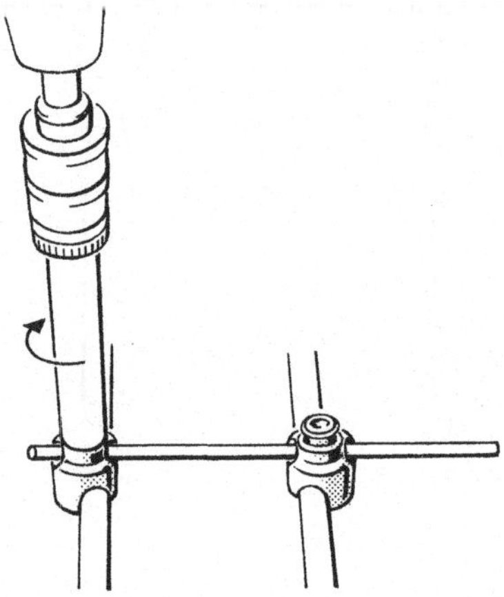

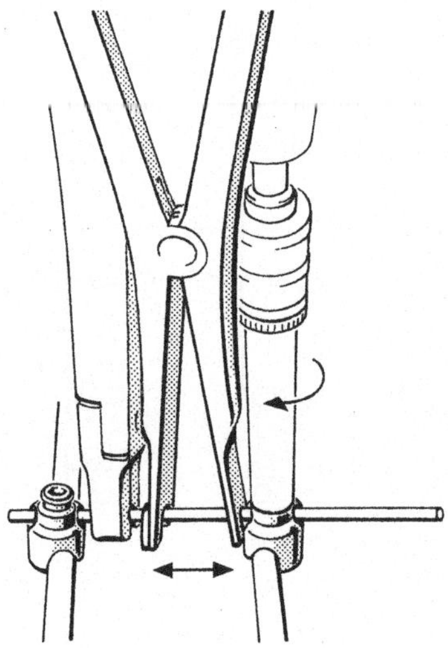

Fig. 8.57 Connecting rod pushed 0.5 cm beyond clamp and hexagonal nut tightened

Fig. 8.58 3.5-mm rod holder reattached near to a clamp and the USS distractor used to apply distraction. The nut is tightened

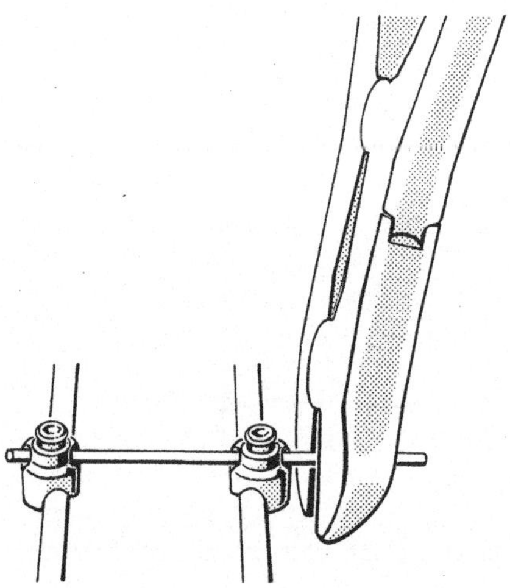

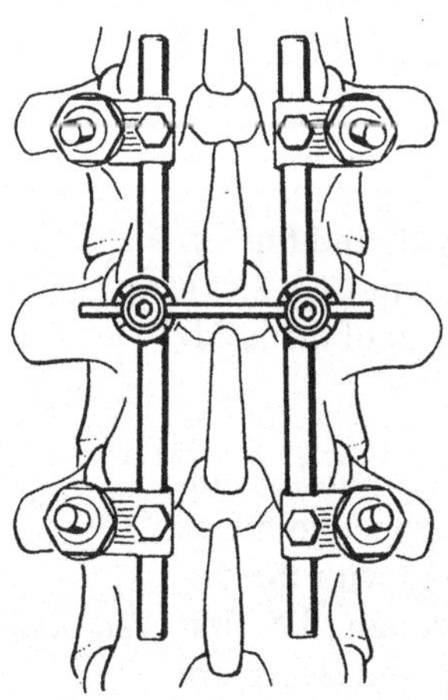

Fig. 8.59 Cutting the rod

Fig. 8.60 Final position of the cross-link system

Cross-link with Wire

If there is no space for either cross-link to be attached to the 6-mm rod, then a wiring technique can be applied. Security screws are placed into the posterior aspect of the screws already attached to the 6-mm rod. A figure-of-eight wire is attached to diagonally opposite screws. The AO wire tightener is used to tighten the wire and, after cutting the excess wire, the security screws are tightened.

8.2.2 USS for Deformity

The design of the USS allows new concepts to be used in the correction of scoliosis. *No distraction or compression* is used in the reduction of the deformity; the spine passively finds its own length. The USS instrumentation includes:

- The apical vertebrae, via hooks or pedicle screws anchored to the vertebrae.
- The spine is reduced to the rods by segmental manipulation.
- Emphasis is placed particularly on the application of the convex rod, which allows translation of the apex towards the mid-line.
- The concave implants are finally attached to the rod, the attachment of the implants to the vertebral body allowing derotation of individual vertebra.

8.2.2.1 Basic Principles

- Soft tissue release (posterior ± anterior)
- Anchorage of implants to individual vertebra including the apex
- Contour of rod in correct sagittal plane
- Reduction of spine to the 6-mm rod
- Derotation of individual vertebra, (translative and pulling posteriorly)
- End vertebrae are used to build the construct
- Cross-linkage of rods
- No distraction or compression

8.2.2.1.1 Basic Principle of Construct

The cranial and caudal neutral vertebrae are used as cornerstones of a virtual frame which are instrumented (Fig. 8.61a). The end vertebrae are instrumented using the caudal end vertebrae as a base on which to build the construct. Pedicle screws are inserted (Fig. 8.61b, c). The cranial end is instrumented with the specialized pedicle hook into the upper end on the concave side (Fig. 8.61b, c) and a claw construct with laminar hook and specialized pedicle hook one vertebra below on the convex side (see Fig. 8.65). The upper convex hook must be a laminar hook and *not a transverse process hook*; otherwise when the convex rod is used to translate the spine to the mid-line it will pull off the transverse process.

Figs. 8.61–8.74 Principles of reduction in scoliosis

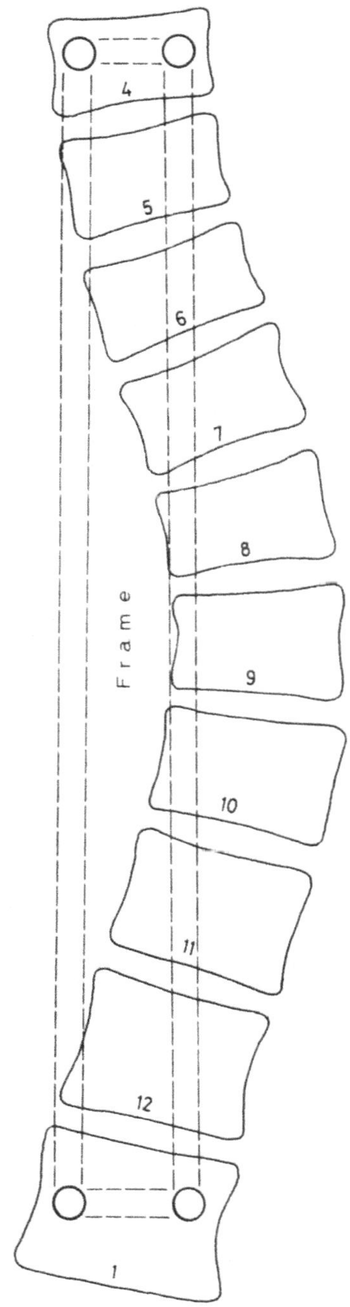

Fig. 8.61
a The scoliosis frame

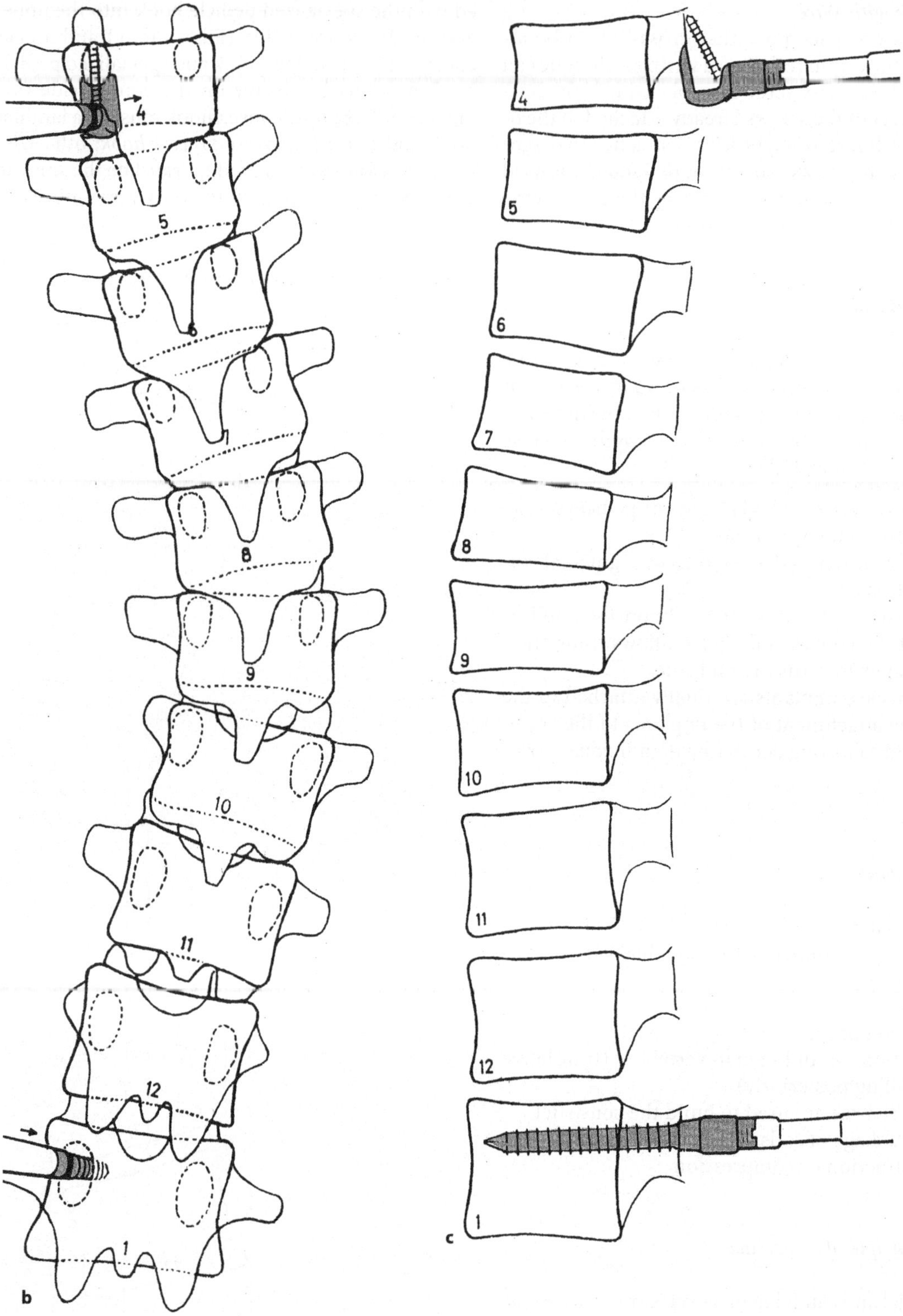

(Fig. 8.61)
b,c Cranial and caudal neutral vertebrae are instrumented
b Frontal view
c Sagittal view

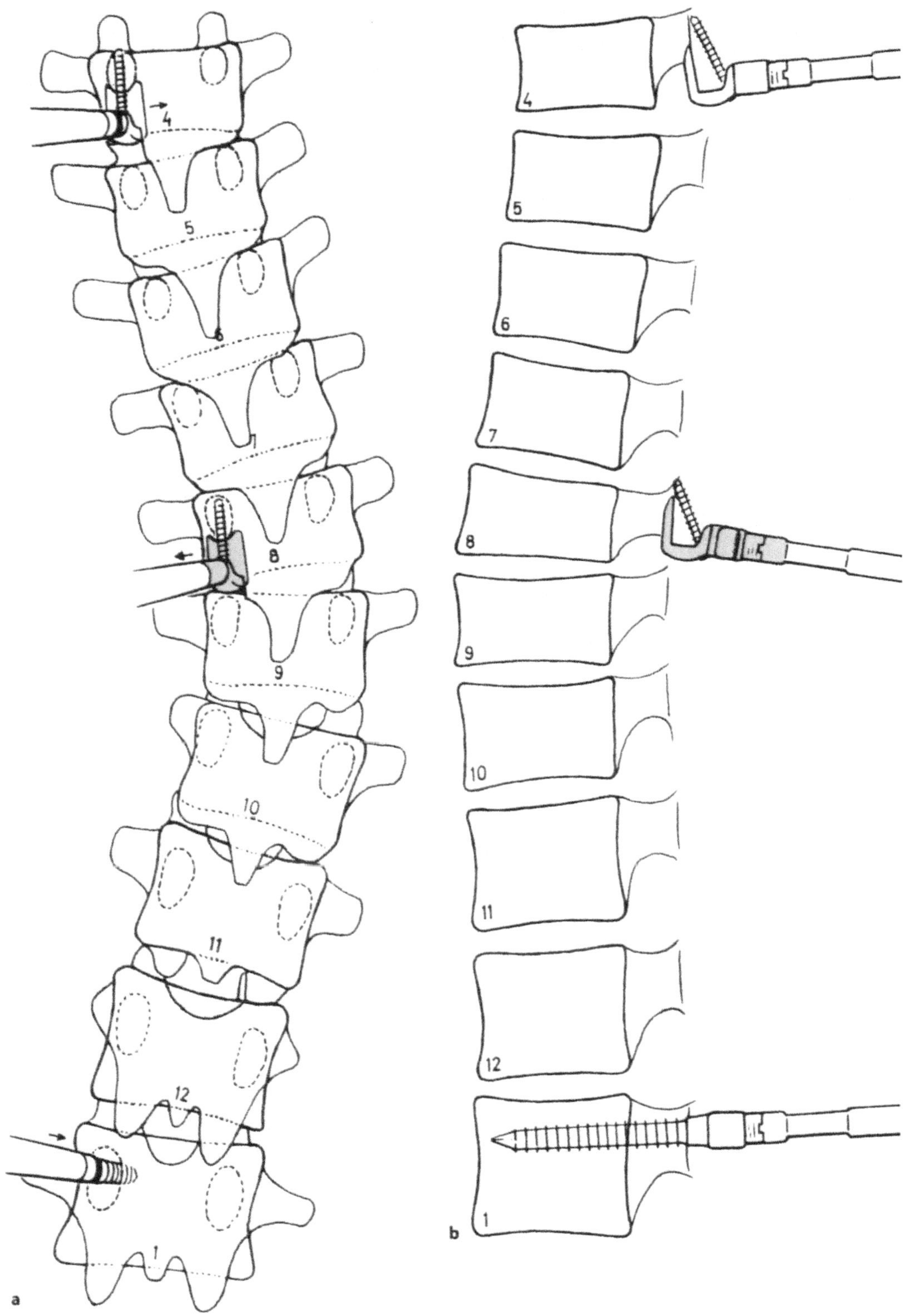

Fig. 8.62 Apex is instrumented
a Frontal view
b Lateral view

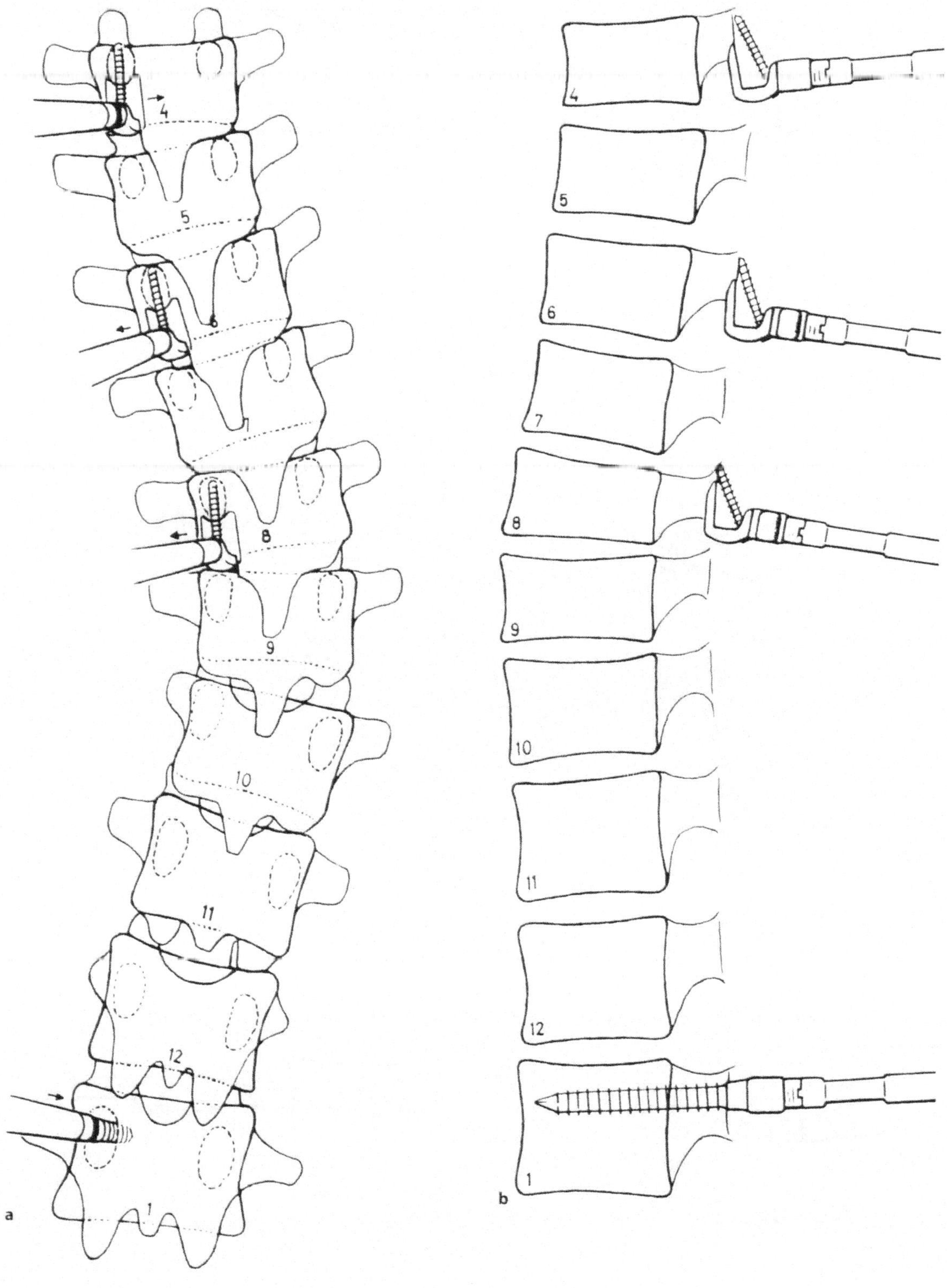

Fig. 8.63 The concave hook construct hooks/screws to alternative vertebrae between apex and end vertebrae

a Frontal view
b Lateral view

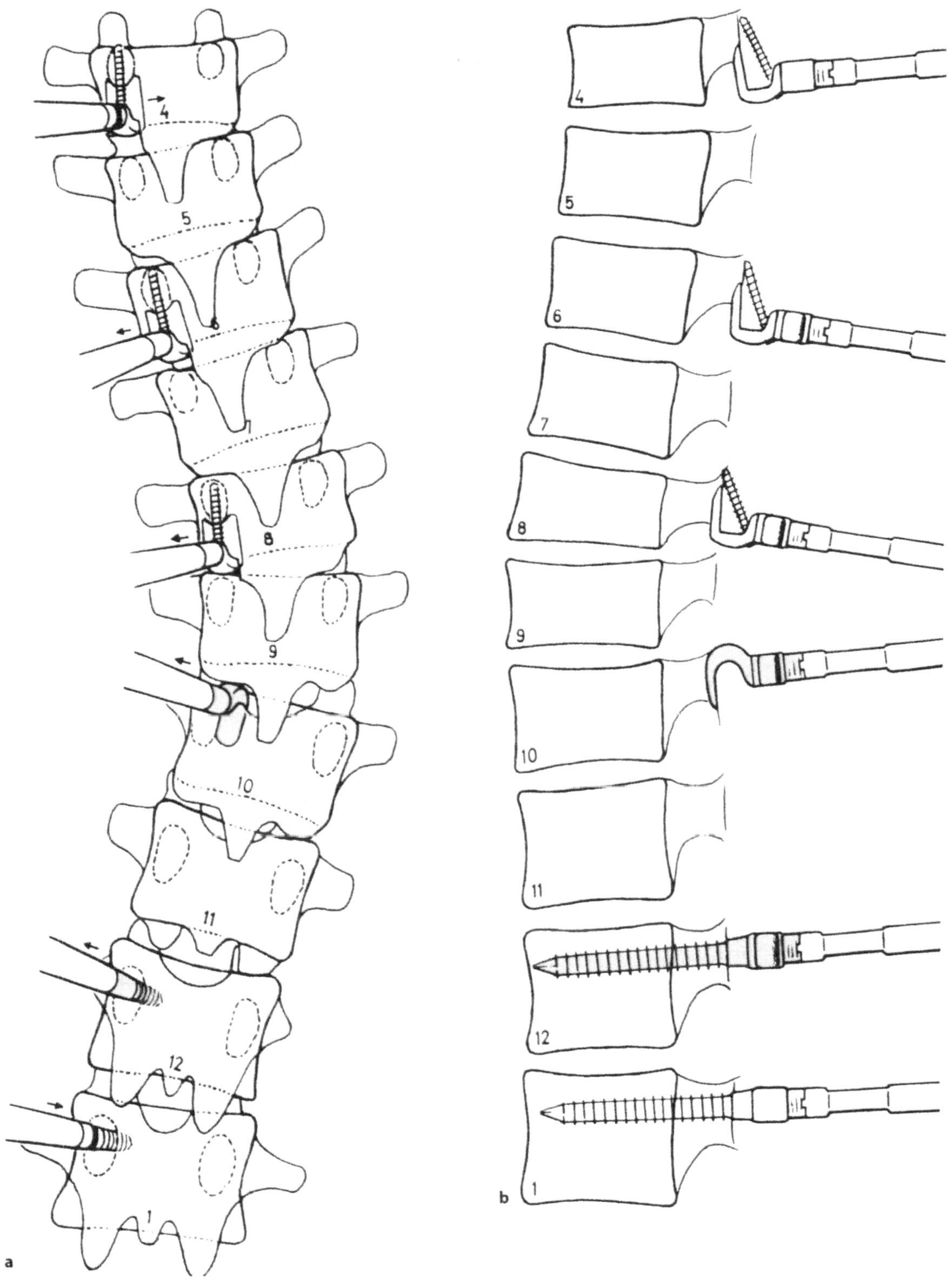

Fig. 8.64 Insertion of laminar hook at T10
a Frontal view
b Lateral view

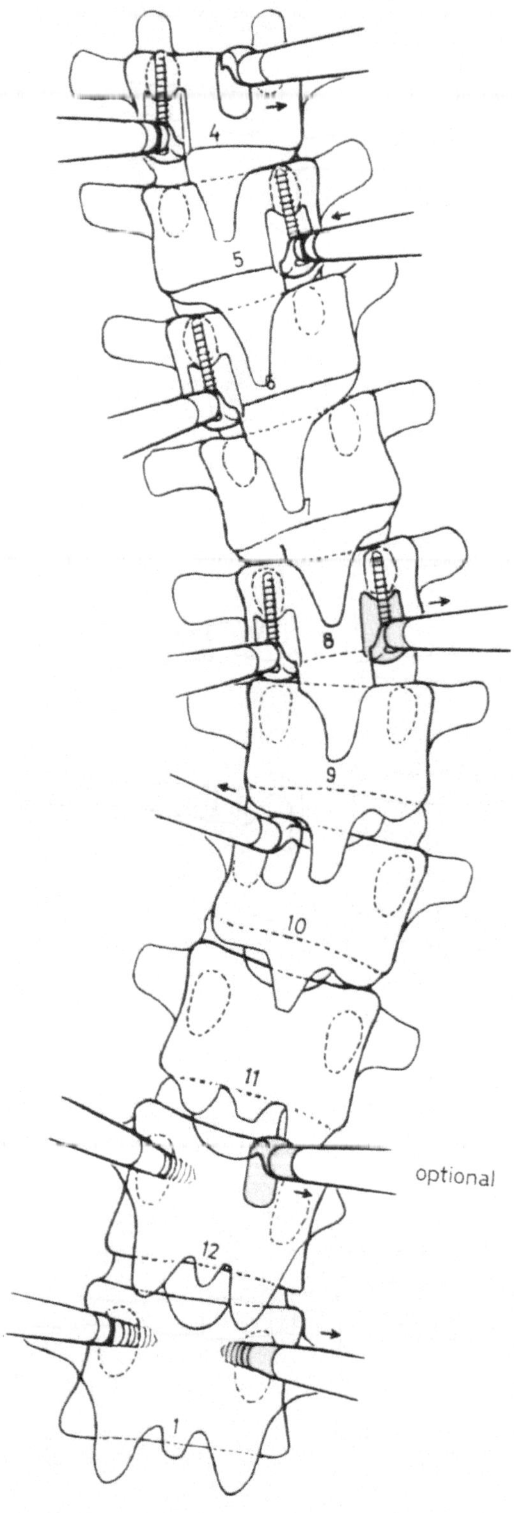

Fig. 8.65 Convex side construct – apical specialized pedicle hook and optional implants in stiff curve

8.2.2.1.2
The Concave Curve

The apical vertebra is instrumented on both sides with specialized pedicle hooks with the concave hook opening laterally and the convex hooks also opening laterally (Figs. 8.62a, b, 8.65). The intervening vertebrae are instrumented at alternative levels (Fig. 8.63a, b); at T10 level, either a laminar hook or pedicle screw may be used (Fig. 8.64a, b), *the latter only by experienced surgeons.* If the curve is stiff then each vertebra next to the apex can be instrumented.

8.2.2.1.3
The Convex Side

The convex side is instrumented at the apex, and if a stiff curve is encountered extra implants can be added. The other implants are the claw construct proximally and the pedicle screw distally (Fig. 8.65).

8.2.2.1.4
Insertion of Rod and Reduction of Spine

The concave rod, contoured in the required sagittal plane according to the template (Fig. 8.66a, b), is inserted in the *sagittal plane* and locked at the distal end; the proximal end must remain loose (Fig. 8.67a, b). The concave implants are then reduced to the concave 6-mm rod beginning proximally and distally working towards the apex. The spine passively elongates (Fig. 8.68a). No significant force should be used at this stage – if force is required STOP – transfer your surgery to the convex side.

The convex rod *having been contoured* is now placed in the superiorly instrumented vertebrae and locked in the claw construct (Figs. 8.69, 8.70a–d). The convex rod is then reduced to the spinal apical pedicle hook and loosely attached and then attached to the distal screw (Fig. 8.71). This maneuver translates the spine to the mid-line. Finally the hooks on the concave side are lifted and attached to the concave rod (Fig. 8.72). The vertebrae are derotated through the use of the stick on the specialized endplate hook and screw, working towards the apex (Fig. 8.73). Cross-links are applied and the nuts tightened (Fig. 8.74).

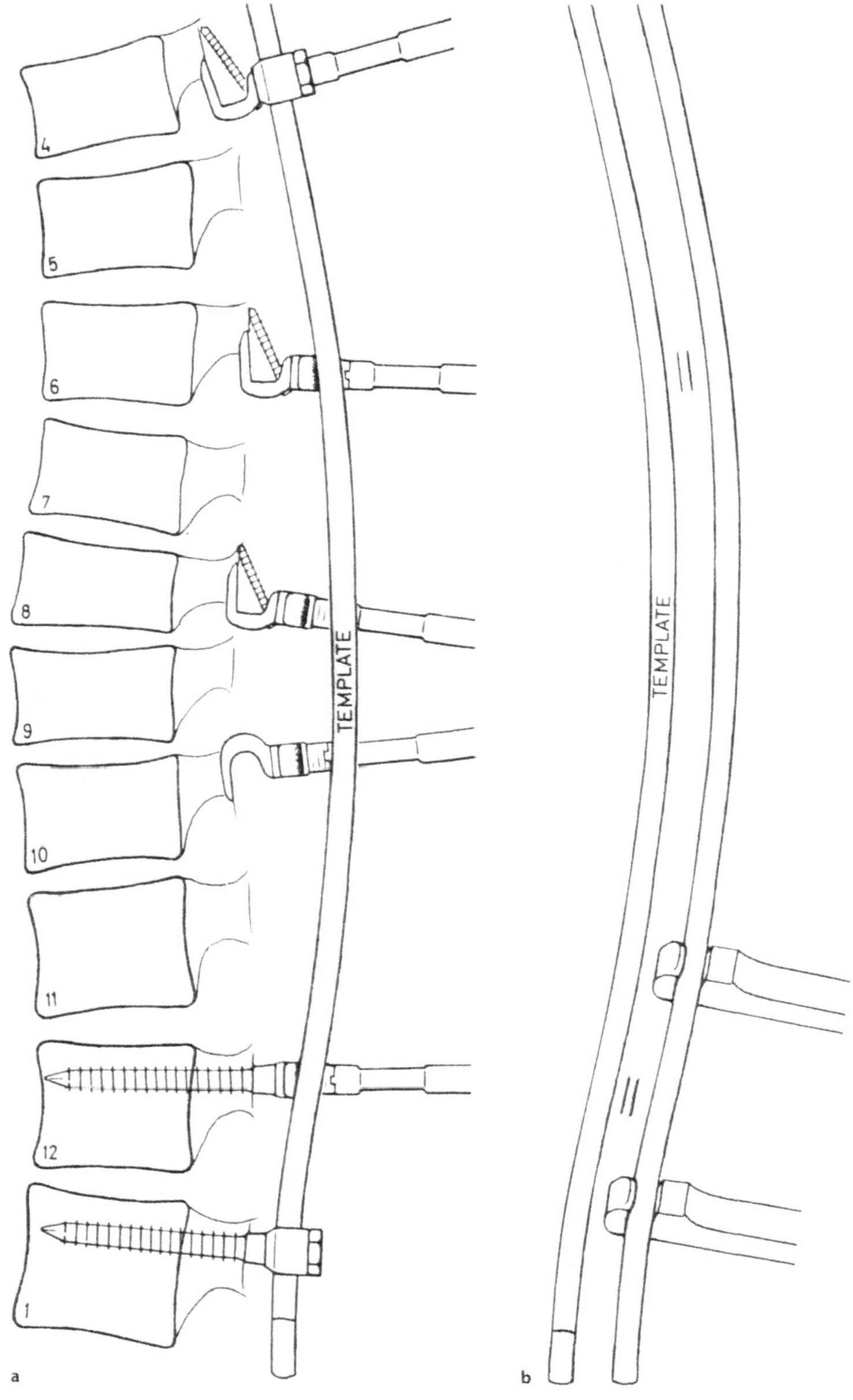

Fig. 8.66 Bending of the rod (**a**) according to the sagittal template contouring (**b**)

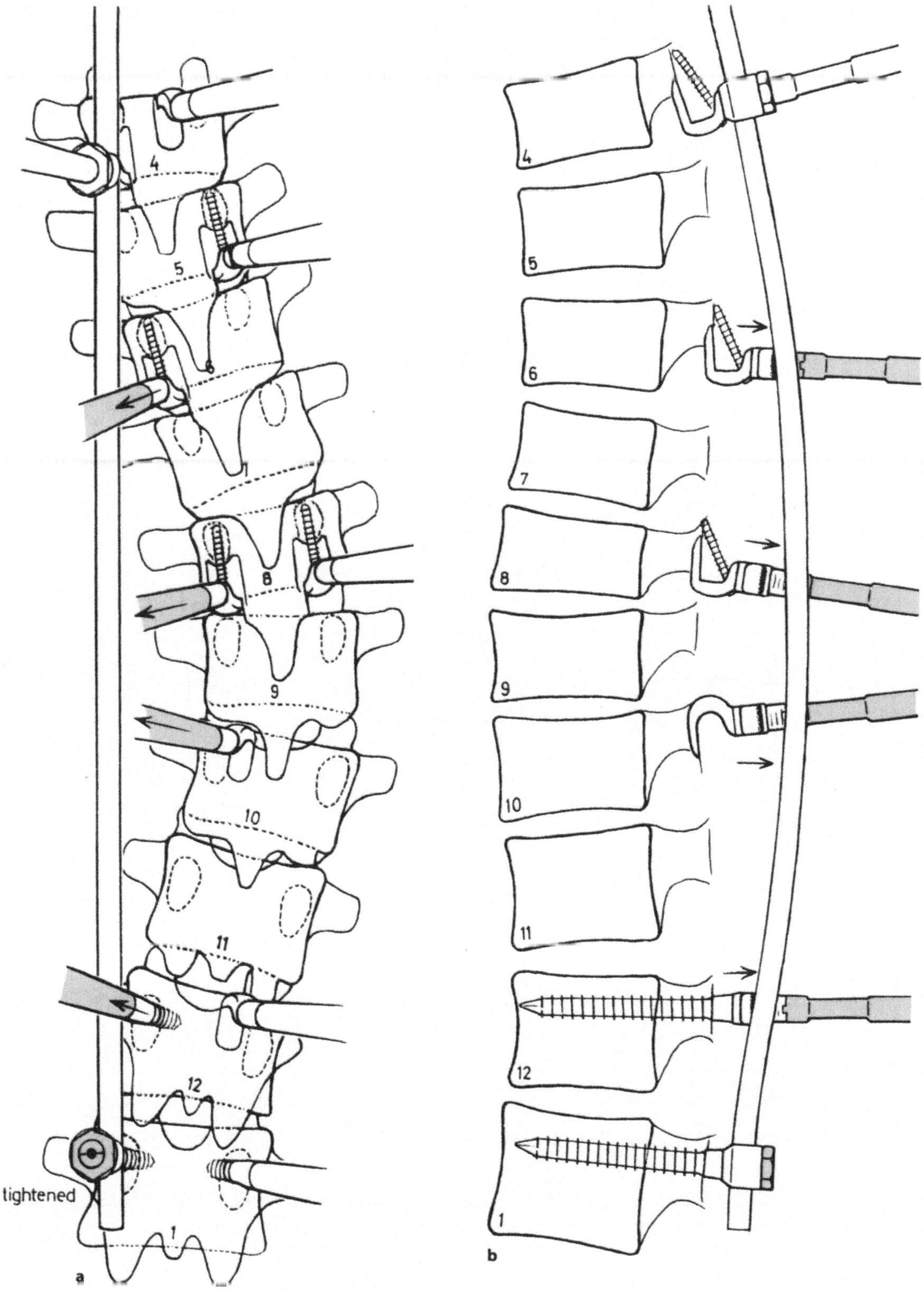

Fig. 8.67 Application of concave rod (**a**) corrects sagittal profile (**b**)

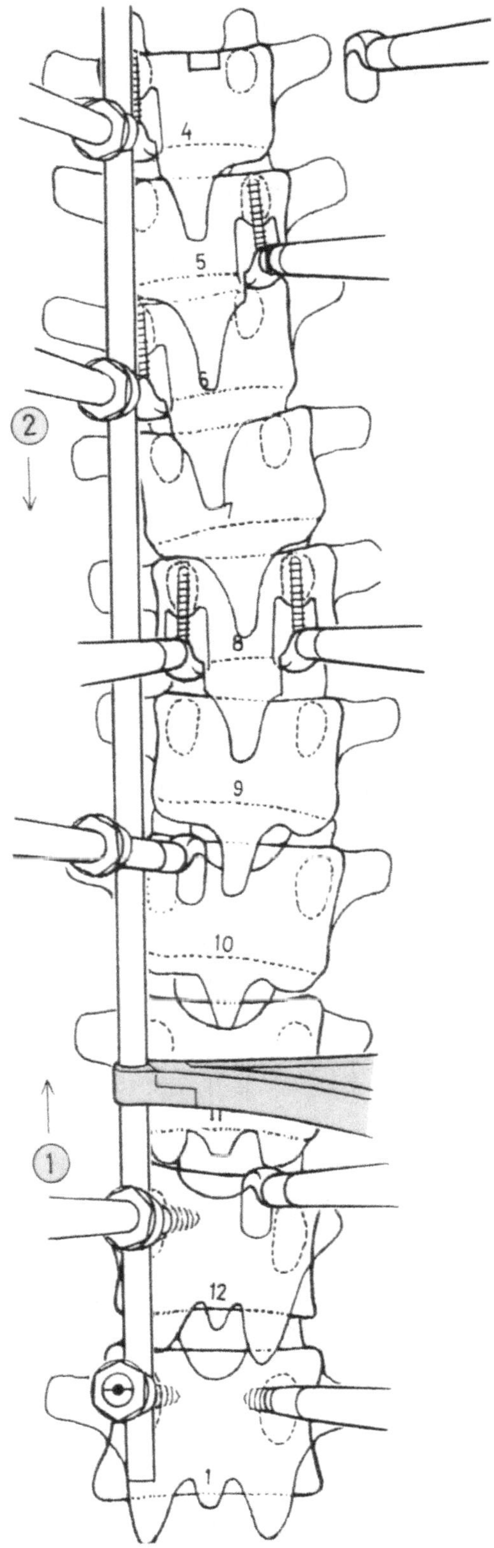

Fig. 8.68 The spine is reduced starting caudally (1) and then cranially (2) working towards the apex. The apical hooks/ screws are not reduced to the rod at this stage

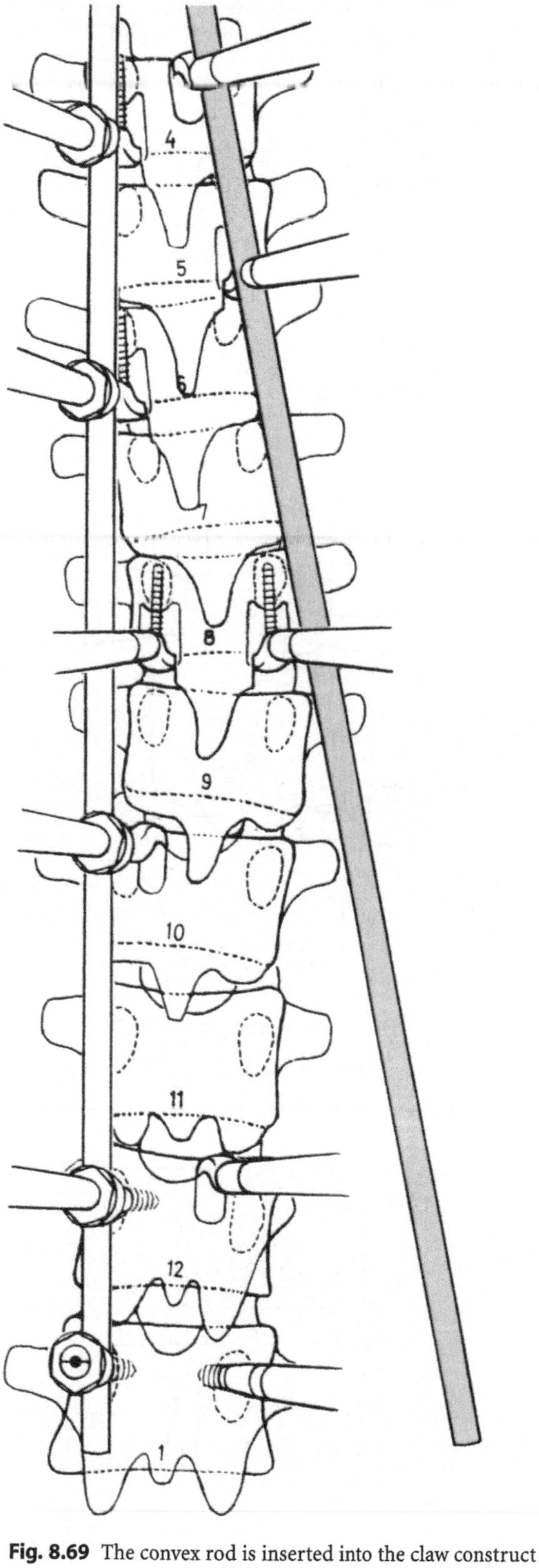

Fig. 8.69 The convex rod is inserted into the claw construct

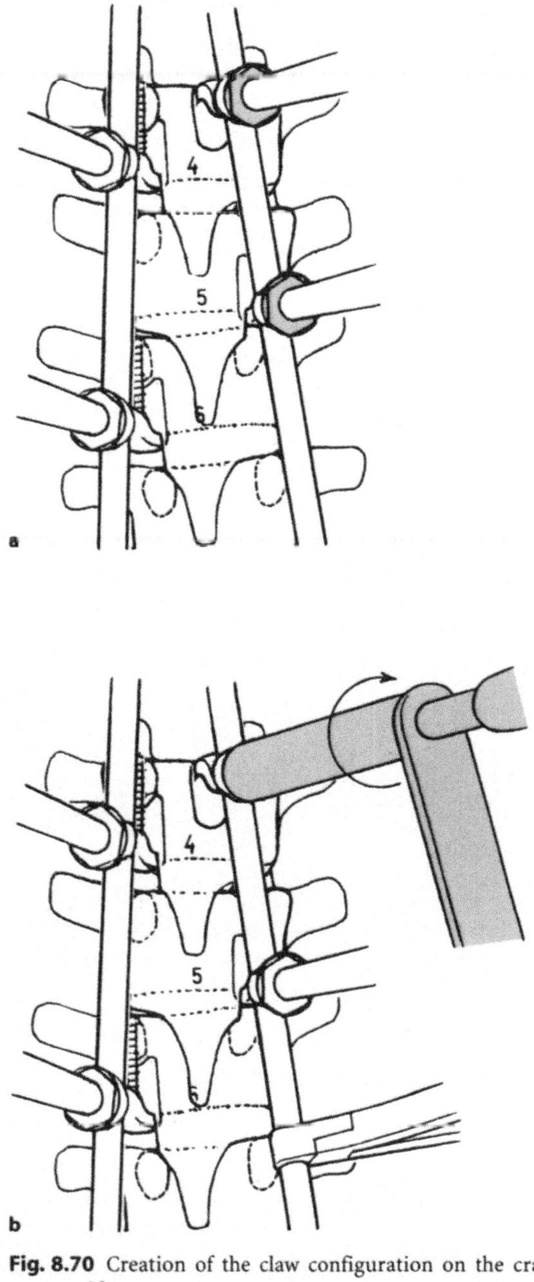

Fig. 8.70 Creation of the claw configuration on the cranial convex side:

a Insertion of the 6-mm rod into the claw configuration

b Tightening of the nut at the top hook

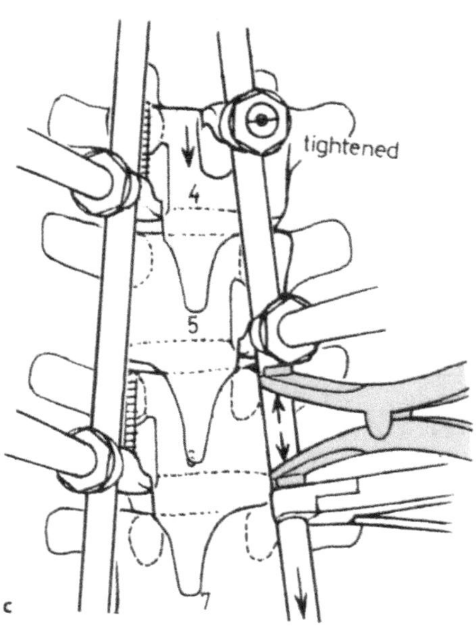

c

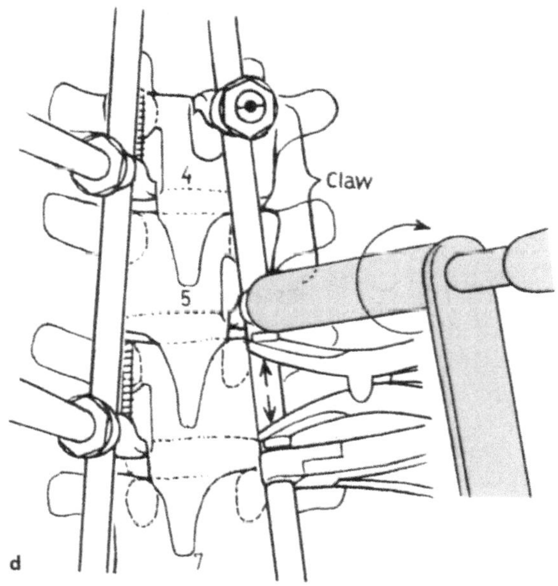

d

(Fig. 8.70)
c Loading the distal pedicle hook with the distractor, thus compressing the claw configuration
d Tightening of the nut of the distal hook of the claw configuration

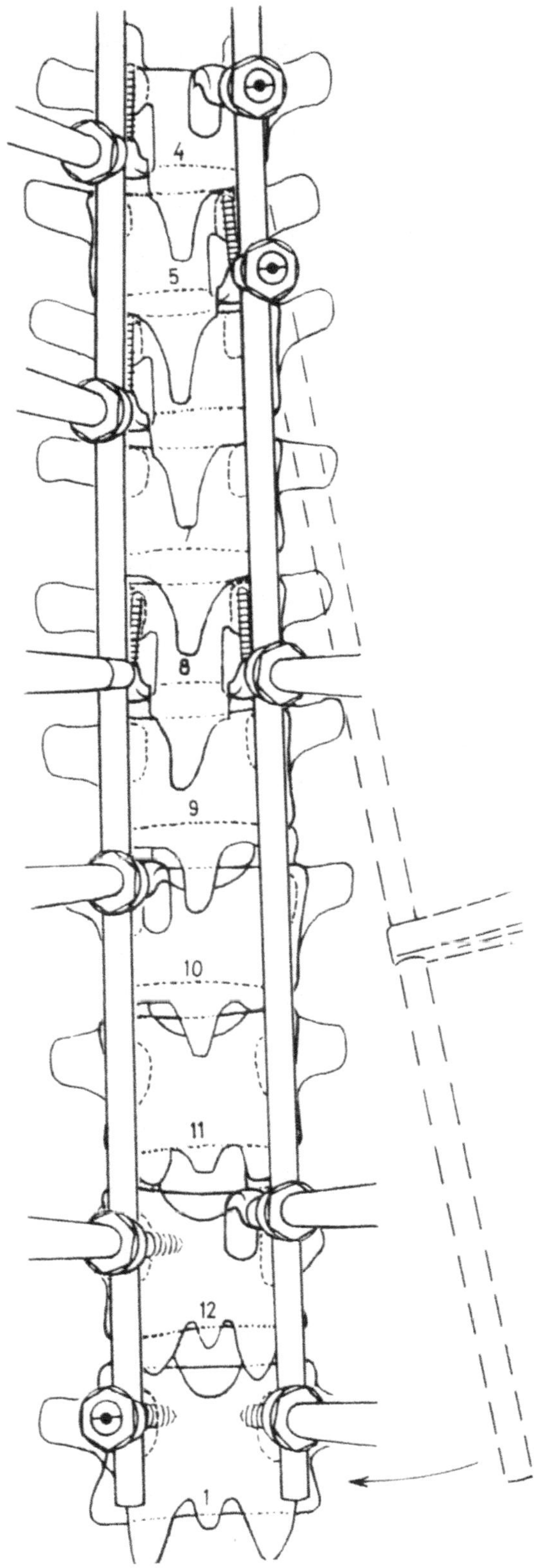

Fig. 8.71 The apex is translated to the mid-line and then the rod attached to the distal screw

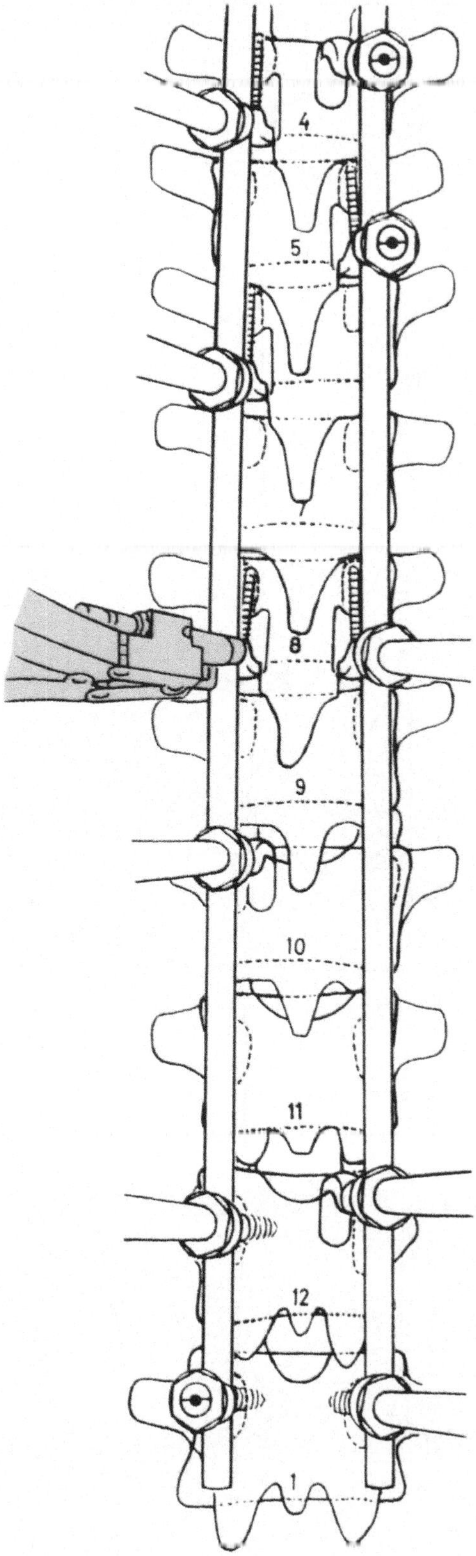

Fig. 8.72 The remaining hook/screws on the concave side are now reduced to the rod using the persuader

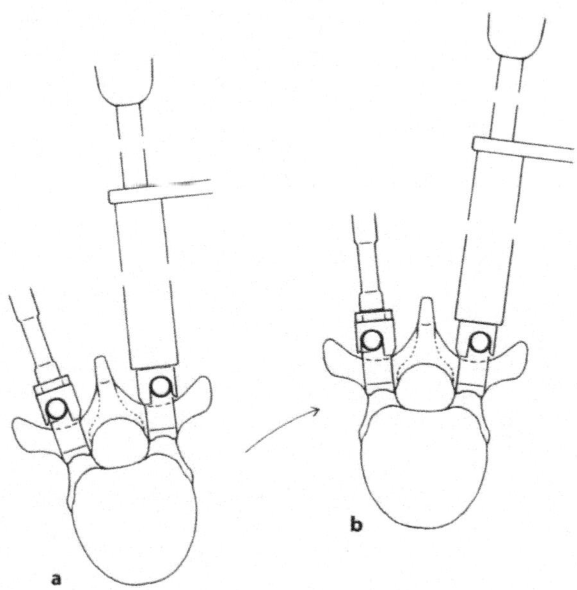

Fig. 8.73 The extension sticks are used to support the individual derotation of rotated vertebrae **(a)** in end position **(b)**

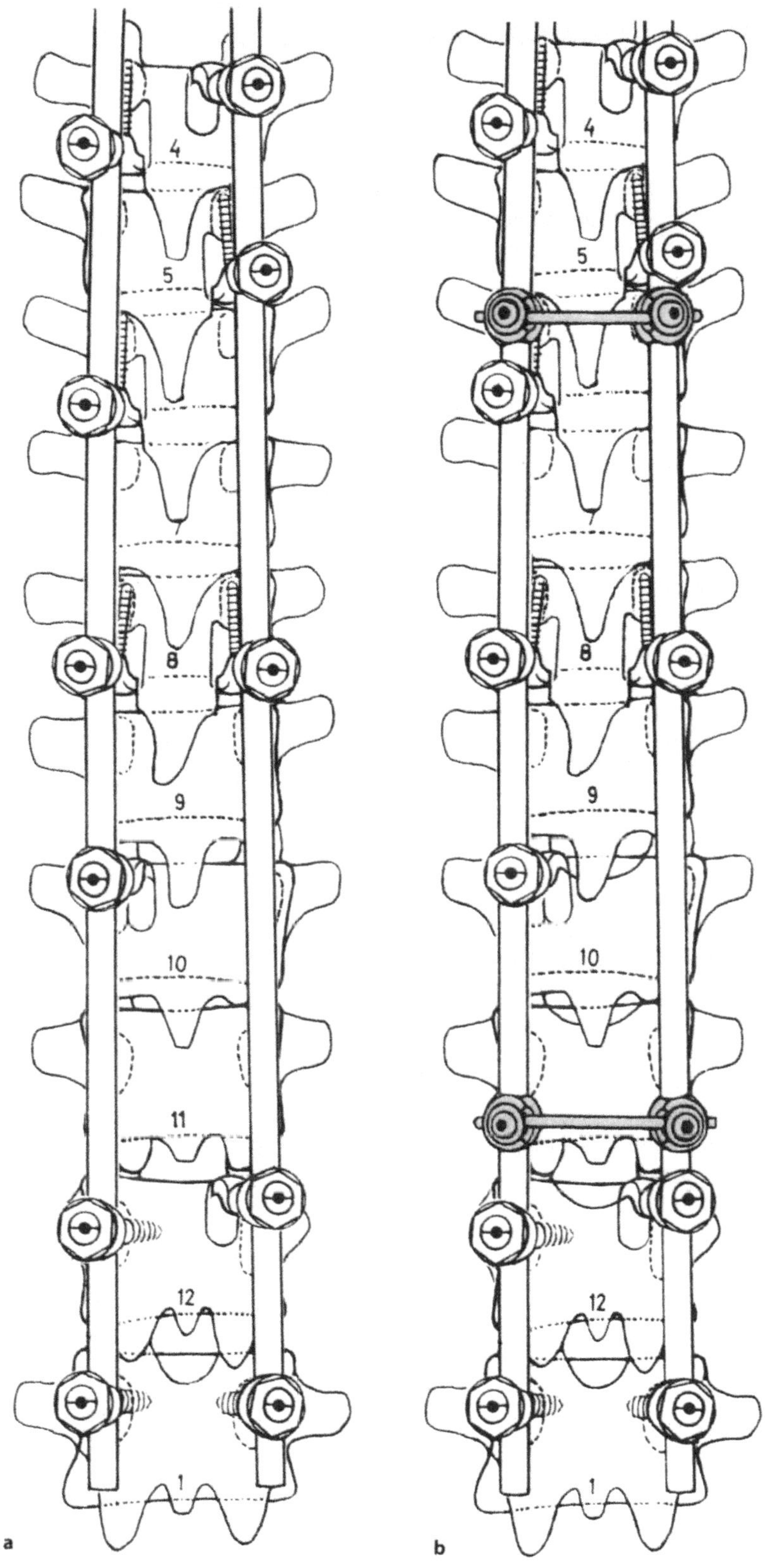

Fig. 8.74
a The final construct
b with crossbars, one cranially and one distally

8.2.2.2
Scoliosis: Posterior Correction and Stabilization

8.2.2.2.1
Right Thoracic Late Onset Scoliosis

Preoperative Plan
The proximal and distal end vertebrae are identified on an anteroposterior standing radiograph and anteroposterior lateral bending film. The classical instrumentation is from Th4 to L1.

Concave Side
The foundation of the construct is made with a pedicle screw in L1. The cranial vertebra, Th4, is instrumented with a specialized pedicle hook with an end-plate screw with the opening facing medially (Fig. 8.75). The apical vertebra is either Th8 or Th9 depending on which is most rotated. The specialized pedicle hook and end-plate screw are inserted with the opening facing laterally (Fig. 8.76). Cranially a specialized pedicle hook is placed between the apical vertebra and the end-plate vertebra (Fig. 8.77). Caudally the Th10 vertebra is either implanted with a pedicle screw or a laminar hook. A pedicle screw can also be inserted into Th12 as well as L1 (Fig. 8.77), especially in a stiff curve.

Convex Side
A proximal claw is constructed at Th4 and Th5. A downward laminar hook with the opening laterally is placed into Th4; a specialized pedicle hook with an end-plate screw is placed in Th5 with the opening facing medially (Fig. 8.75). At the apex a specialized pedicle hook and end-plate screw are inserted with the opening laterally (Fig. 8.76). A pedicle screw is inserted in L1 (Fig. 8.75) (a hook can be used as an alternative). An optional laminar hook/screw can be placed into Th12 if a stiff curve and a kyphotic deformity is present (Fig. 8.77).

Figs. 8.75–8.82 Right thoracic late-onset scoliosis (see also Figs. 8.61–8.74).

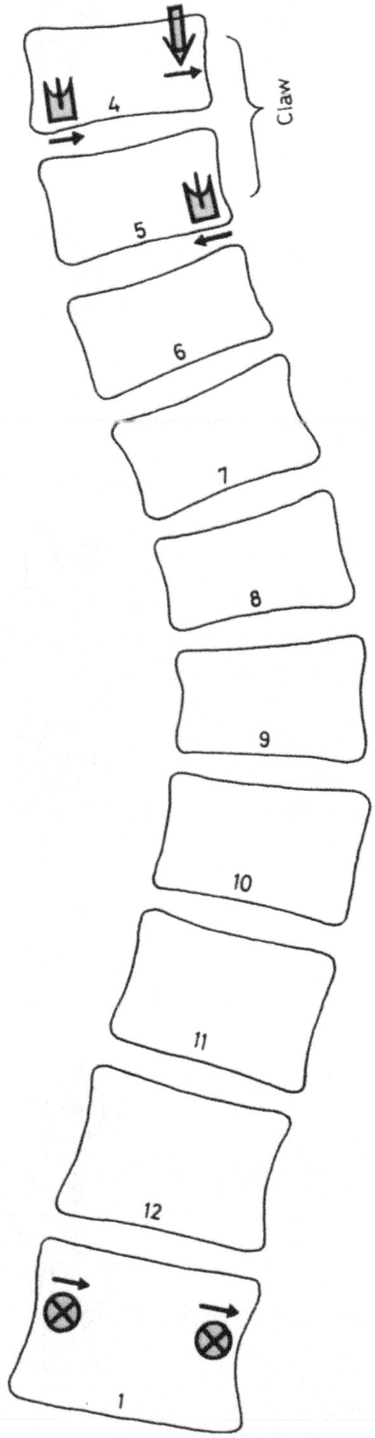

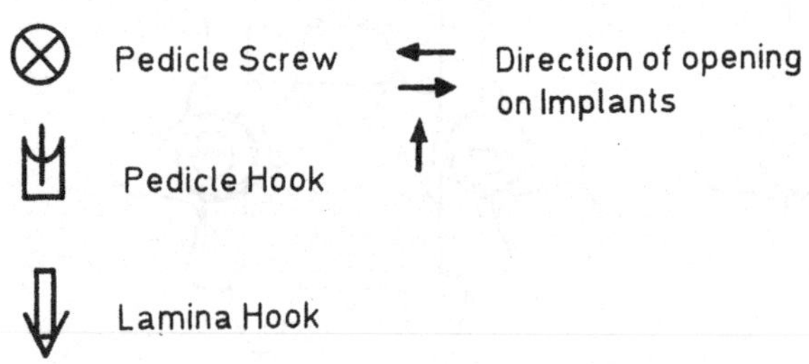

Fig. 8.75 Pedicle screw is inserted into L1 and the special pedicle hook with end-plate screw is inserted into Th4. A proximal claw construct between Th4 and Th5 is made on the convex side. Th4 laminar hook opening laterally and at Th5 a special pedicle hook with end-plate screw opening medially. The L1 pedicle screw is also inserted on the convex side

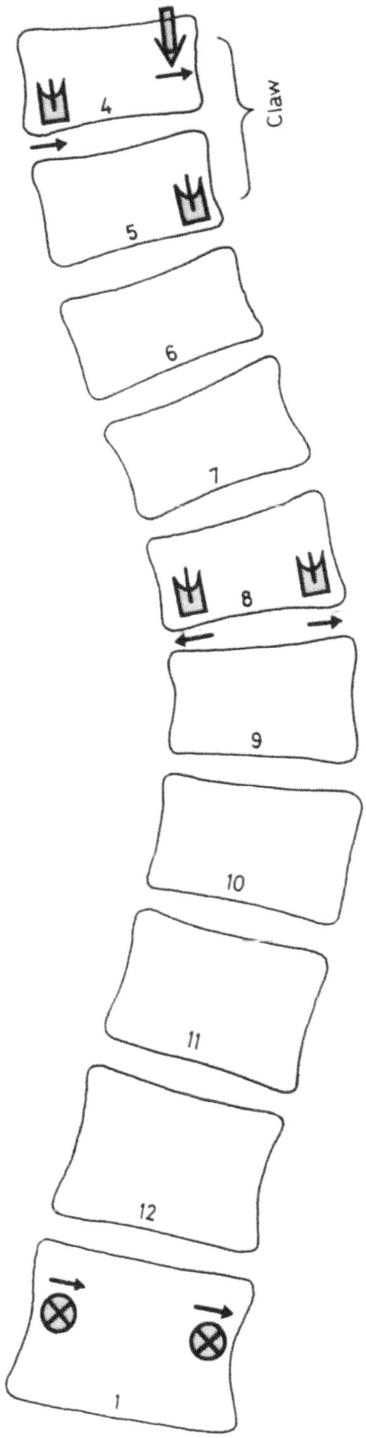

Fig. 8.76 The apical vertebrae are instrumented at Th8 with the special pedicle hook and end-plate screw on the concave as well as the convex side

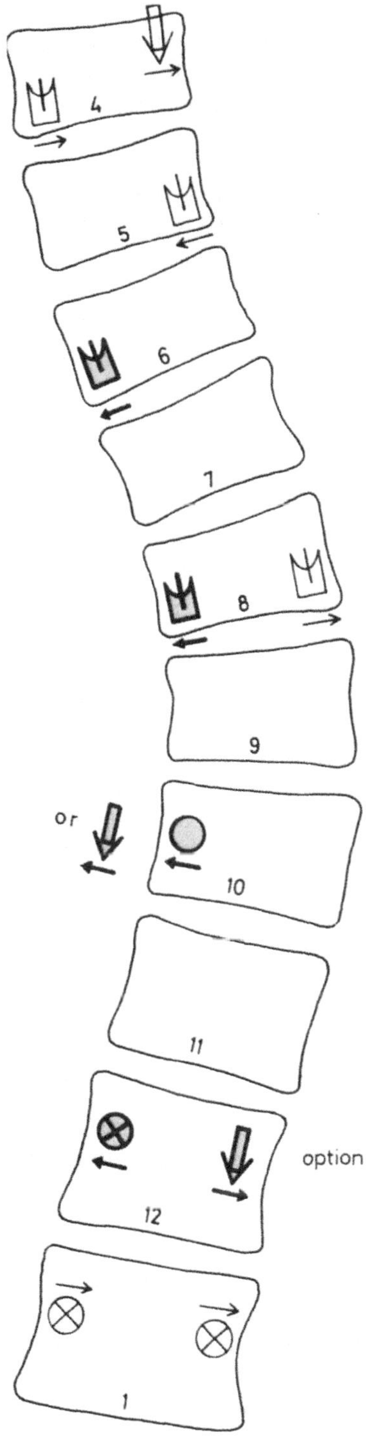

Fig. 8.77 Special pedicle hook and end-plate screw are inserted into Th6. Either a laminar hook or pedicle screw is placed into Th10 and a pedicle screw is placed into Th12 (a hook may be used) on the concave side. Insertion of the apex hook and an apical Th12 laminar hook – the opening facing laterally on the convex side

Surgical Technique

The spine is exposed with subperiosteal dissection and the levels identified with a radiograph. The implants are inserted as previously described.

Reduction

Once all the implants are attached to the vertebra, before beginning the reduction with the rods, decorticate the spine in the usual manner. A 6-mm rod template is placed in the sagittal plane on the concave side between the Th4 hook and L1 screw. The sagittal profile is then bent into the template rod (see Fig. 8.66a). The template rod is removed and a *hard* 6-mm rod is cut to the appropriate length and contoured in the sagittal plane (see Fig. 8.66b). The rod is inserted into the Th4 and L1 screw and only tightened to the L1 screw (Fig. 8.78). A 6-mm rod holder is held onto the 6-mm rod to maintain its position also in the sagittal plane (see page 138 Fig. 8.41, 8.42, 8.43)

Using the complex reduction forceps (Fig. 8.72), the Th6 and Th10 implants are brought to the rod. *Do not use too much force!* If the curve is tight do not proceed, direct your attention to the convex rod. If Th6 and Th10 implants are brought to the rod *do not reduce the apical hook to the rod* (Fig. 8.79). The contoured convex 6-mm rod is now inserted (Fig. 8.80).

The laminar hook is held in place with the hook holder and universal handle, which is loaded with nut and sleeve. The 6-mm rod is placed into the pedicle hook on Th5 and the laminar hook Th4 (see page 154 Fig. 8.70a). The sleeve and nut are dropped onto the laminar hook and the nut tightened with the L-shaped handle and 6-mm socket wrench (see Fig. 8.70b). A sleeve and nut are dropped onto the Th5 pedicle hook. A 6-mm rod holder is attached to the 6-mm rod below the Th5 hook and with the use of the distractor the bar is pushed caudally, which allows the laminar hook to fit snugly under the lamina (see Fig. 8.70c). The Th5 pedicle hook nut is tightened with the L-handed socket wrench and the 6-mm socket wrench. The claw construct is now complete (see Fig. 8.70d).

The 6-mm rod is pushed toward the mid-line using the 6-mm rod holder, first engaging into the apical hook; a sleeve and nut are added but left loose. Using the 6-mm rod holder and a rod pusher the 6-mm rod is now inserted in L1 and a sleeve and nut added but not tightened (Fig. 8.81). The laminar hook is added to Th12 if required. The apical hook on the concave side will now have been translated toward the concave rod. The complex reduction forceps are used to attach the pedicle hook to the 6-mm rod (see Fig. 8.41, 8.42, 8.43, 8.72). The spine will have pas-

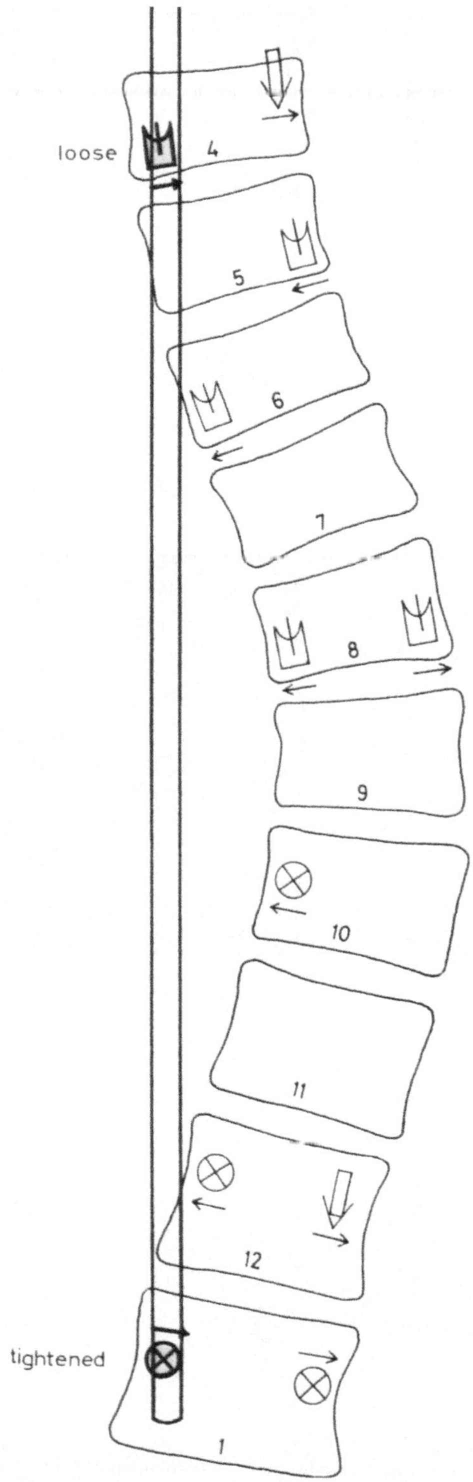

Fig. 8.78 The contoured 6-mm USS rod is inserted into Th4 pedicle hook and L1 pedicle screw (see also Figs. 8.66 and 8.67)

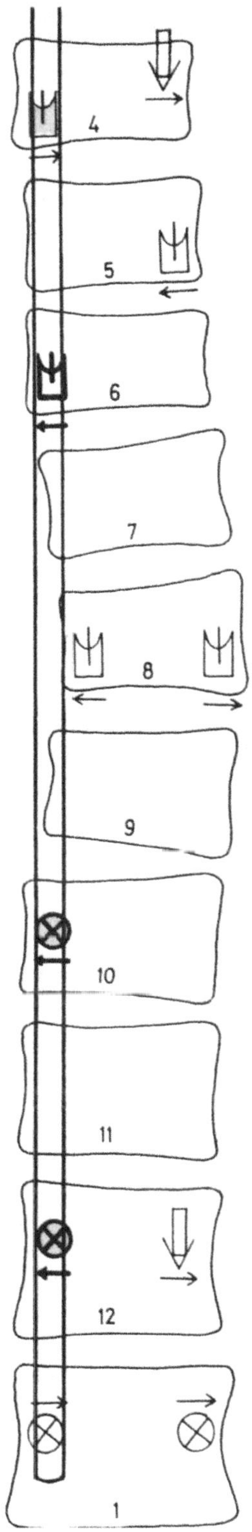

Fig. 8.79 Approximation of Th6 and Th10 implants to the 6-mm rod. *Do not force Th8 towards the rod!* (see also Fig. 8.68)

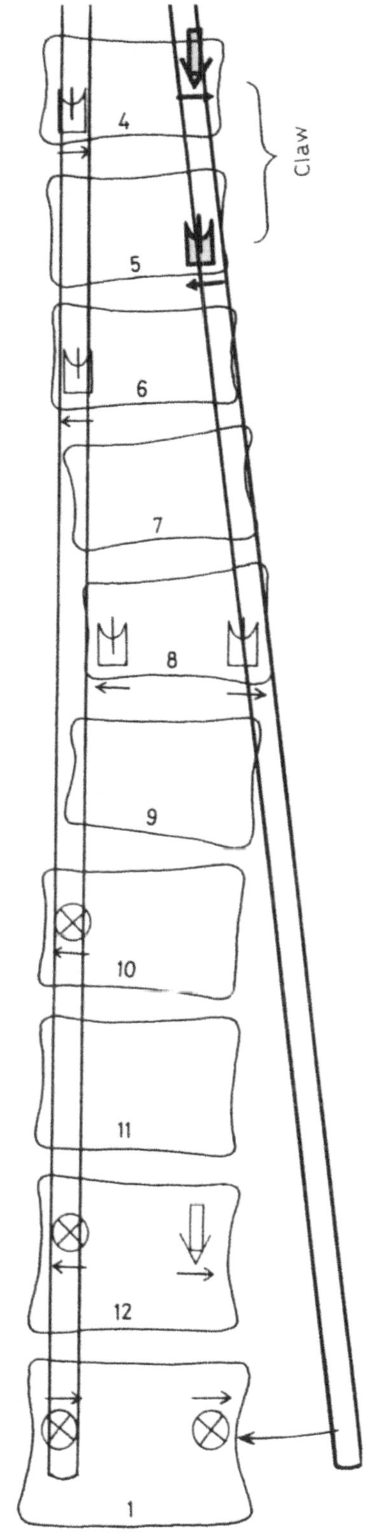

Fig. 8.80 The convex 6-mm rod which has been contoured to the sagittal plane is inserted into the claw construct (see also Fig. 8.69)

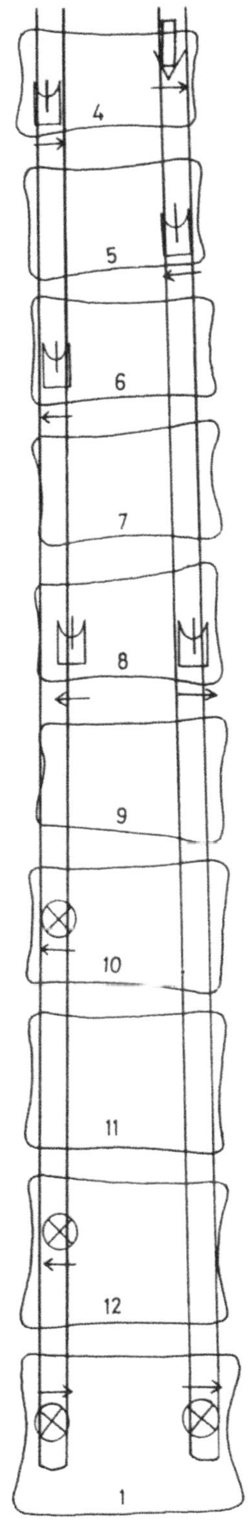

Fig. 8.81 The 6-mm rod is pushed with the rod holder medially and inserted into the pedicle hook at Th8 and the pedicle screw at L1. The sleeves and nuts are added but not tightened

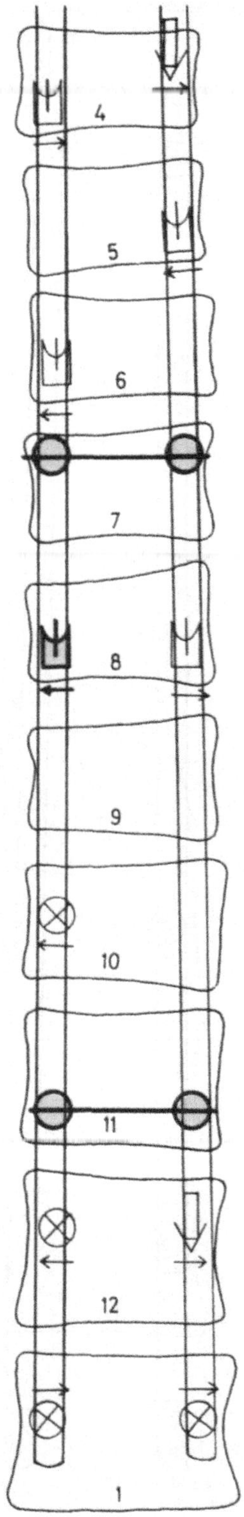

Fig. 8.82 The two cross links are added

sively found its own length. The screw holders are now attached to the pedicle screw hooks (see Fig. 8.73a) and starting from each end, the vertebrae are derotated and the nuts tightened (see Fig. 8.73b). Hold the end vertebrae in a normal position while derotating the intermediate vertebrae. Two cross-links are applied and all the nuts are now tightened (see Figs. 8.74b, 8.82). A bone graft is applied to the decorticated spine.

8.2.2.2.2
Double Curve

Principle

The same basic concept of reduction in a single curve is applied to double curves (Fig. 8.83a). The foundation is made on the neutral vertebrae between the curves rather than an end vertebra (Fig. 8.83b). Each curve is considered separately so, in fact, the neutral vertebra will act as an end vertebra.

Pedicle screws are inserted into the neutral vertebra (Fig. 8.83b). The upper curve is instrumented as previously described in the single right thoracic curve (Fig. 8.84a) and the end of the lower curve is also instrumented in a similar way with pedicle screws (Fig. 8.84b). The rods are contoured to create a normal sagittal profile in the thoracic and lumbar spine. The rod is inserted into the upper concave side of the curve, Th4 and Th12 and locked to the neutral vertebra (Th12) (Fig. 8.85a). The concave side of the thoracic curve is reduced as described in a single curve but do not use force (Fig. 8.85b). Using the caudal part of the rod it is placed on the convex portion of the lumbar curve and the curve is translated to the mid-line and the rod attached to L4 (Fig. 8.85b).

The second rod is inserted into the convex claw of the upper curve and is then pushed medially to translate the apex of the upper curve to the mid-line – the Th8 pedicle hook with end-plate screw is attached to the rod (Fig. 8.86a) and the rod then reduced to the T12 pedicle screw. The caudal part of the rod is then attached to the distal pedicle screw (L4) (Fig. 8.86b). The remaining hooks/screws and both apices are reduced to the rods with the complex reduction forceps or crimper forceps. Finally the cross-links are attached and bone graft applied (Fig. 8.87).

Figs. 8.83–8.87
Double curve

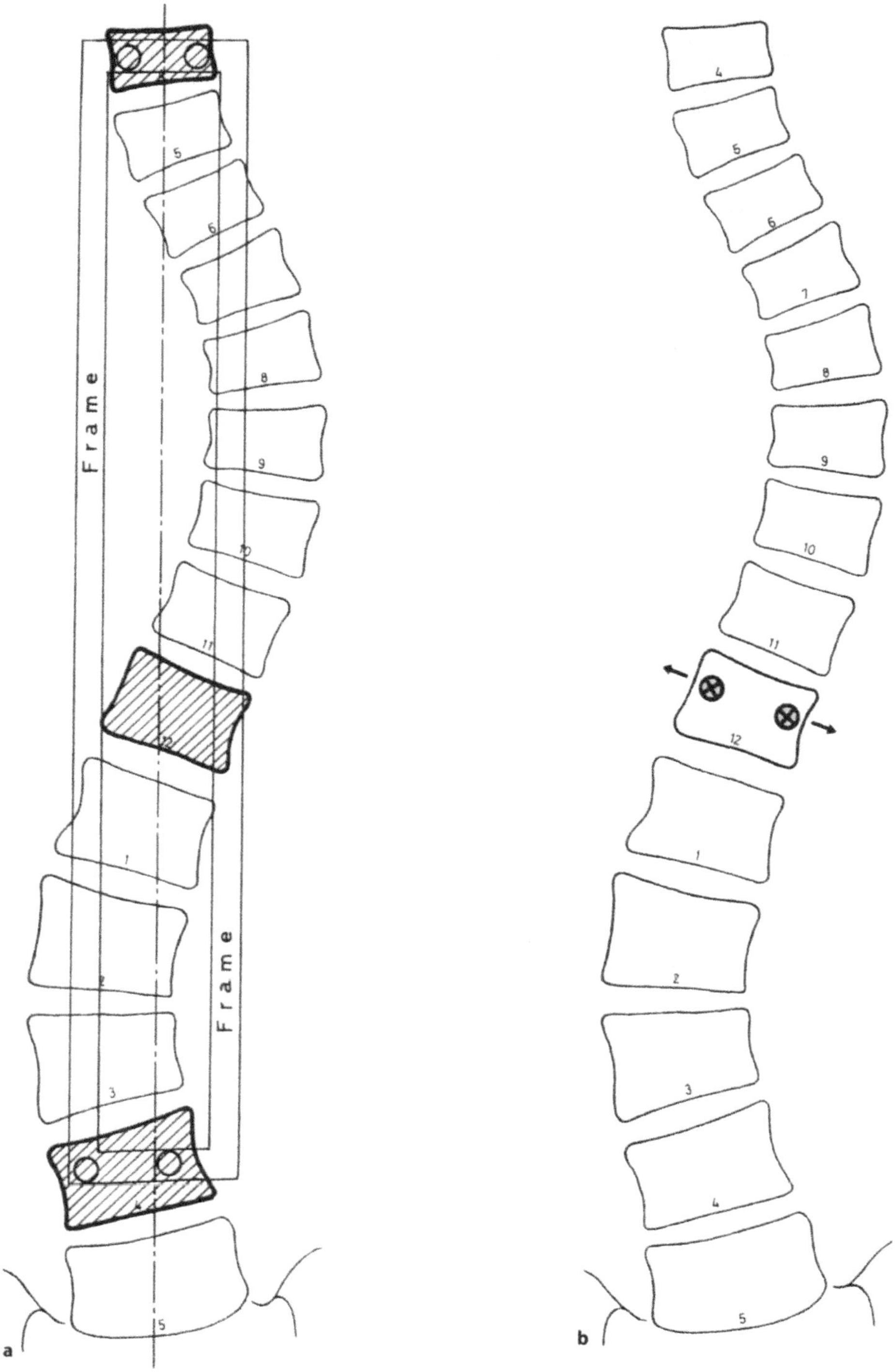

Fig. 8.83
a Double curve identified by the neutral vertebra and end vertebra. The frame concept is added **b** Insertion of pedicle screws into Th12

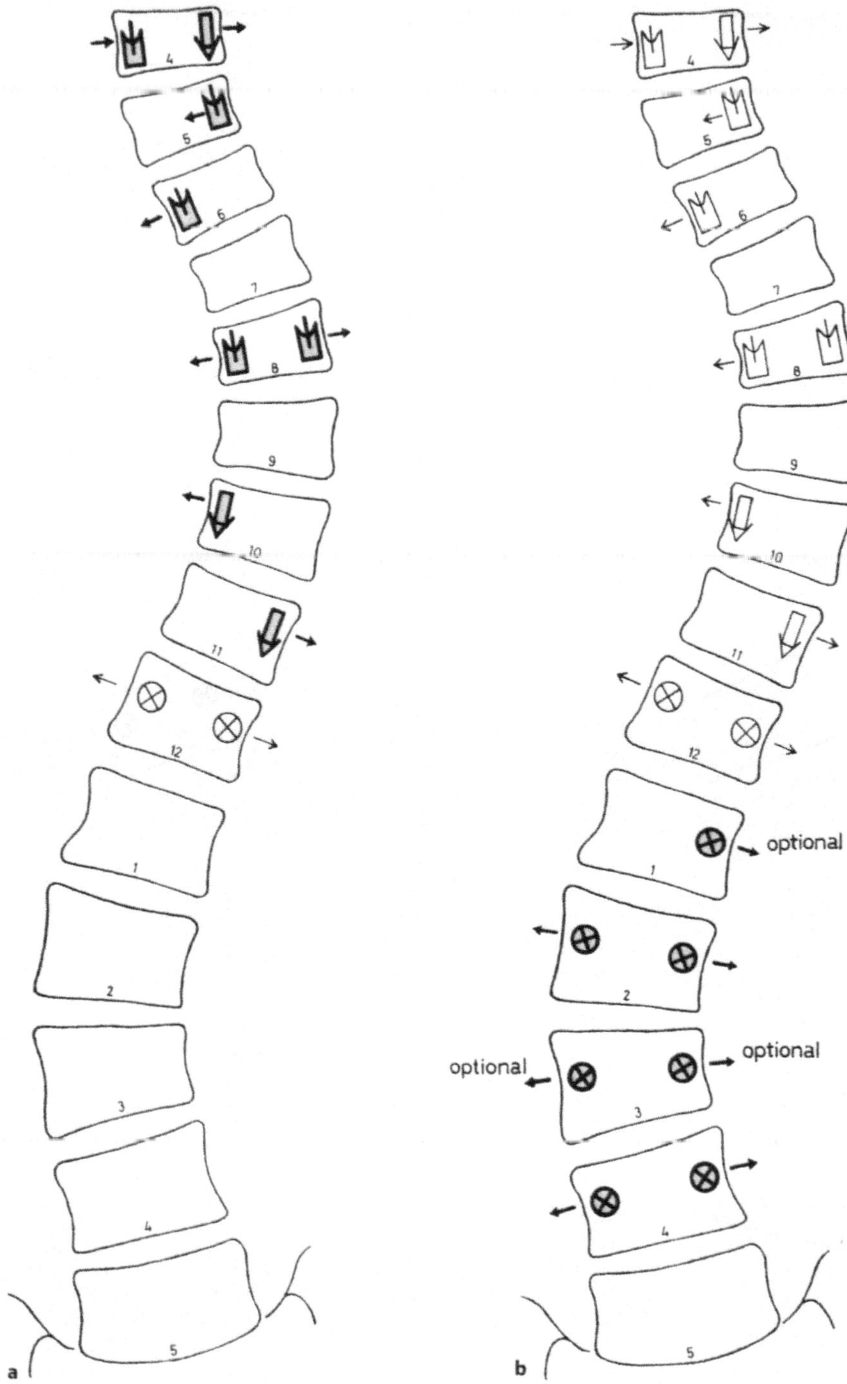

Fig. 8.84
a The upper curve instrumented
b The lower curve instrumented

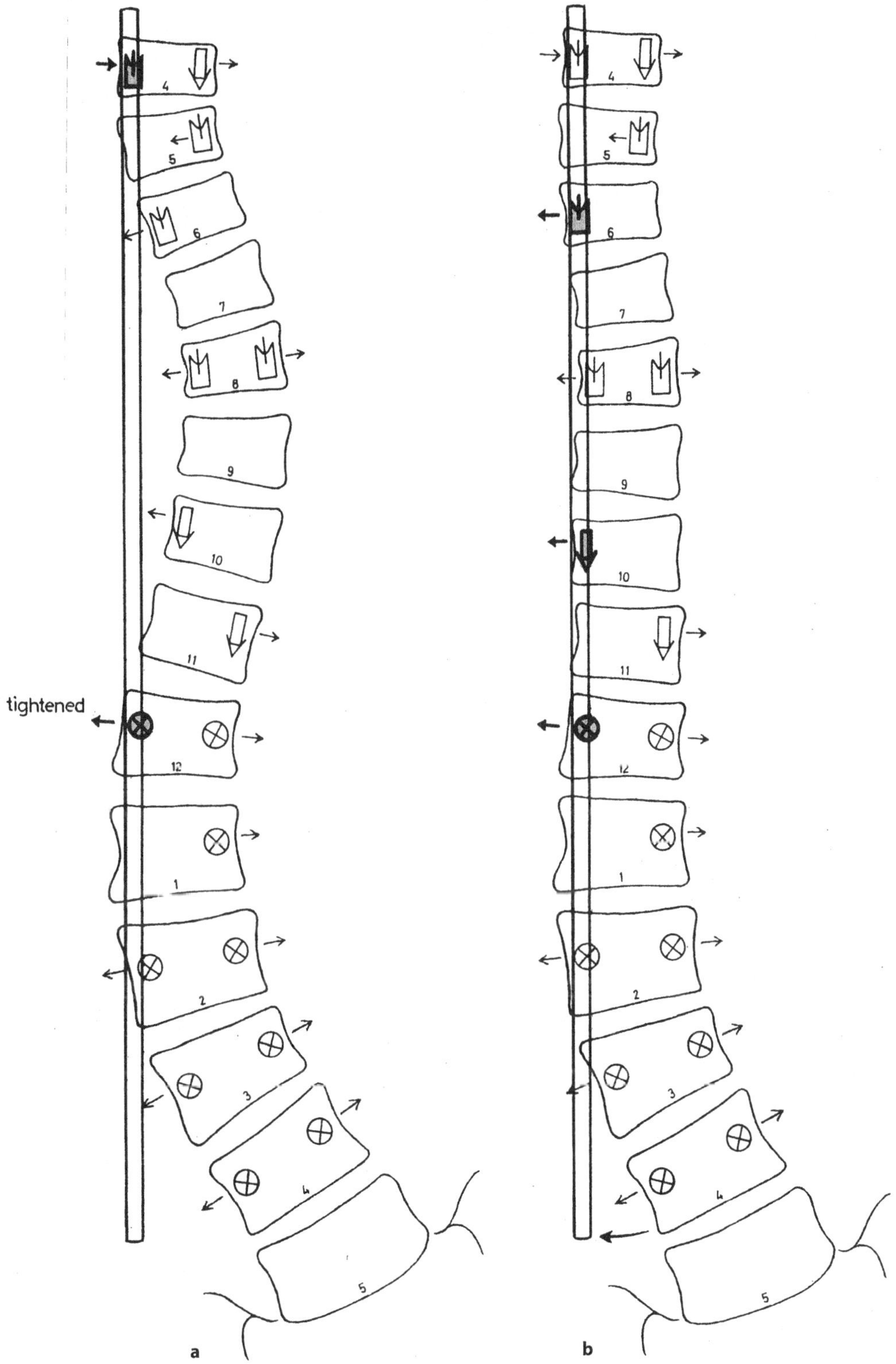

Fig. 8.85
a The rod is inserted into the concave upper curve and fixed to Th12
b The concave curve is partly reduced to the rod

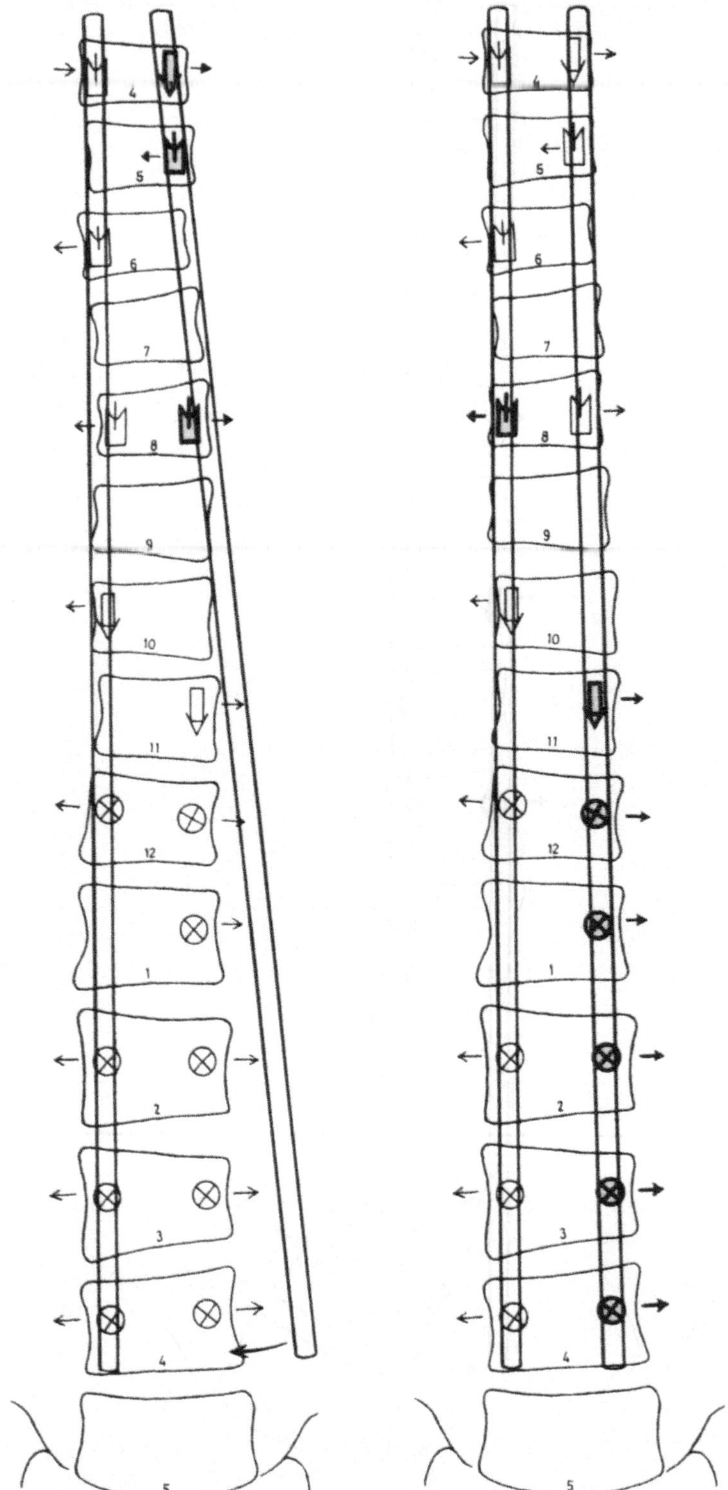

a b

Fig. 8.86

a The second rod is added

b The remaining hooks/screws are reduced to the rod

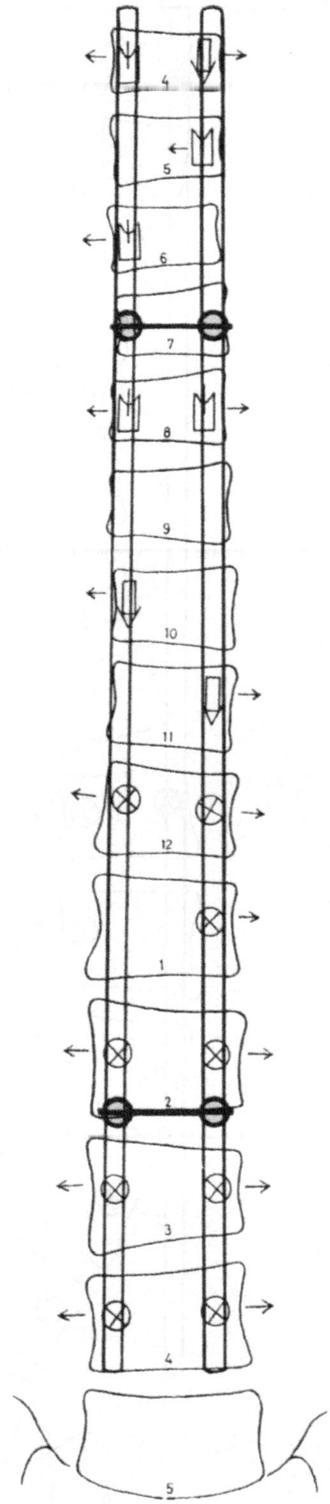

Fig. 8.87 Cross links are added

8.2.2.3
Scoliosis: Anterior Correction and Stabilization

The USS also makes it possible to address a scoliotic deformity from an anterior approach.

Concept
The pedicular screws – 5-mm and 6-mm screws – can be used for anterior anchorage into the vertebral bodies. The ordinary 6-mm hard rod is usually used in combination with the screws. The concept of correction is the same as in posterior surgery. The pre-bent rod is inserted into the screws, anchored in the end vertebrae and all the included vertebral bodies are then gradually pulled onto the rod, resulting in a three-dimensional correction of the deformity. The anterior approach to the spine at any level of the thoracic and lumbar spine is more demanding for the surgeon and patient, but the correction of the deformity is likely to be superior to posterior surgery. A combination of anterior surgery and posterior correction is indicated in severe and rigid curves; in such cases an anterior release is necessary, without anterior instrumentation; if anterior instrumentation is performed it would prevent the balancing potential of the secondary posterior instrumentation for definitive correction.

Principles
All the vertebrae involved in the deformity from the end vertebra above to the end vertebra below are instrumented with USS laterally, using open screws – 5 or 6 mm in diameter. The screws are inserted into the vertebral body from the lateral convex side of the vertebral body. The rod is pre-bent in the form of the sagittal plane, i.e., with a lordosis in the lumbar and kyphosis in the thoracic spine.

The pre-bent rod is attached to the end screws, one of them being completely tightened in order to avoid rotating of the rod, and the other kept loose so the rod can glide during the corrective measures, i. e., the spine can elongate naturally. The vertebrae between both end vertebrae are then gradually rotated to the rod with the persuader, alternating from the top and the bottom of the construct, working towards the middle.

Indications
- Lumbar scoliosis.
- Thoracolumbar scoliosis.
- Thoracic scoliosis in bony immature individuals.

Advantages
- Derotation is best achieved by anterior instrumentation.
- Instrumentation can be shorter than with posterior instrumentation.
- Prevents crank-shaft phenomena in skeletally immature patients.

Disadvantages
- The surgical approach is more demanding, and may need the collaboration of an abdominal and/or thoracic surgeon. The patient may need to stay in an intensive care unit postoperatively.
- Rigid curves cannot be controlled and balanced by anterior surgery alone.

Technique
Depending on the curve, either a thoracotomy, a retroperitoneal approach or a combination of both with reflection of the diaphragm is performed on the convex side of the curve in order to obtain good access to the spine area. The exposure of the spine in preparation for the instrumentation is well described in standard textbooks.

The parietal pleura and/or the parietal peritoneum is mobilized well into the concavity of the curve, starting from the lateral aspect of the vertebral body, in order to gain access with the finger to the contralateral side of the vertebral bodies (concave side of the curve). All the disks between the end vertebrae are removed, and the cartilage removed in order to have bare, bleeding end plates.

The entry point of the USS 5 or 6-mm screw is preferred at the junction of the pedicular origin and the vertebral body (Fig. 8.88) and directed perpendicular to the contralateral side. At the end-vertebrae location a staple is inserted with a special staple holder (Fig. 8.89c). This small implant provides a fixed angle between the staple and screw, preventing the pull out and/or tear out of the screw (Fig 8.89b). Once the staple is inserted (Fig. 8.89d), the cortex is opened through the staple with the short, sharp awl followed by the long, blunt awl (feeler) (Fig. 8.90), which is pushed with one hand through the vertebral body and the contralateral cortex until it can be felt with the index finger of the other hand when penetrating the cortex. The definite length of the screw is chosen 5 mm longer than necessary in order to enable the positioning of a plastic washer of 4.5 mm diameter as a counterfit to the screw. The screw will be turned into the washer, which is held compressed towards the contralateral vertebral cortical wall and prevents the pulling out of the screw from the vertebra. This technique is specifically used for the screws set into the

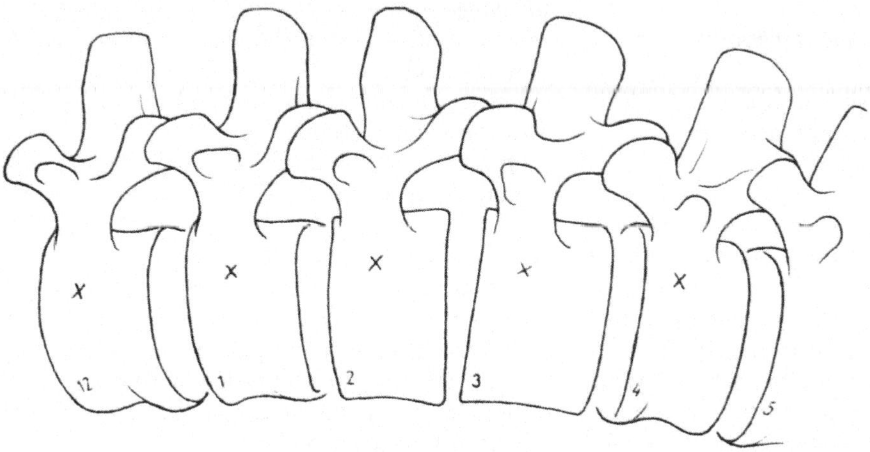

Fig. 8.88 Entry point for the 5- or 6-mm USS laterally open screw in the vertebral body

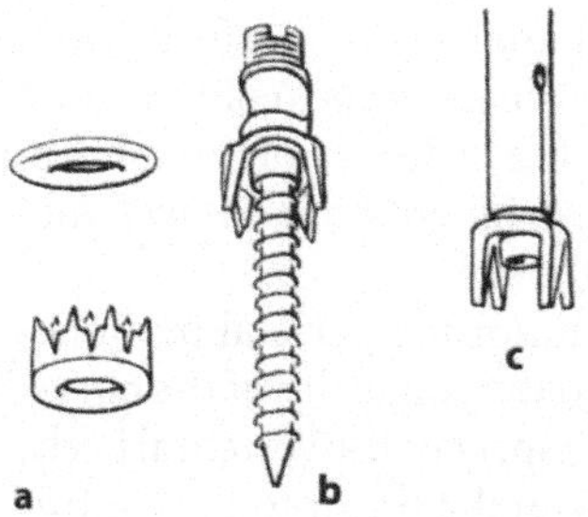

Fig. 8.89 Special implants
a Metal washer and 45-mm plastic washer
b Fixed angle between screw and the metal staple
c Metal staple attached to the staple introducer
d Insertion of the staples at the carnial and caudal end

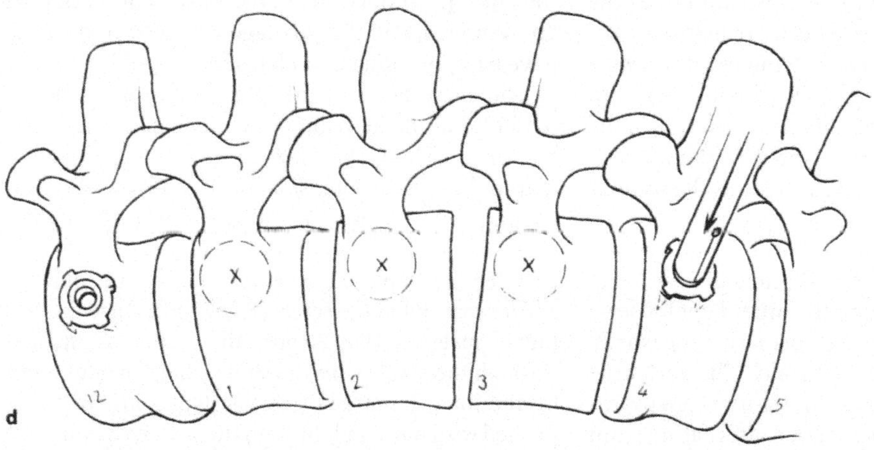

end vertebrae (Fig. 8.91). All the remaining vertebrae which have been chosen to be included in the montage are now instumented but, instead of using staples, washers are used with the convex side resting on the concavity of the vertebral body. It is optional for the surgeon to also mount the screw tips of the intermediate vertebrae with a plastic washer since the stress of these screws is less than on those in the end vertebrae and the apical vertebrae. They should only be used if the bone is osteoporotic.

The rod length and contour is chosen with the help of the template (Fig. 8.92a, b). The rod needs to be about 2 cm longer than measured in order to allow the lengthening of the spine along the rod. The appropriate-length hard rod is matched to the template by bending the rod with the rod bender or the bend-

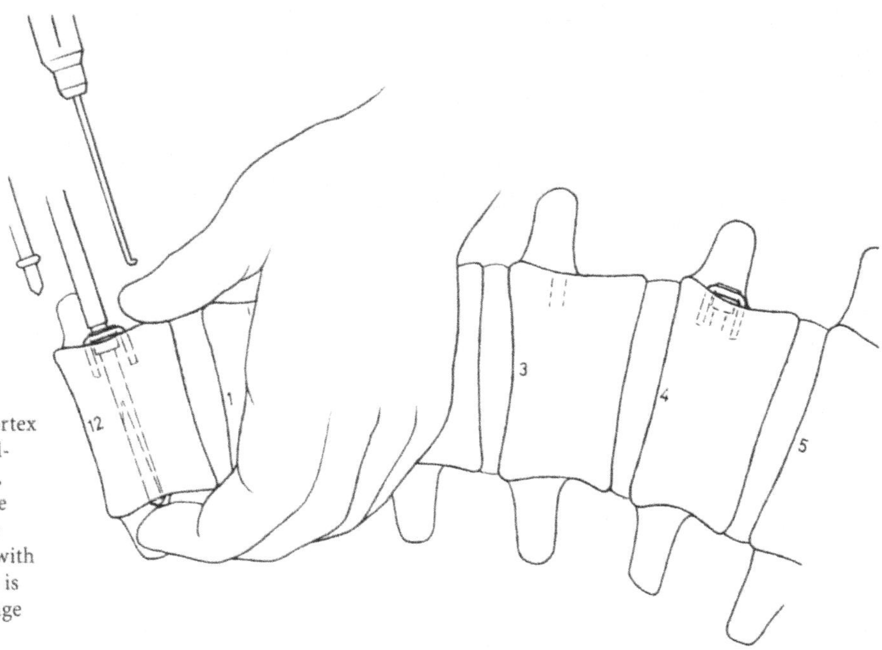

Fig. 8.90 Opening of the cortex with the short sharp awl, followed by the long blunt awl, which is pushed through the contralateral cortex and the penetrating awl can be felt with the index finger. Screw hole is measured with the depth gage

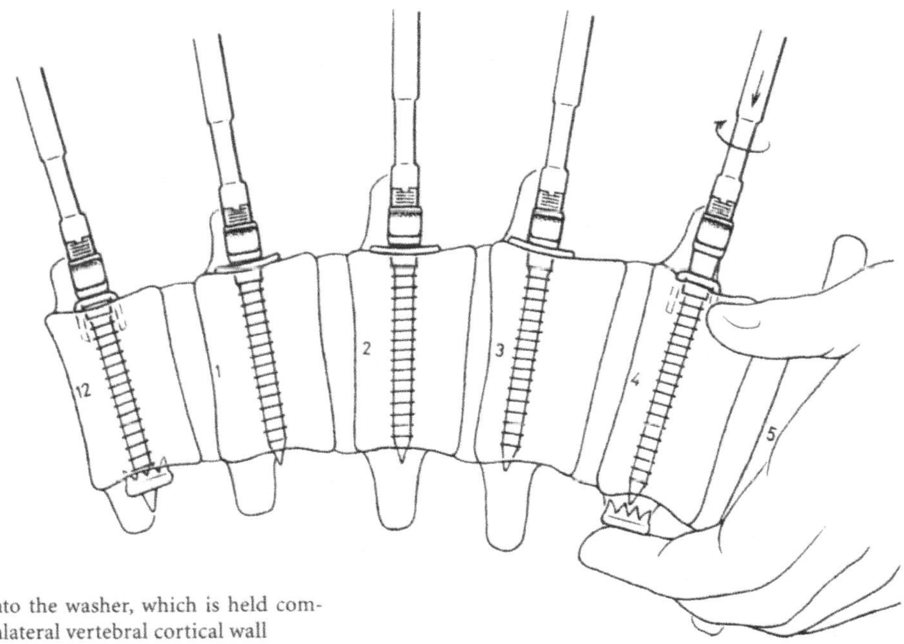

Fig. 8.91 Screw turned into the washer, which is held compressed towards the contralateral vertebral cortical wall

ing irons (Fig. 8.92c). The prepared rod is introduced into the most cranial and caudal screws. The most cranial screw is tightened with the rod in the position of the planned correction. The most caudal screw is left loose so that the rod can glide during the correction maneuver (Fig. 8.93). The remaining screws are now reduced to the rod using the complex reduction forceps beginning from the cranial (Fig. 8.94) and caudal end working towards the apex. The screw of the apex vertebra of the curve is therefore gradually brought close to the rod so that it becomes possible to lock this screw to the rod with the persuader. Bone grafts are inserted into the disk spaces to maintain the lordosis (Fig. 8.95). The spine elongates during the correction procedure and usually there are two disks which are

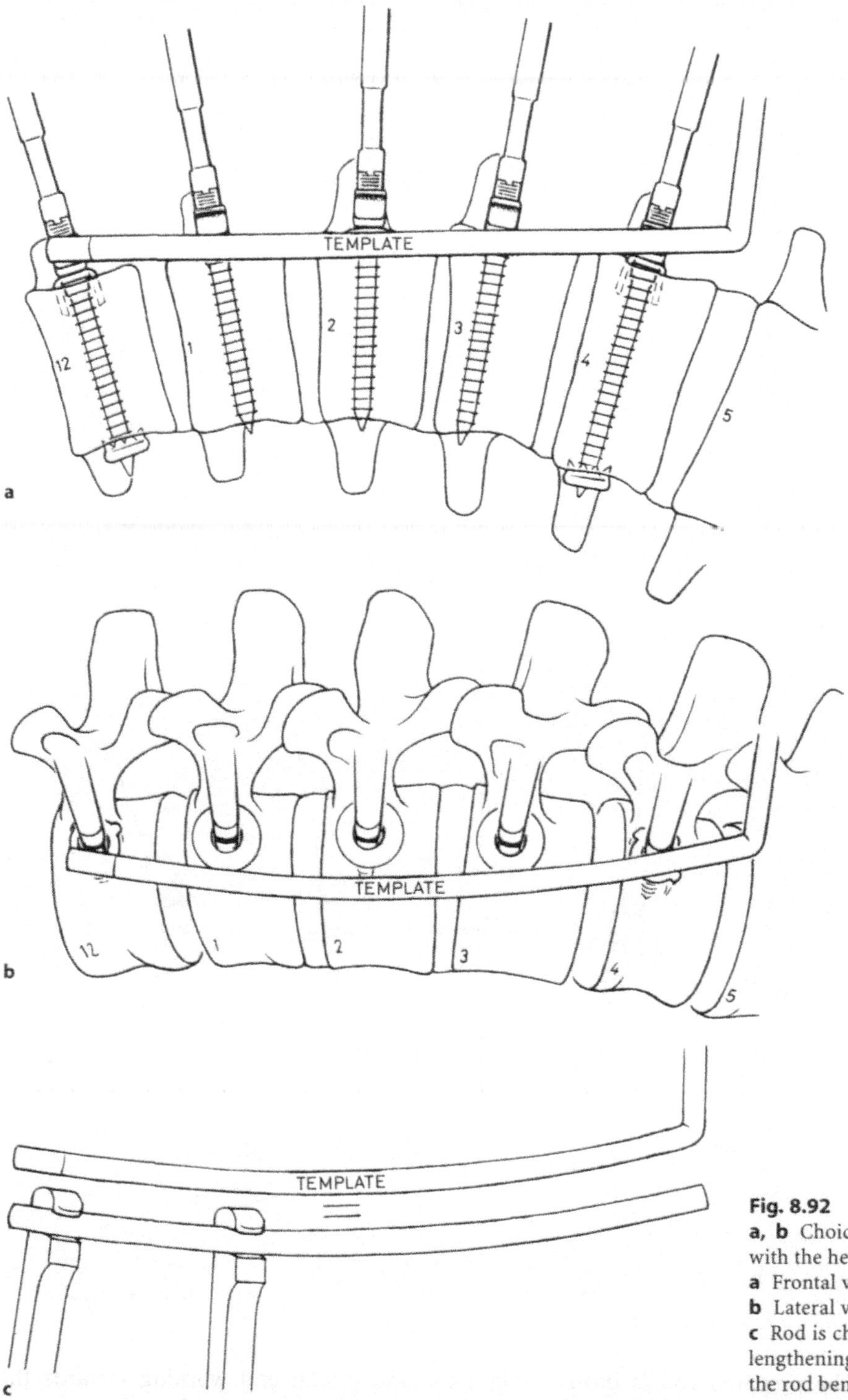

Fig. 8.92
a, b Choice of rod length and contour with the help of the template rod
a Frontal view
b Lateral view
c Rod is chosen 2 cm longer to allow the lengthening of the spine along the rod and the rod bent according to the template

gaping significantly; these can be filled with wedge-shaped femoral rings or titanium cages. The wedge-shaped grafts guarantee a good mechanical support.

The final step is to compress the grafts. It is necessary to have all screw heads loose except the top end-screw. In order to achieve this objective, the second cranial-screw is compressed against the locked end-screw (Fig. 8.96) by means of the rod holder in place and the distractor. *It is important not to allow the*

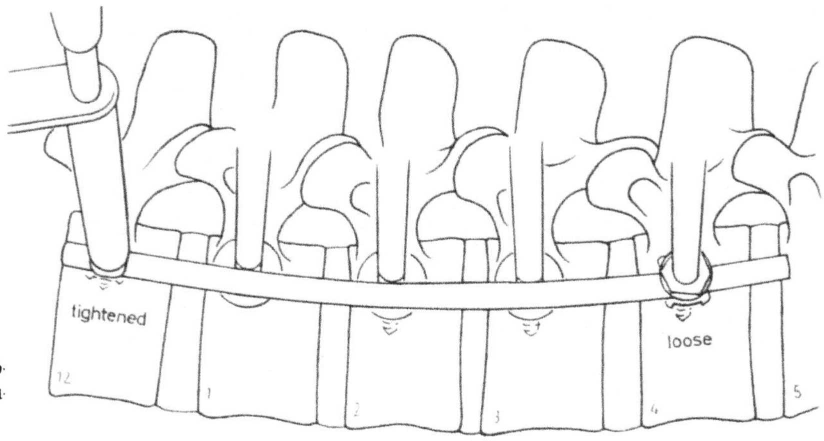

Fig. 8.93 The prepared rod is introduced into the most cranial and caudal screw

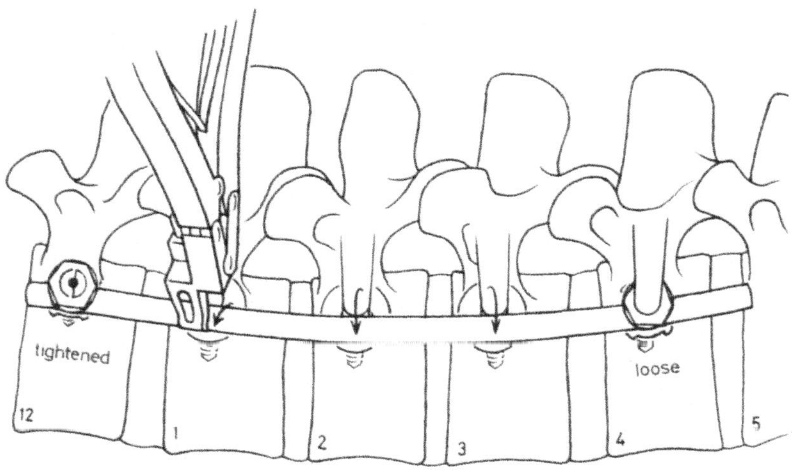

Fig. 8.94 Progressive reduction of all the screws to the rod with the crimper or the persuader. The open screw locks to the rod with the persuader

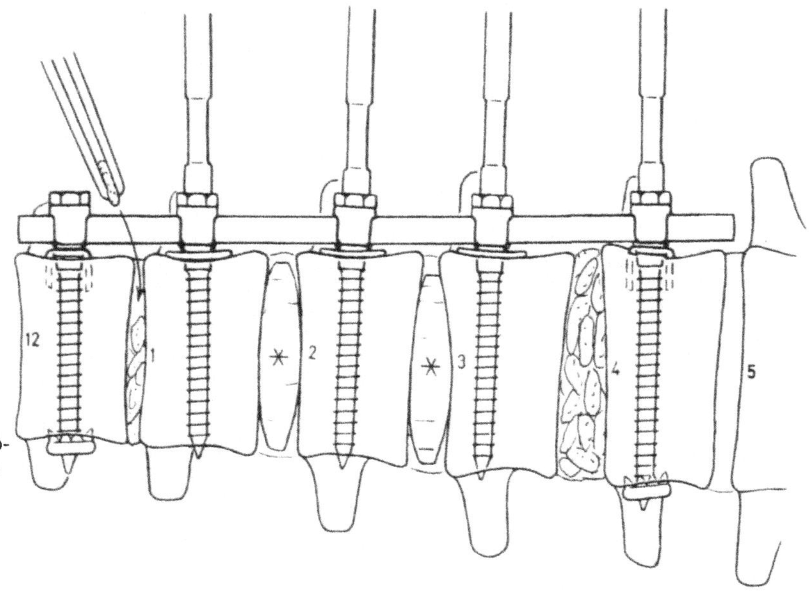

Fig. 8.95 Bone grafting with femoral rings (or titanium cages) of the widest disk spaces (*). The rest is filled with cancellous bone

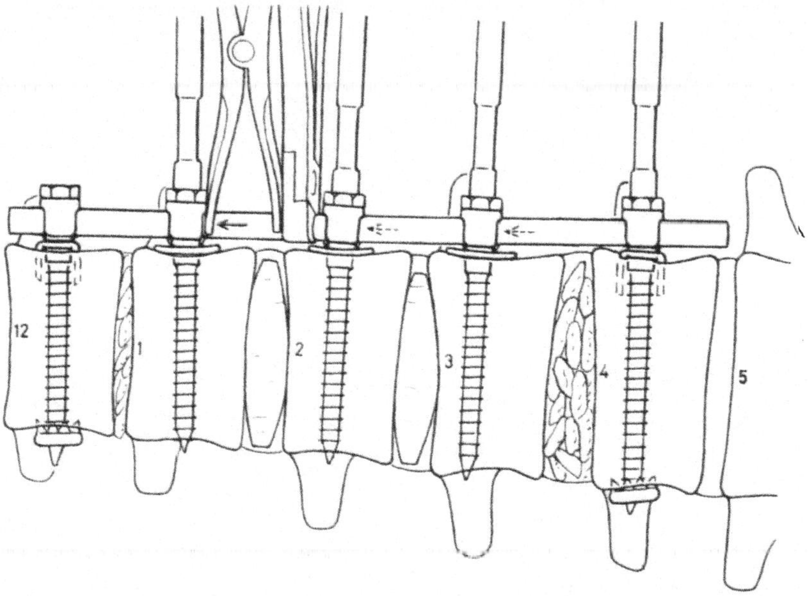

Fig. 8.96 Compression of the disk space with the grafts, using the distractor against the rod holder in place

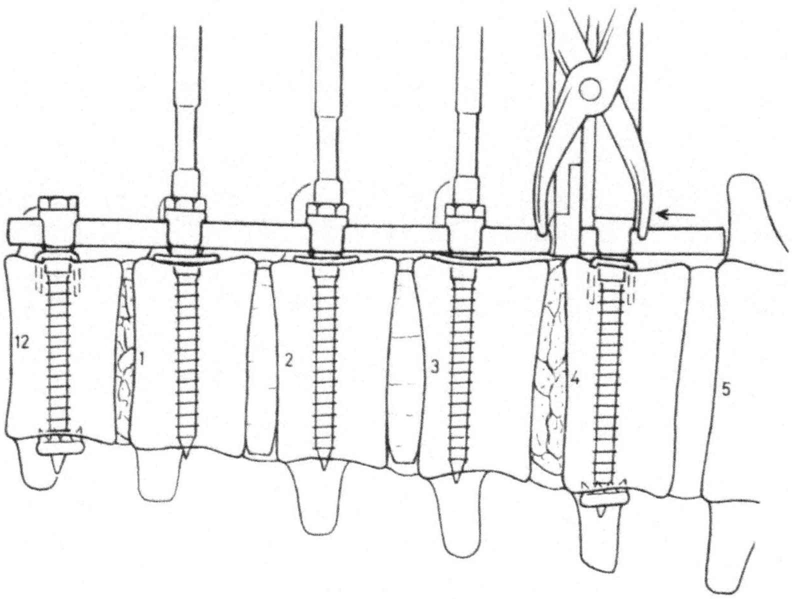

Fig. 8.97 Avoid angulation of the screw during compression and compression across the whole graft: the last screw is compressed against the rod holder with the compression clamp

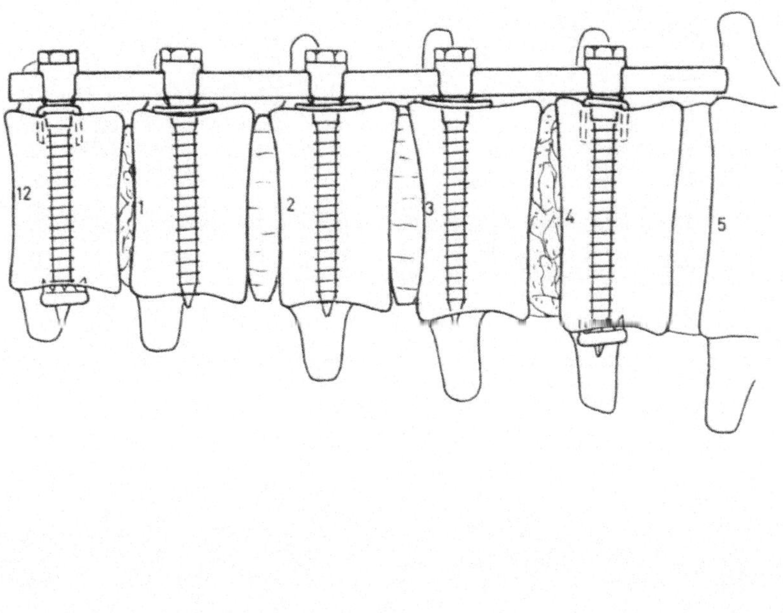

Fig. 8.98 Final rod screw configuration

screw to angulate during compression; the L-handle socket wrench and 6-mm socket must keep the screw parallel with the first screw, as this will allow compression across the whole graft. Each vertebra is derotated. The last screw is compressed against the rod holder with the compression clamp (Figs. 8.97, 8.98).

This technique restores the normal sagittal plane of the spine. If the rod is too long in the distal screw it can be cut with the rod cutter.

8.2.2.4
Kyphosis: Posterior Correction and Stabilization

Principles

The construct that is applied posteriorly acts like a tension band. Compression causes shortening of the spine, and distraction is not recommended in the correction of kyphotic deformities as this may cause elongation of the cord contents, which may affect cord perfusion with neurological consequneces. The side-opening hooks and screws make the assembly and correction of the deformity relatively simple. Preoperative planning of the insertion of the implants must be made. The standard construct for a thoracic Scheuermann's kyphosis would be between Th2 and L1. However, the exact area to be instrumented will be determined by the whole spine sagittal standing view and a forced extension view of the deformed area. The hooks are placed on alternate sides of the upper thoracic spine, spreading the load more evenly throughout the posterior lamina and allowing bone graft application at each level.

Preoperative Plan

The area of instrumentation is dictated by the length of the curve and flexibility. Anterior release through an open or endoscopic transthoracic approach may be necessary. For a standard kyphotic instrumentation we choose the thoracic spine between Th2 and L1. Cranial implants begin with a claw construct on each side (Fig. 8.99), one at Th2–Th3, the other at Th3–Th4. Pedicle hooks are inserted at alternate levels, the number depending upon the stiffness of the curve (Fig. 8.100a, b). It is possible to put pedicle hooks or screws on the same level above the apex of the kyphosis, in order to push the curve into correction. The caudal level can be instrumented with either pedicle screw or laminar hooks (Fig. 8.101a, c). If pedicle screws are used they must be protected from pull-out by laminar hooks on each side (Fig. 8.101b or c). Axial compression of the implant along the rods towards the upper claw increases the correction (Fig. 8.102a, b).

Cross-links are applied (Fig. 8.102 b).

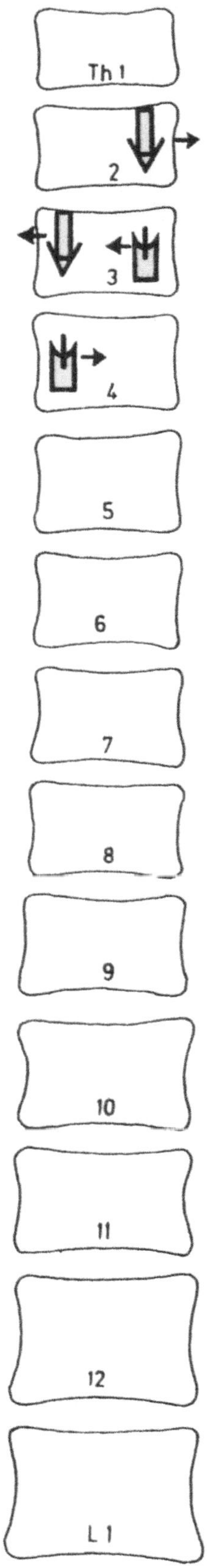

Fig. 8.99 Diagrammatic representation of cranial implants with a superior claw construct (left side T3–T4, right side T2–T3)

Surgical Technique

The spine is exposed with subperiosteal dissection between Th1 and L1. Initially the pedicle hooks with end-plate screws are inserted as in the preoperative plan (Fig. 8.99). The laminar hooks are inserted into left Th3 and right Th4. The ligamentum flavum is carefully removed and with a Kerison bone is removed to allow a close fit of the laminar hook. Pedicle screws are inserted with radiograph guidance into T12 and L1 (Fig. 8.101a). Alternatively a claw construct can be used (Fig. 8.101b, c).

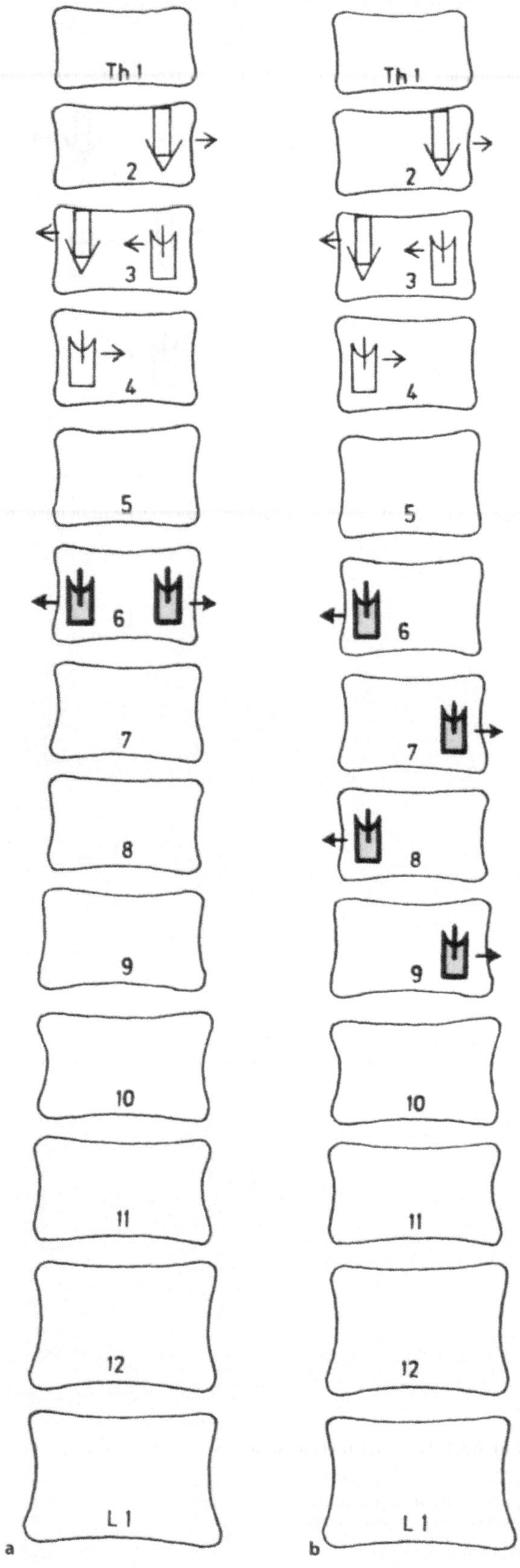

Fig. 8.100
a Insertion of pedicle hooks at the apex
b Alternative hook configuration

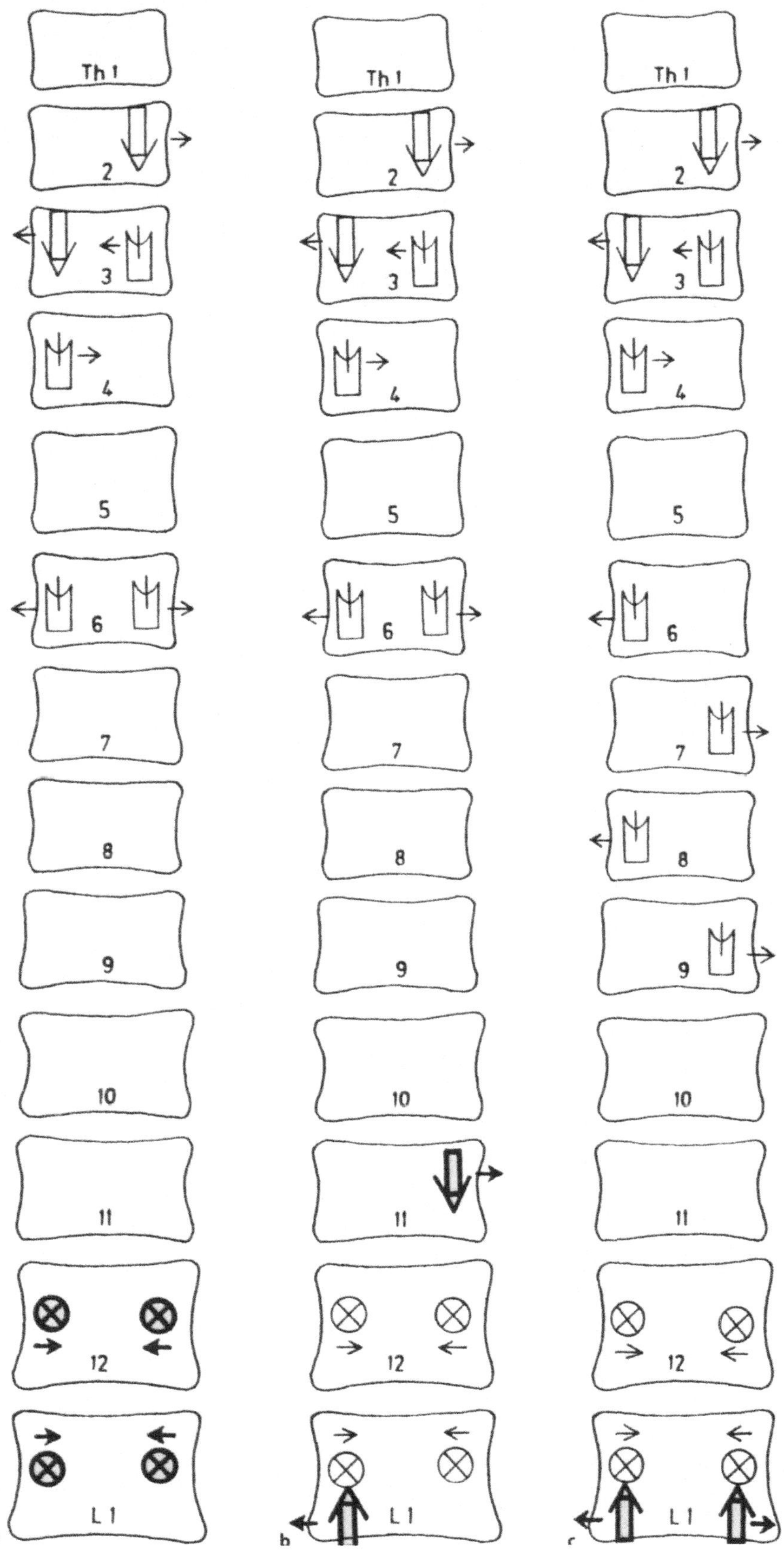

Fig. 8.101
a Caudal insertion of pedicle screws
b Protection of caudal pedicle screws with laminar hooks
c Alternative screw/hook configuration

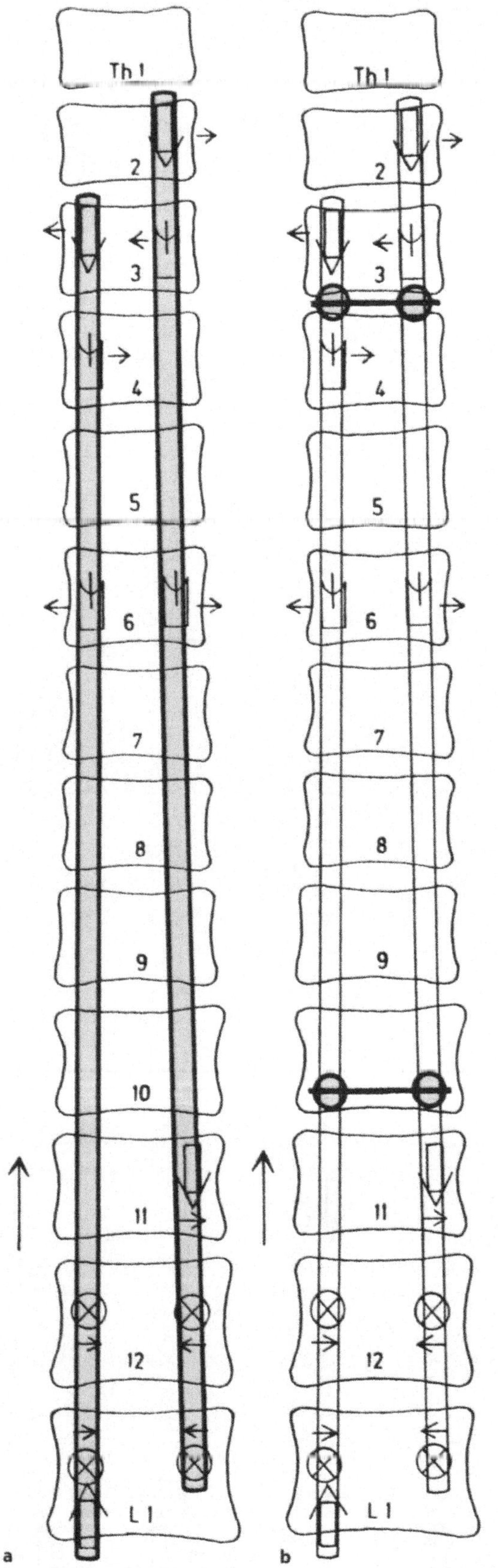

Fig. 8.102 Final construct:
a Compression along the rods against the top claw configuration
b Two cross-links inserted

A 6-mm rod template is placed between T4 and L1 to identify the length of the rod (Figs. 8.103, 8.104a). A normal sagittal plane kyphosis is built into the rod, using two rod holders to measure the kyphosis. If Titanium rods are used then the sagittal correction on the rods must be less than normal kyphosis as some bend will occur in the rod during correction. The T12–L1 level is straightened to allow a smooth transition from the thoracic kyphosis to the lumbar lordosis (Fig. 8.104b).

The 6-mm rods are now inserted into the upper pedicle hooks and the sleeve and nut dropped onto the hooks (Fig. 8.105a, b). The laminar hook is inserted and attached to the rod and the sleeve and nut dropped into place. The hook is controlled with the 6-mm socket wrench, and the nut is tightened with the 11-mm L-handled socket wrench (see Fig. 70a, b, c, d). The claw is now compressed (Fig. 8.105c), or alternatively a 6-mm rod holder is clamped caudally to the pedicle hook, a distractor is applied to the rod and with gentle distraction the rod is pushed distally and the laminar hook fits snugly around the lamina (see Fig.70a, b, c, d). This is repeated on the opposite side. The 6-mm rod is now inserted into the next caudal pedicle hook, compression is applied to the hook with the spreader, and the sleeve and nut are applied and tightened (Fig. 8.108).

This technique is applied at each level. *If the curve is particularly stiff then to prevent pull-out further laminar hooks can be attached to the rod* (Fig. 8.100b).

Two 6-mm rod holders are applied to the rods and then both are gently pushed down to T12 and L1 pedicle screws (Fig. 8.107a); if the rod is too long it can now be shortened. The rods are inserted into the lower screws and the nut and sleeves are loosely positioned (Fig. 8.107b). Compression is applied to the screws and the nuts tightened (Fig. 8.108). Laminar hooks are applied onto L1 and Th11. *The position of these hooks will vary depending upon available space on the 6-mm rods.* Finally two cross-links are applied (Fig. 8.102b).

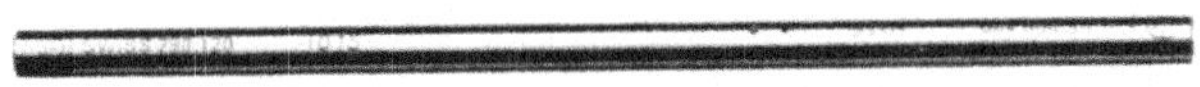

a

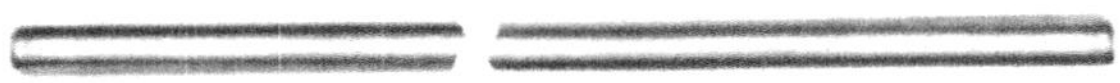

b

Fig. 8.103
a USS rod, 6 mm diameter, hard
b USS bending template

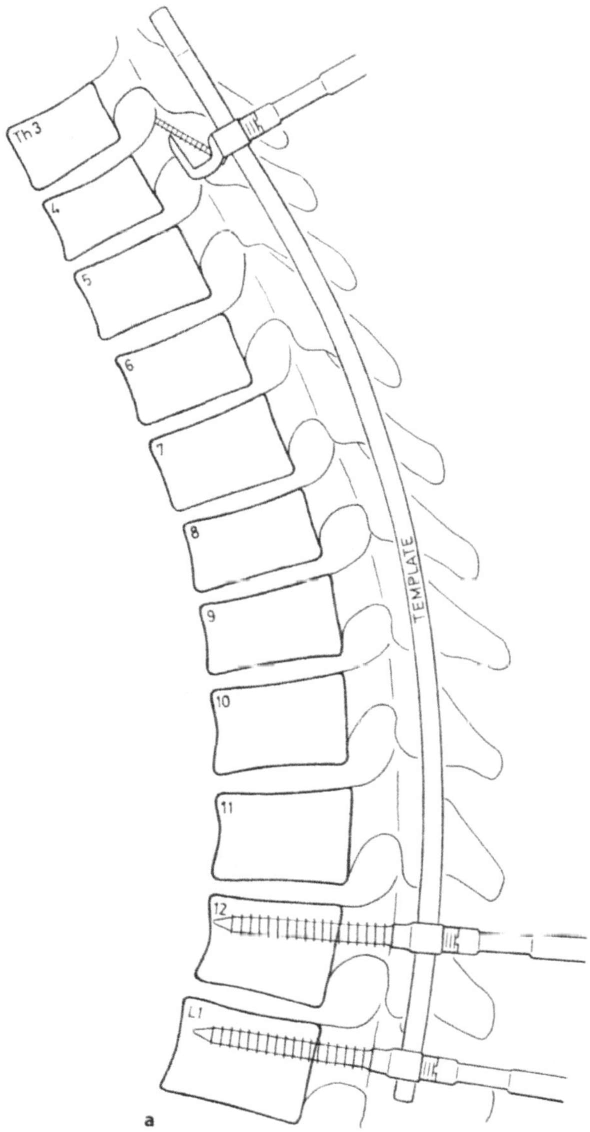

a

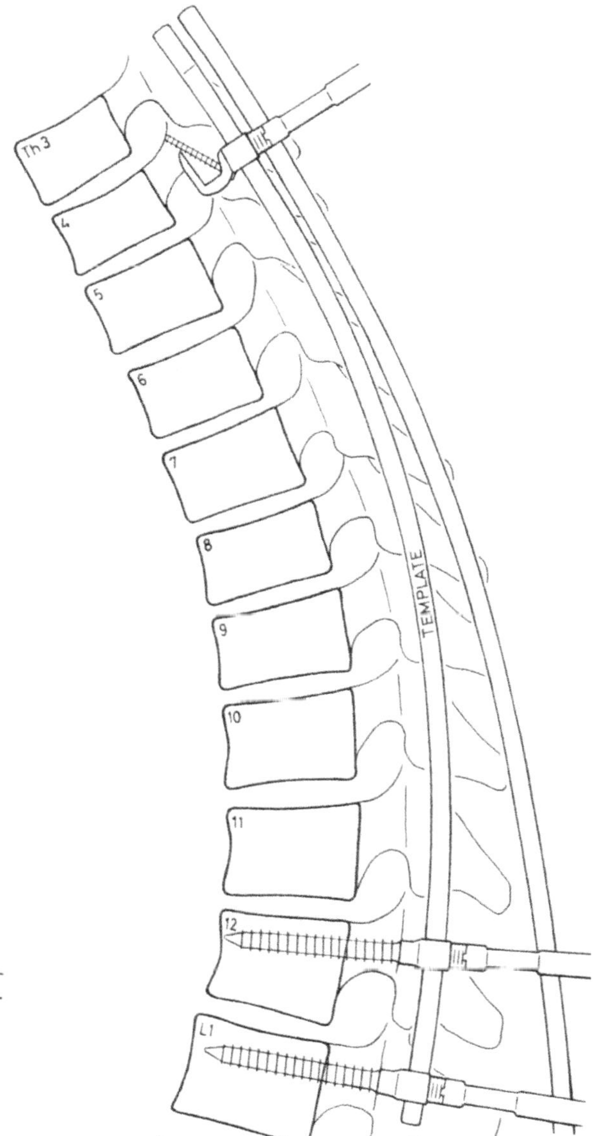

b

Fig. 8.104
a Rod template bent along the spine to fit the hooks and screws
b Definite rod bent less than template, but appropriate to the amount of spine correction

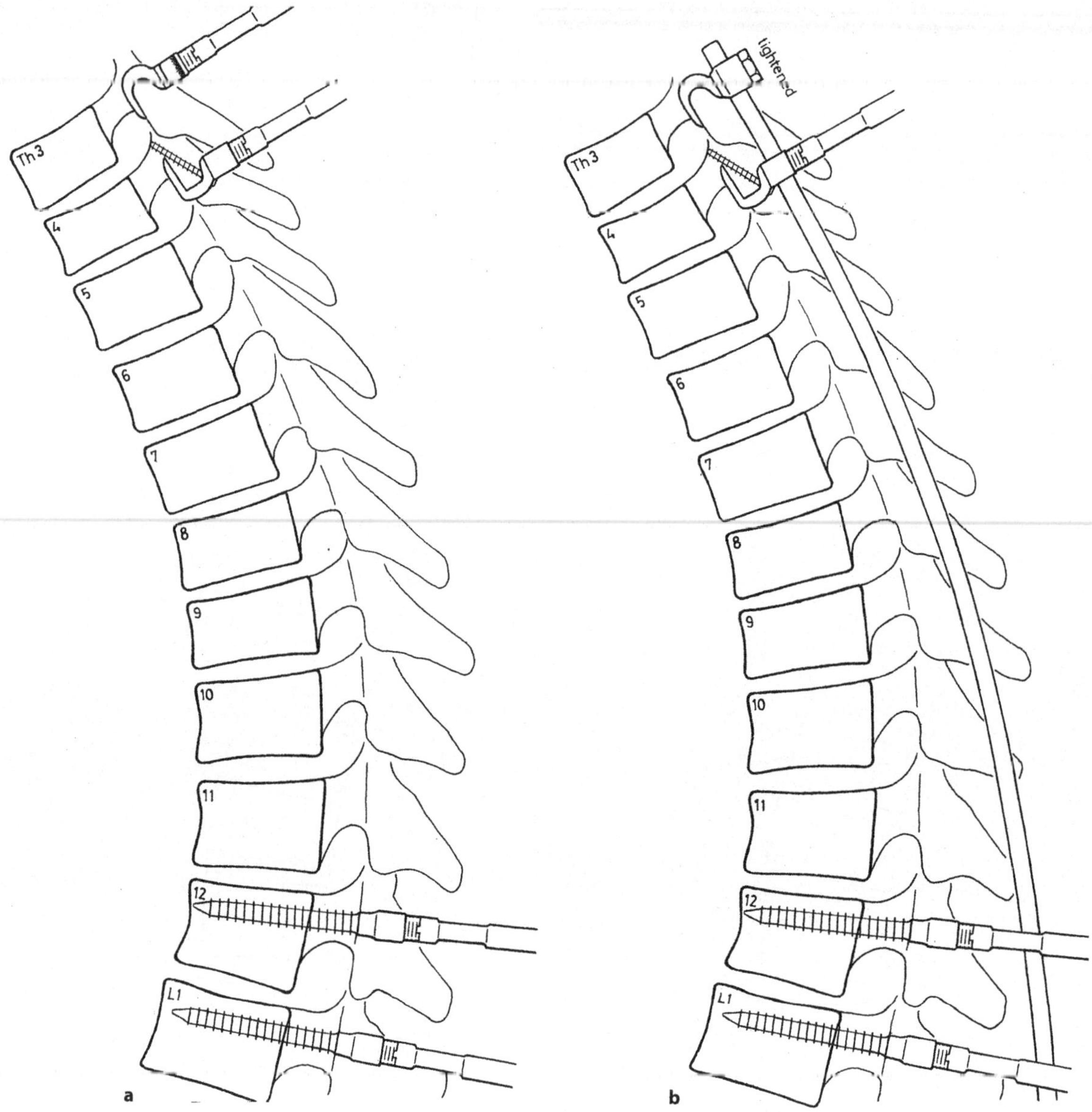

Fig. 8.105a Construction of the cranial claw configuration **b** Application of 6-mm rod into pedicle hook and attachment of hook and sleeve and insertion and tightening of laminar hook

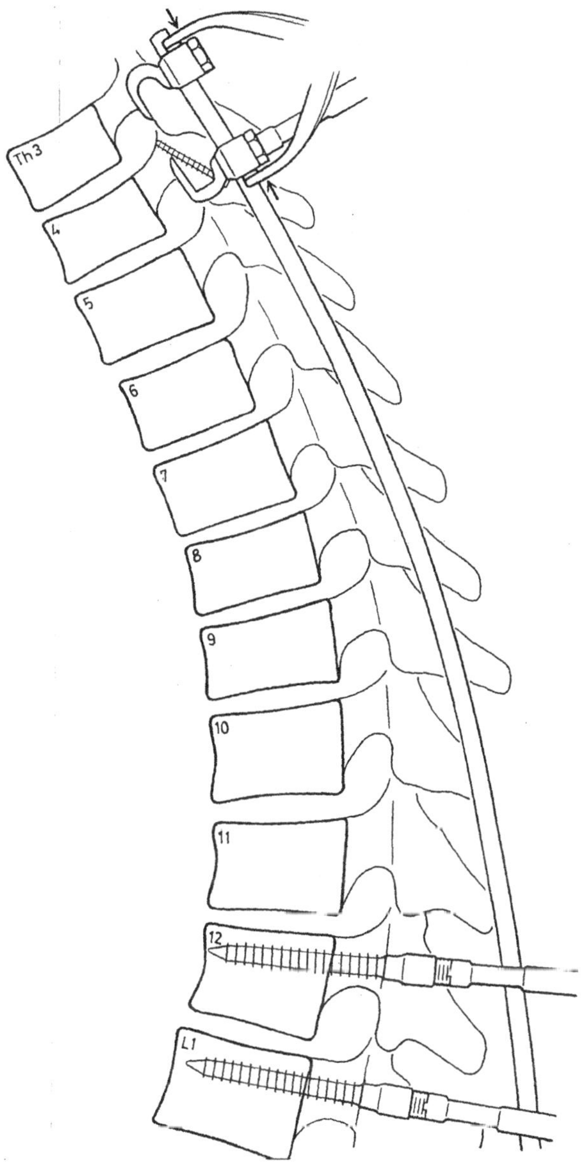

Fig. 8.105c Compression of claw

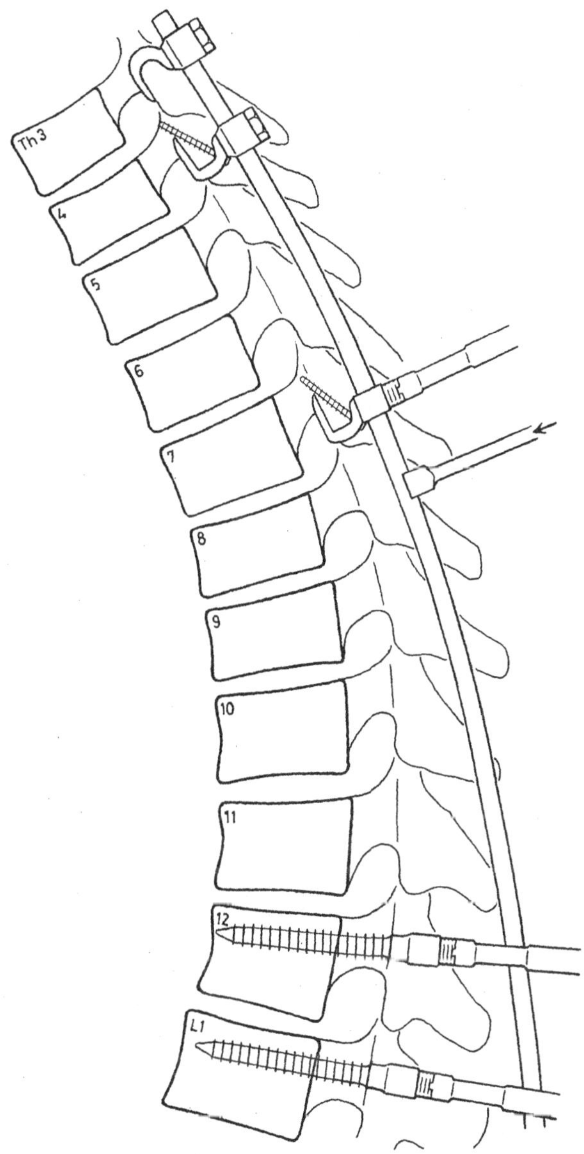

Fig. 8.106 Insertion of the rod into the apical pedicle hook

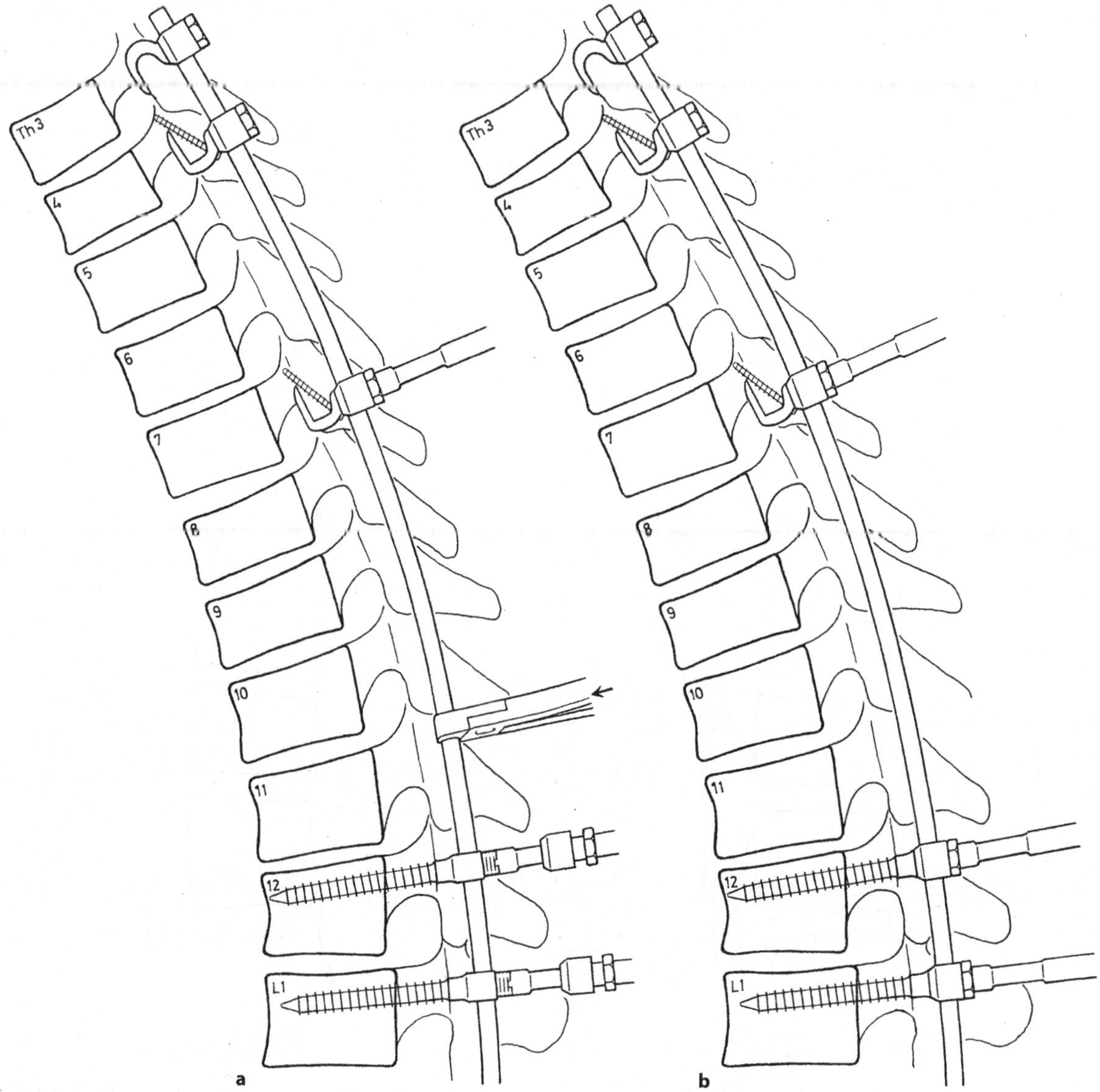

Fig. 8.107

a Reduction of rod to lower pedicle screws

b Attachment to the pedicle screw

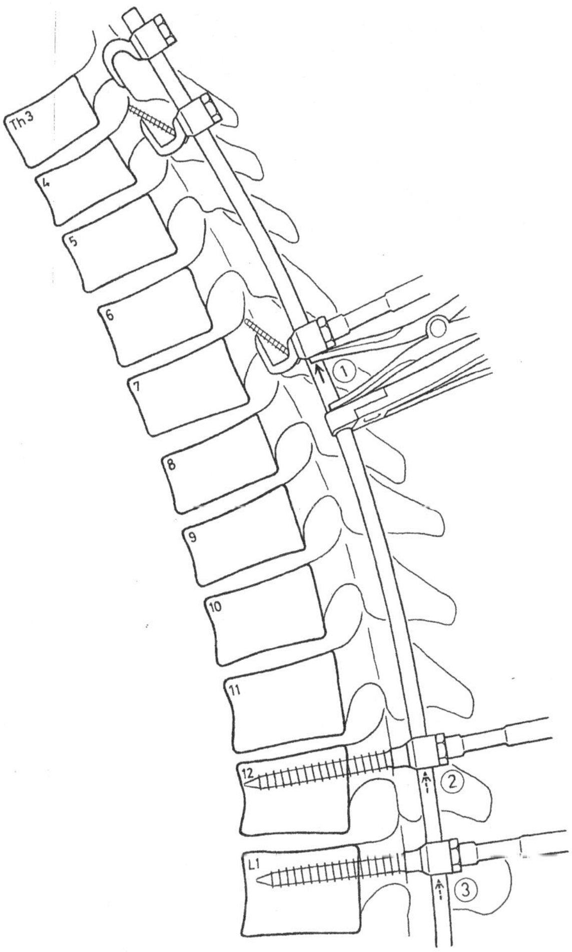

Fig. 8.108 Compression applied to screw

8.2.3 USS for the Degenerative Lumbosacral Spine

8.2.3.1 Standard Fixation

Basic Principles and Instrumentation

In many instances of degenerative lumbar spine disease an internal fixation over one or several segments may be considered as indicated to enhance the posterior fusion, to stabilize the spine area in the position which is recognized as the most balanced, or to stabilize an obvious unstable segment. It is not the purpose of this chapter to discuss the need of internal fixation for degenerative lumbar spine disease, which may still be controversial for certain indications. The goal of this chapter is to provide the appropriate surgical technique to the surgeon when he feels internal fixation is necessary. The reader is referred to the original literature and textbooks for discussion of the position of internal fixation in the treatment of lumbar degenerative spine disorders.

The stabilization of the lumbar and lumbosacral spine is unthinkable today without the use of pedicle screws. Therefore the application of the USS in the degenerative lumbar and lumbosacral spine is based on pedicle screw fixation and we do not think that hooks are any more a valid alternative except in very rare cases. There are a variety of possibilities available for the fixation in the sacrum, either by the same standard pedicle screws or by a special sacral implant (see p. 186, chapter 8.2.3.2).

Indications

- Degenerative instability (uni- to multisegmental), e.g., degenerative spondylolisthesis.
- Iatrogenic instability after decompressive surgery.
- Concomitant procedure when a laminectomy is performed.
- Adult degenerative scoliosis.

Advantages

- Immediate stability for postoperative mobilization.
- Only light orthosis necessary.
- Enhancement of the fusion healing.
- Correction of a deformity possible.
- Preservation of the sagittal profile.

Disadvantages
- Complications from the pedicle screw insertion.
- Complications from the implant (screw breakage, rod breakage).
- Infection rate higher.

Implants and Instruments (Fig. 8.109, 110)
The procedure is typically used for the treatment of the lumbar and lumbosacral degenerative spine.

Pedicle Screws: Side-Opening Screws. The head of the side-opening screw conforms with the head of the hooks. The advantage of these screws is that they can be exchanged, added or removed any time without the need to uncouple the whole montage. This is not possible with back-opening screws. The side-opening screws are available with a 5-, 6- or 7-mm-diameter thread and a length of 30–60 mm. Most of the lumbar pedicles take a 6-mm screw, the S1 pedicle and in tall and heavy people the lower lumbar pedicles can also be instrumented with a 7-mm screw (Fig. 8.109). The screws are self-tapping.

A screwdriver with holding sleeve and universal handle is used for the screw insertion (Fig. 8.110a–c). The screw can be lifted directly from the screw pack. The screwdriver is inserted into the screw head and the holding sleeve lowered and turned clockwise to complete the connection (Fig. 8.111a, b). The sleeve and nut are prepared on the screw rack for loading, into the 11-mm cannulated socket wrench with a straight handle (Fig. 8.112).

The nut and sleeve is loaded onto the 11-mm cannulated socket wrench. Alternatively, the screw extension stick can be mounted on the screw and used as a screwdriver with the universal handle (Fig. 8.114 or see page 129 Fig. 18.18–18.23). With this handle the stick can be easily removed or the handle itself can be removed separately leaving the extension stick in place. The extension stick can be used as a guide to facilitate the insertion of the nut and sleeve (Fig. 8.115) as well as for the cannulated socket wrench and also for the complex reduction forceps *(persuader)* (Fig. 8.116). When the socket wrench is loaded and the screws have been prepared the rod is inserted into the screw heads. The rod has to be exactly 90° to the head of the screw. With the rod in place the sleeve and nut are released (Fig. 8.115) and the socket wrench is used to bring down the sleeve and nut. The smaller side of the sleeve comes down onto the rod and the nut is then tightened.

The rod-crimping pliers are used if there is difficulty introducing the rod into the side-opening (Fig. 8.117). In situations where the rod tends to jump off the screw head before the sleeve and nut

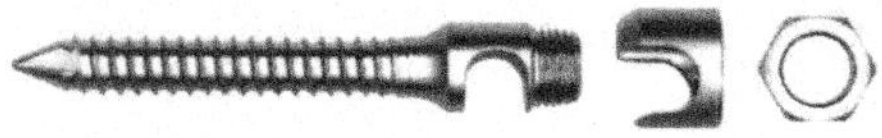

Fig. 8.109 Side-opening pedicle screws. 5, 6 and 7 mm in length and 30–60 mm in diameter

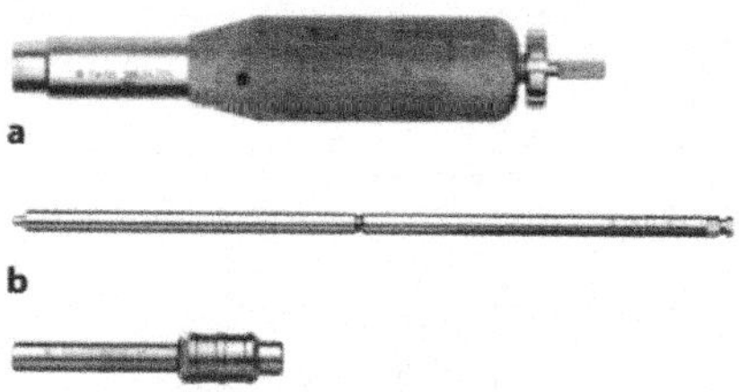

Fig. 8.110
a The U.S.S universal handle
b The screwdriver insert for the side-opening pedicle screws
c The holding sleeve for the screwdriver

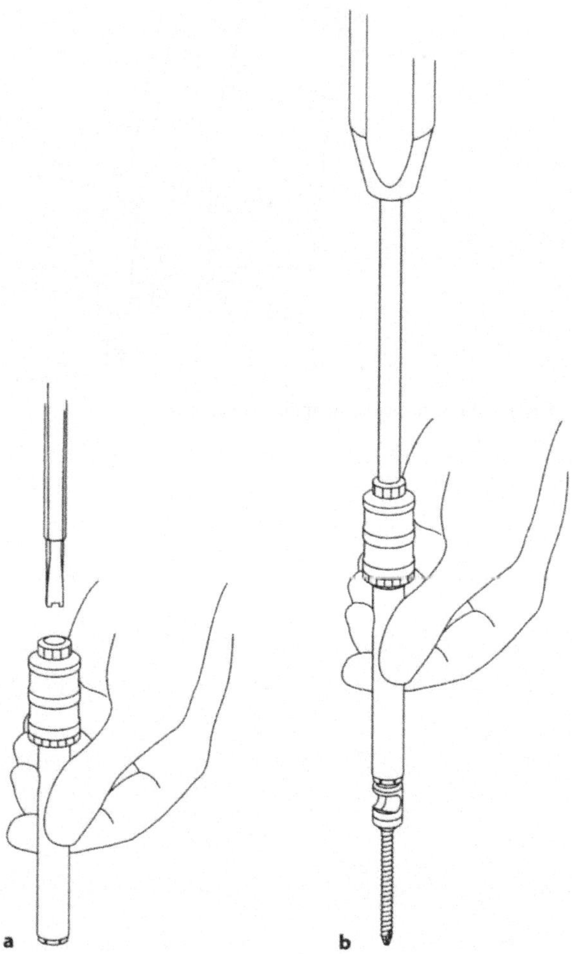

Fig. 8.111
a Screwdriver with mounted holding sleeve
b The screw is held by the sleeve on the screwdriver, which fits firmly to the screwhead when the sleeve is tightened clockwise to complete the connection

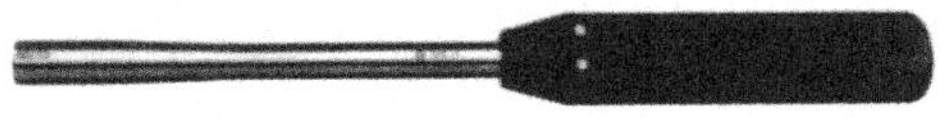

Fig. 8.112 Socket wrench with a spring mechanism at the bottom to hold the sleeve and nut in place

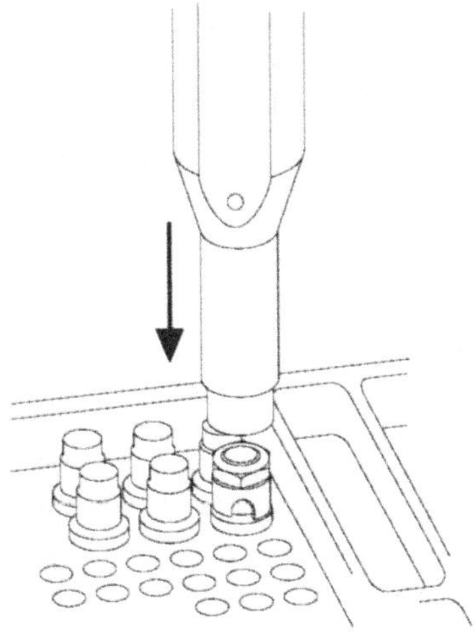

Fig. 8.113 Insertion for nut and sleeve: First the nut and then the sleeve can be directly loaded to the insertion instrument

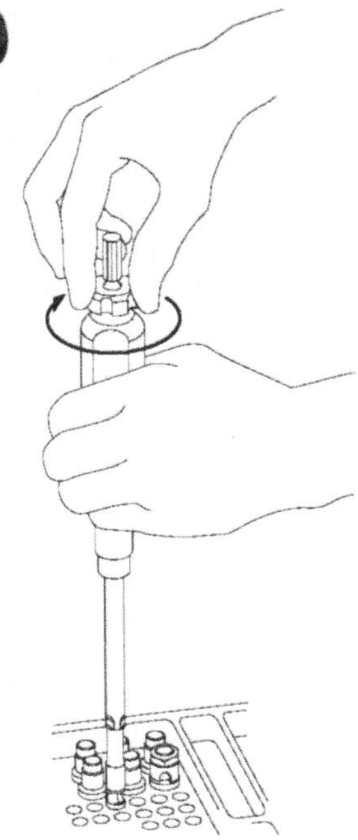

Fig. 8.114 Extension stick for holding the screws and hooks which is screwed onto the screw/hook head. While holding the handle, the nut on the top is rotated to attach the extension stick to the screw

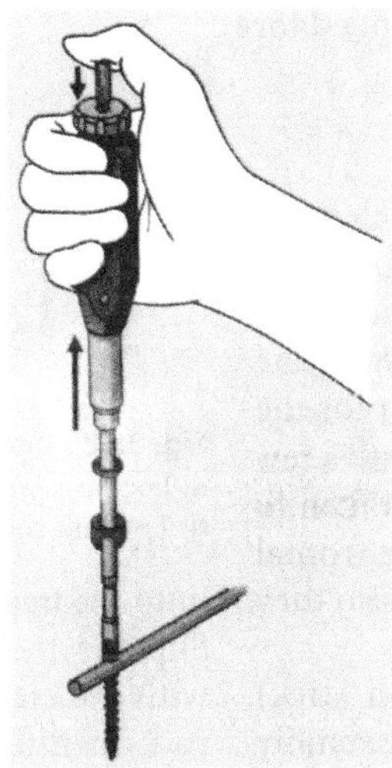

Fig. 8.115 Compression of the nut on top of USS universal handle releases the nut and sleeve and the extension stick acts as a guide

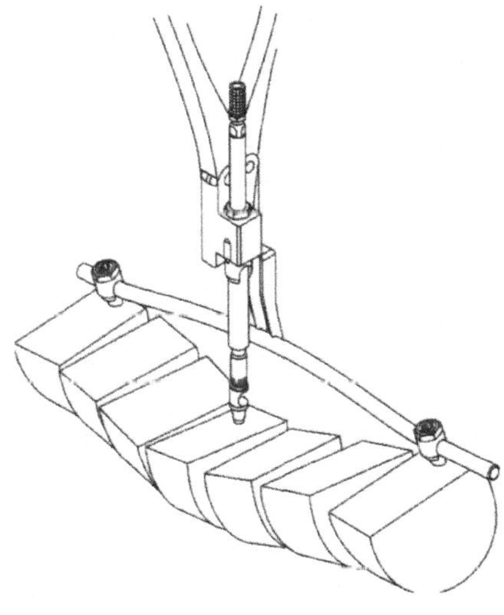

Fig. 8.116 The complex reduction forceps used over the extension stick to reduce the anchorage to the 6 mm USS rod

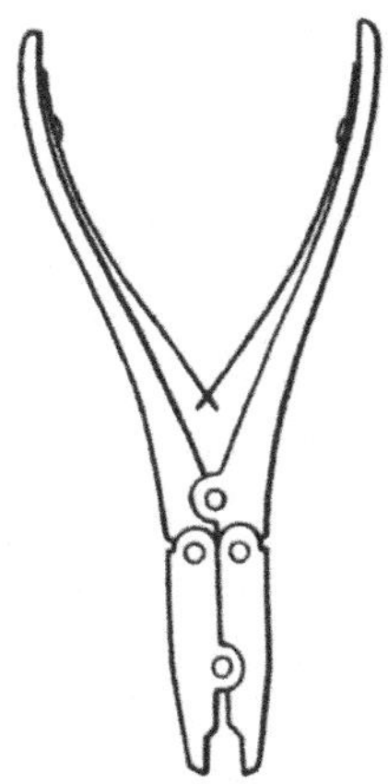

8.117a

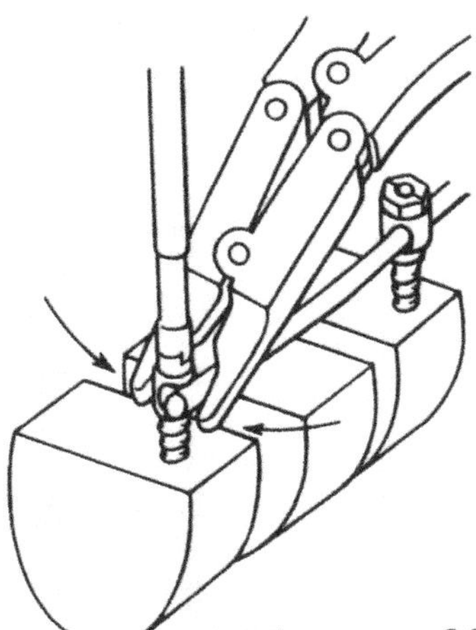

8.117b

Fig. 8.117 a, b The USS rod crimply pliers with which the rod can be brought into the lateral open screw head and extension stick

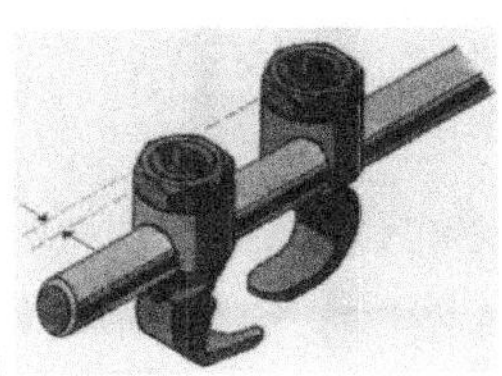

8.118

Fig. 8.118 If the rod is connected to the screws from opposite sides, they can compensate for a hooks 4-mm anatomic offset without having to bend the rod can be lowered down onto the screw head/rod compound, the *persuader* (complex reduction forceps) can be used (Fig. 8.116).

If the rod is connected to the screws from the opposite sides, they can compensate for a 4-mm anatomic offset without having to bend the rod (Fig. 8.118). The pedicle can be compressed or distracted with the compression or distraction forceps and the hexagonal rods tightened (see page 154 Fig. 8.70).

Pedicle Screws: Variable Axis Screw. This screw has the same thread dimensions as the standard side-opening pedicle screw and is available in 6-mm, 7-mm and 8-mm thread diameters, and 30–60 mm lengths (in 5-mm increments). The variable axis screw consists of the titanium nut, collar, locking ring and rod-screw connector (Fig. 8.119a). It is colour coded deep blue to differentiate it from the side-opening screws. The variable axis allows 36° of angulation of the screw (72° of angulation in any plane) to facilitate rod-to-screw connection (Fig 8.119b). The angulation minimises the need for rod contouring.

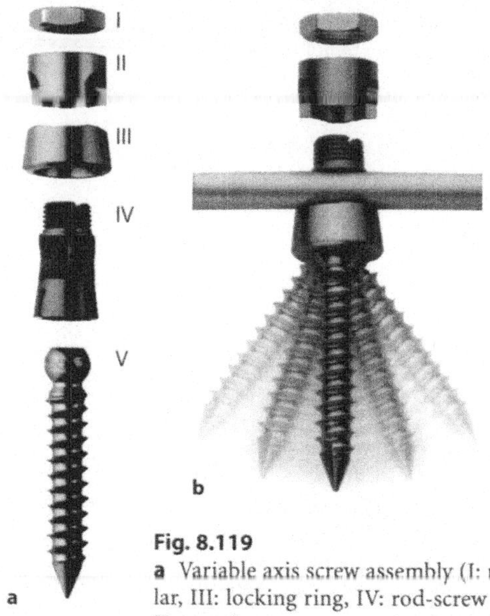

Fig. 8.119
a Variable axis screw assembly (I: nut, II: collar, III: locking ring, IV: rod-screw connector, V: screw)
b 36° angulation around the axis of the screw

Special Instruments (Fig. 8.120 b)
Surgical technique: The appropriate pedicles are prepared with the awl and probe. The length of the required screw is obtained by measuring the depth with a depth gauge. It is important to decorticate around the head of the screw to allow room for the locking ring to seat properly over the rod and screw connector and screw head. Care should be taken to align the screws along the same axis in the frontal plane. This may require adjusting the screws so they are all at approximately the same height.

Fasten the hook/screw holder (extension stick) onto the rod/screw connector. Snap the assembly onto the head of the variable axis screw (Fig 8.121a). Slip the locking ring over the hook/screw holder with the etching on the locking ring parallel to the rod opening in the rod or screw connector. The

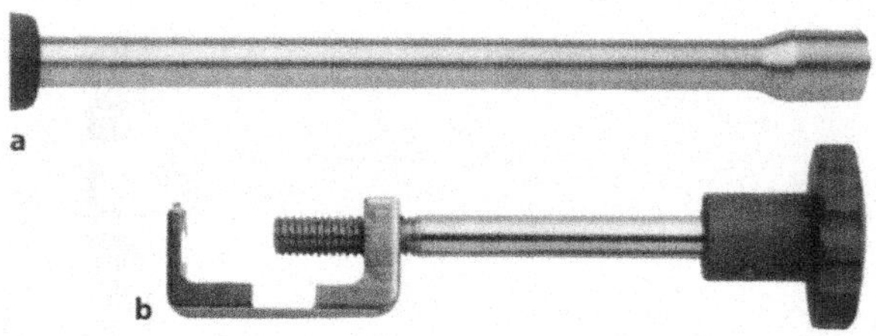

Fig. 8.120 Special Instruments
a Locking ring impactor
b Locking ring extractor

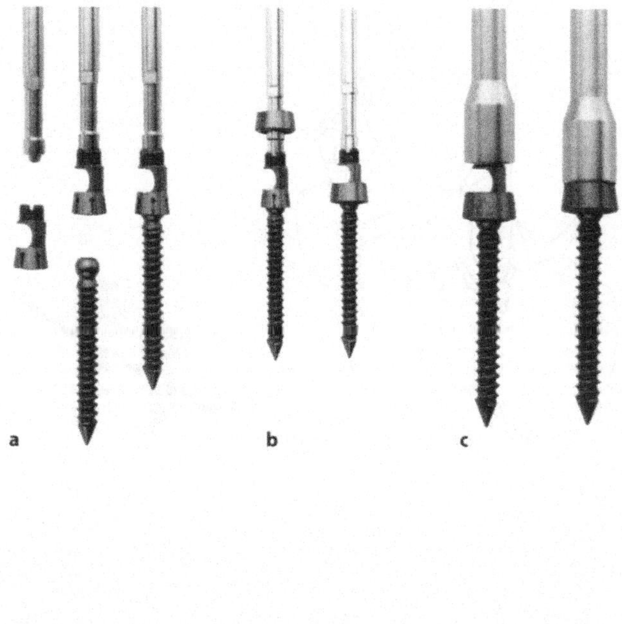

Fig. 8.121
a Hook/screw holder (extension stick) is attached to the rod and screw connector and is snapped onto the variable axis screw
b Slip the locking ring over the hook/screw holder, with the etching on the locking ring parallel to the rod opening in the rod/screw connector
c The locking ring is impacted onto the head of the screw using the locking ring impactor

hook/screw holder is used to guide the ring into position (Fig. 8.121b). *Prior to rod insertion the locking ring may be impacted onto the head of the screw using the locking ring impactor* (Fig. 8.121c). Impaction of the ring ensures the rod screw connector is securely placed over the screw head prior to manipulation. The rod template is used to determine the length and contour of the rod. The *soft* 6-mm titanium rod (Fig. 8.122) is contoured in the usual way (Fig. 8.123a, b).

Orientate the side-opening screws parallel to the rod (Fig. 8.124a) and use the rod crimping pliers to approximate the rod into the side opening screw (Fig. 124b). Load the collar for the variable axis screw and a hexagonal nut onto the loading posts in the tray and align the 11-mm socket wrench over the loading post and apply pressure (Fig. 124c). Place the loaded wrench over the head of the implant and turn clockwise to tighten the nut and secure the assembly (Fig. 8.124d). At this stage compression or

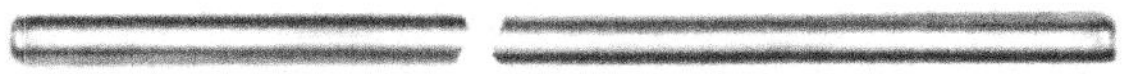

Fig. 8.122 6 mm rod comes in two different types: soft rod, length 50 – 150 mm; hard rod, length 200 – 500 mm

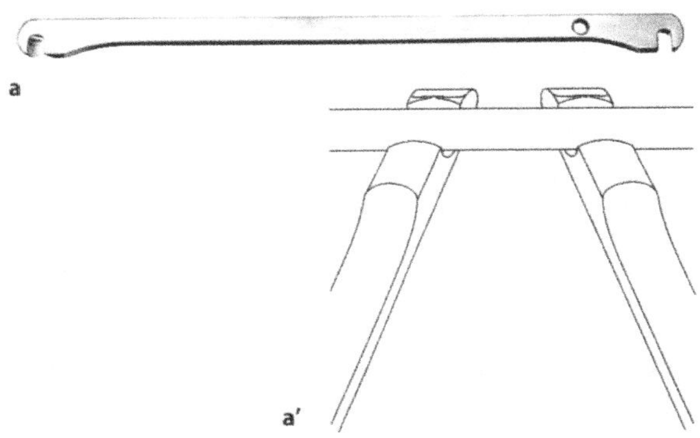

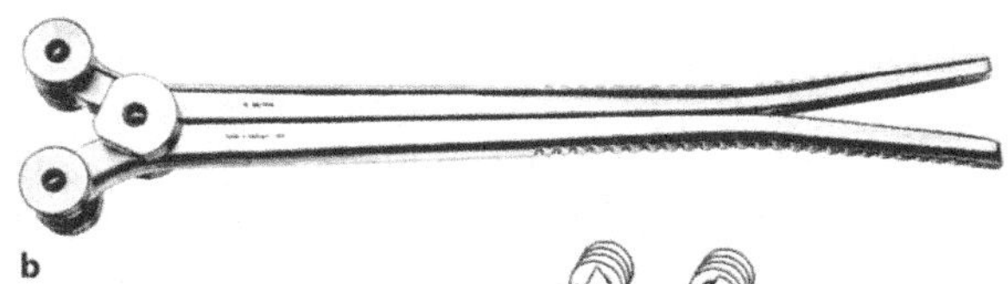

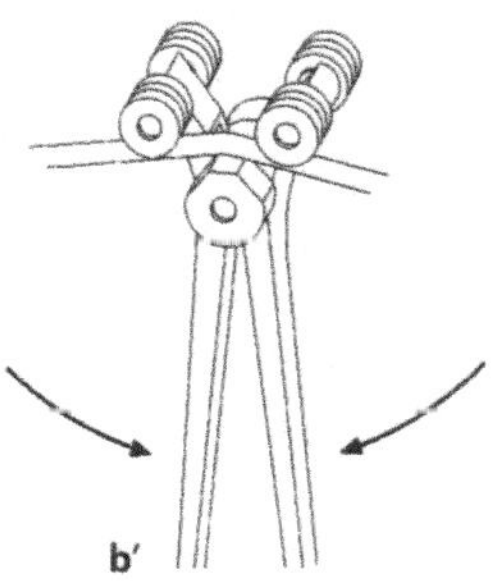

Fig. 8.123
a Bending iron
b Bending pliers

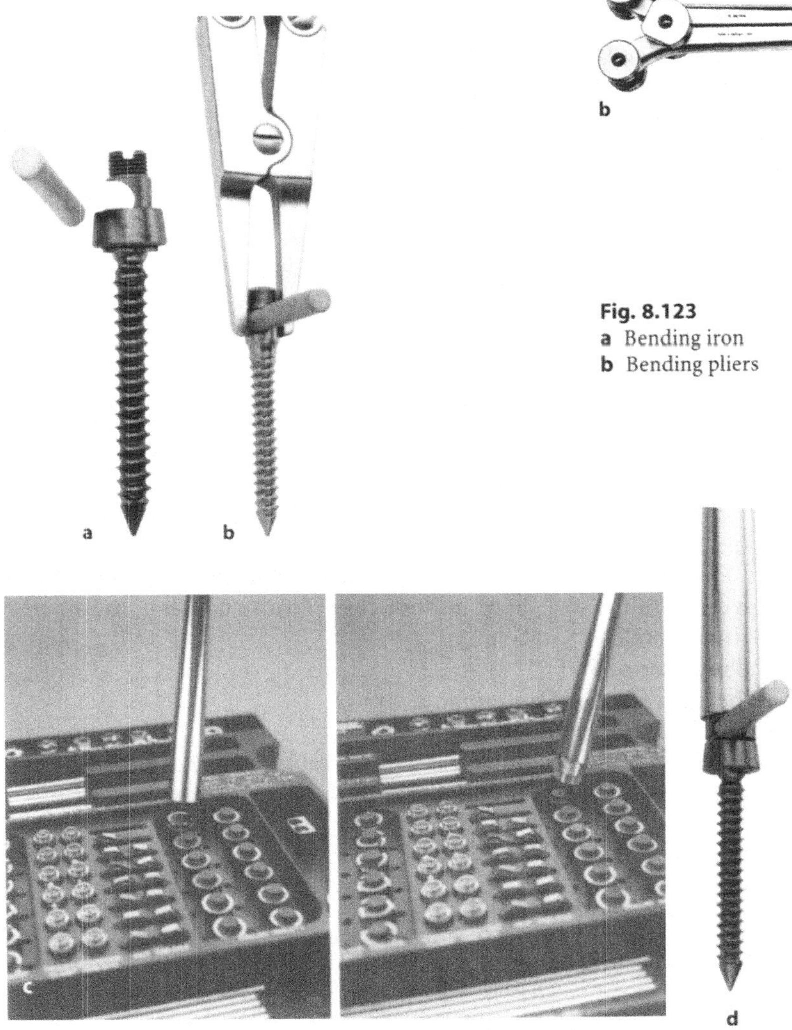

Fig. 8.124
a Orientate the side opening screw parallel to the rod
b Use the rod crimping pliers to approximate the rod onto the side-opening screw
c 11-mm socket wrench is applied over the hexagonal screw and sleeve
d The 11-mm loaded socket wrench is placed over the head of the implant

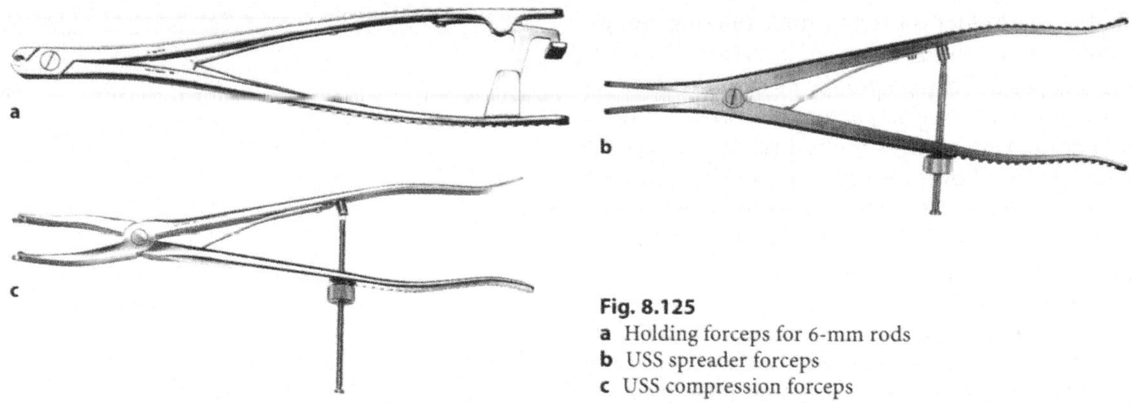

Fig. 8.125
a Holding forceps for 6-mm rods
b USS spreader forceps
c USS compression forceps

distraction can be applied with the holding forceps and either the USS spreader forceps, USS compression forceps as previously described (Fig. 8.125). The 11-mm L-handle socket wrench is used with 6-mm socket wrench over the straight hook/screw holder (extension stick) to tighten the hexagonal nut (page 131, Fig. 8.24).

Alternatively remove the holding sleeve for the screwdriver and place it with the 11-mm L-handle socket wrench onto the hexagonal nut and tighten. This prevents torque on the screw. A cross-link is finally added to the construct. The locking ring extractor (Fig. 120b) is used to dislodge the locking ring of the variable axis screw from the skirt of the connector to allow for removal or replacement of the variable axis screw.

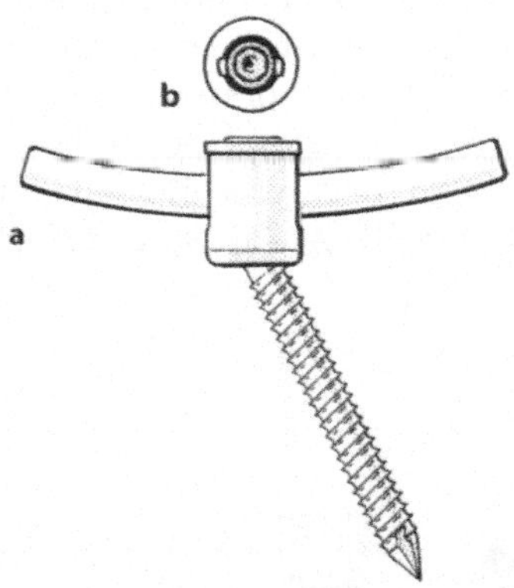

Fig. 8.126
a The pedicle screw with the 3D-head which allows ± 25 ° of freedom of movement in all directions
b The locking cap

Pedicle Screws – Back Opening Screws (Click'X)
The new polyaxial pedicle screw system has been developed for low back surgery. The screw consists of cylindrical pedicle screws, 3D-heads which are clicked on the pedicle screws and locking caps. The pedicle screw have a 'double thread' which doubles the speed of insertion while keeping the thread properties of the USS Pedicle Screws. Once the 3D-head is clicked on, it offers ± 25 ° of freedom in all directions (Fig. 8.126a). This allows sagittal as well as lateral screw offset which reduces the need for precise rod contouring or even allows the use of pre-bent rods simplifying the handling. The pre-bent rods are heat treated after the bending process (normalised) to guarantee the same physical properties as straight rods.

The locking cap consists of a ring to close the back opening screw head and an inner (blue) set screw to fix the rod and the polyaxial freedom of the 3D-head (Fig. 8.126b)

Indications
- Degenerative spinal instabilities (uni-multisegmental) e.g. degenerative spondylolisthesis.
- iatrogenic instability after decompressive surgery
- fractures with intact posterior wall or with stable bone graft or cage reconstruction of the anterior column.

Contraindications
- Deformities
- Fractures with unstable interior column support[1]
- Tumours[1]

1 Pedicle screws should only be used to supplement anterior column reconstruction with bone graft or cages.

Implants (Fig. 8.127a, b)

Instruments (Fig. 8.128)

Surgical technique
The pedicle is opened as decribed earlier and the depth measured. The appropiate pedicle screw is picked up directly from the screw rack using the self-holding screwdriver and inserted into the pedicle (Fig. 8.129a). Make sure there is enough space und and around the ball top of the pedicle screw to be able to click on the 3D-head. Take care to align the top of the crews in one plane.

Pick up the 3D-head directly from the screw rack using the self-holding positioning holder. Click the 3D heads on each inserted pedicle screw (Fig. 8.129b).

Use the rod template to predeterminate the correct length and contour of the 6 mm USS soft rod (Fig. 8.129c). Note, the ± 25 ° of freedom of the 3D-head compensates a certain lateral screw offset which reduces the need for precise rod-contouring.

Note: Titanium rods must not be bent more than 45 °. Care must be taken that rods are not bent forwards and backwards (danger of breakage).

Insert the rod into the aligned 3D-heads using the USS rod holder (Fig. 8.129d). Use the rod pusher to push the rod into the 3D-head (Fig. 8.129e). In constructions with more than two pedicle screws per side, start with the most central 3D-head.

Pick up the locking cap from the screw rack using the self-holding screwdriver, slide it through the already placed rod pusher onto the 3D-head and tighten it (Fig. 8.129f). The rod is now secured in the 3D-head which still has its polyaxial freedom. Repeat for all remaining 3D-heads before tightening the blue set screws using the hexagonal screwdriver. The rod pusher is used to counteract the tightening moment (Fig. 8.129g).

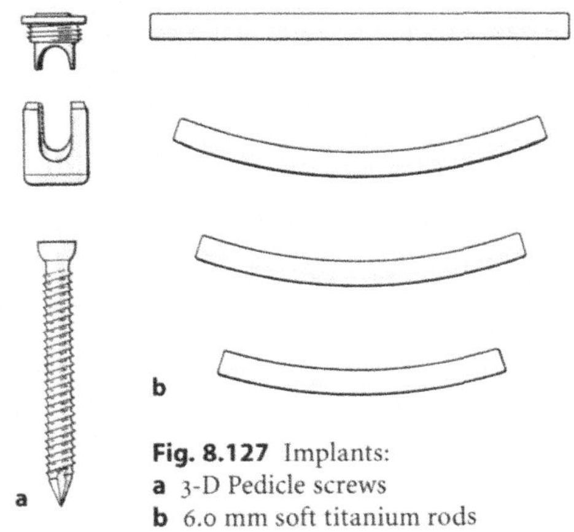

Fig. 8.127 Implants:
a 3-D Pedicle screws
b 6.0 mm soft titanium rods

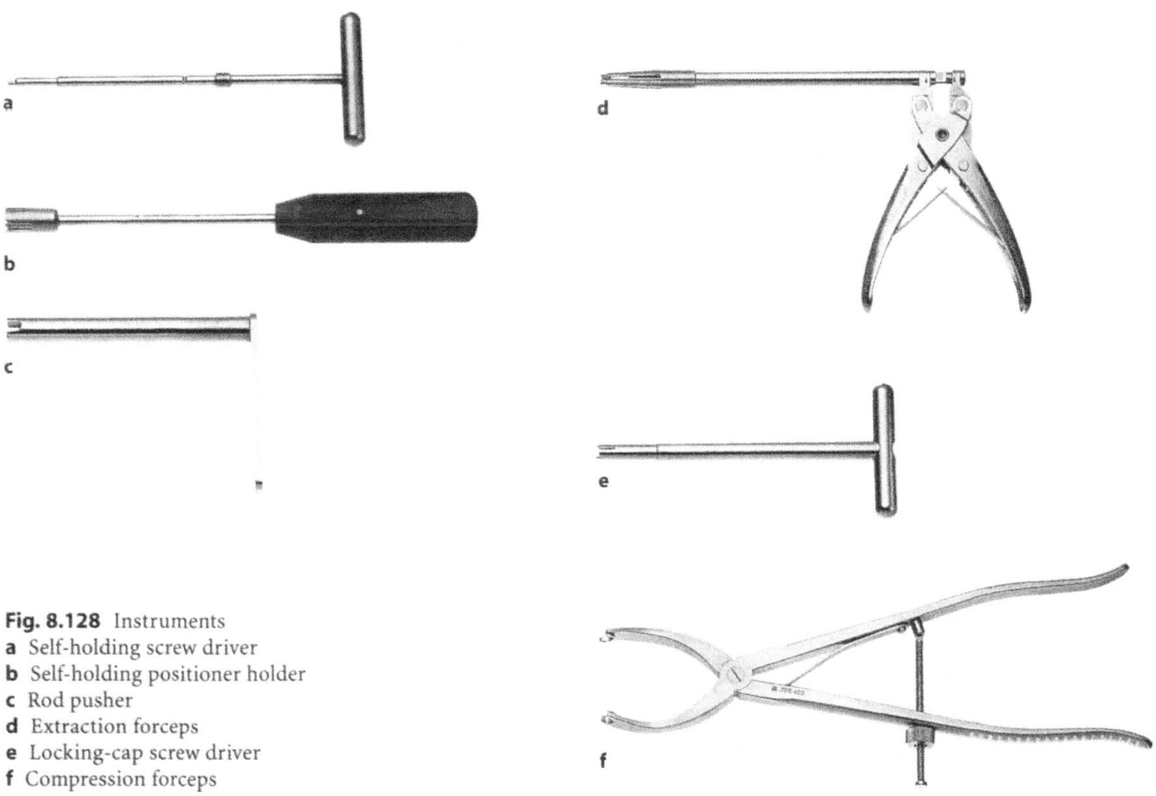

Fig. 8.128 Instruments
a Self-holding screw driver
b Self-holding positioner holder
c Rod pusher
d Extraction forceps
e Locking-cap screw driver
f Compression forceps

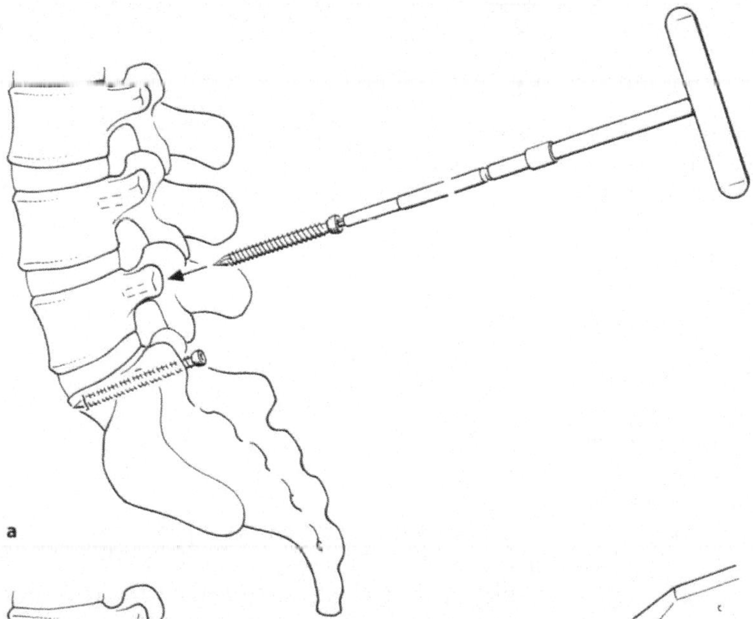

a

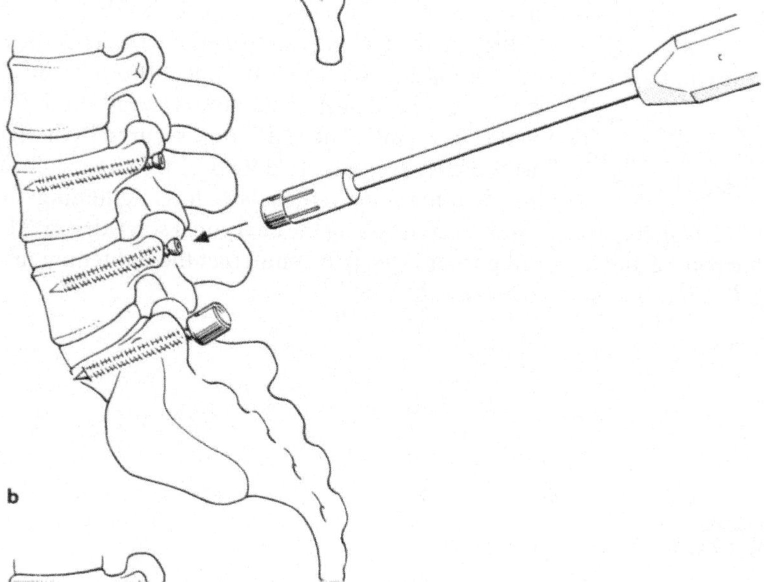

b

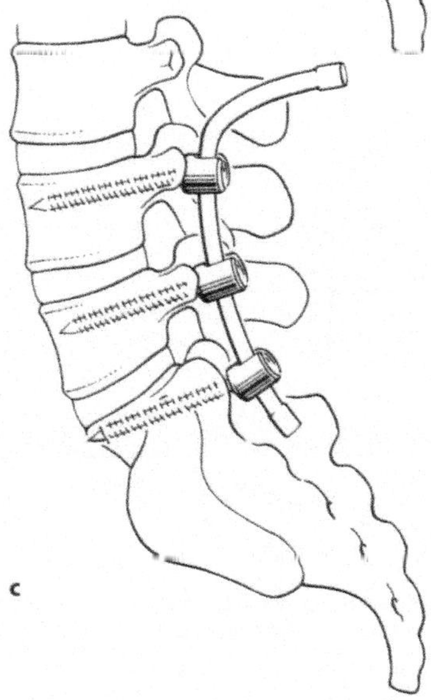

c

Fig 8.129
a Insertion of screw with the self-holding screwdriver
b 3D-head in the self-holding positioner holder
c Rod-template to predetermine the correct rod length

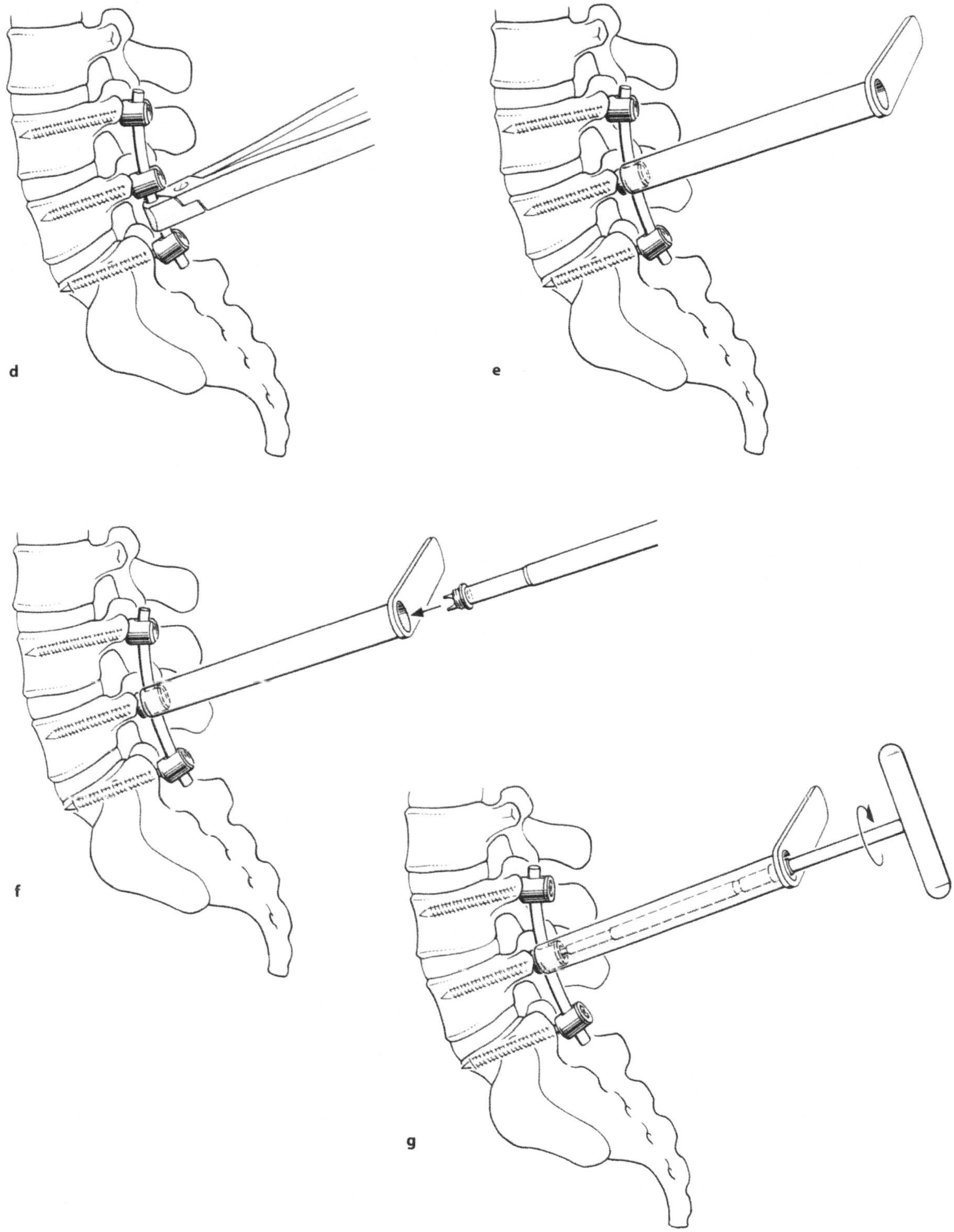

(Fig 8.129)
d Insert the rod with the 6 mm USS rod holder
e Use the rod pusher to push the rod into the 3D-head
f Insert locking cap with the self-holding screwdriver and insert it down the already placed rod pusher
g The hexagonal screwdriver is used to tighten the set screws, the rod pusher is used to counteract the tightening moment

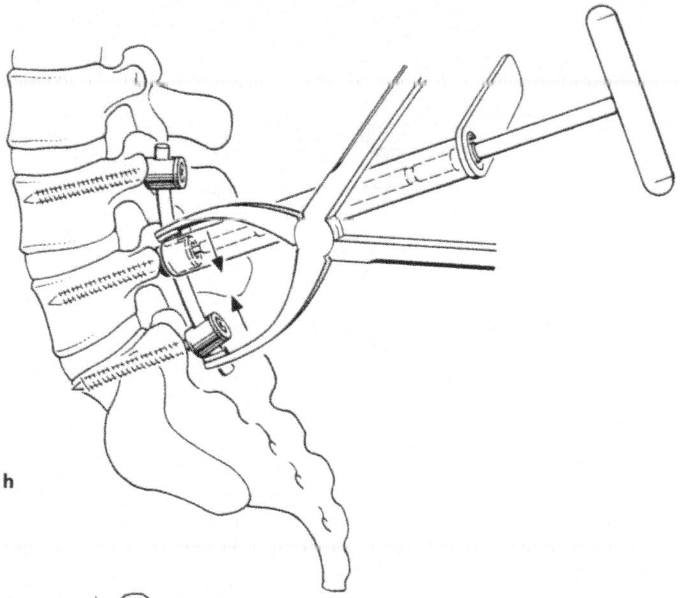

h

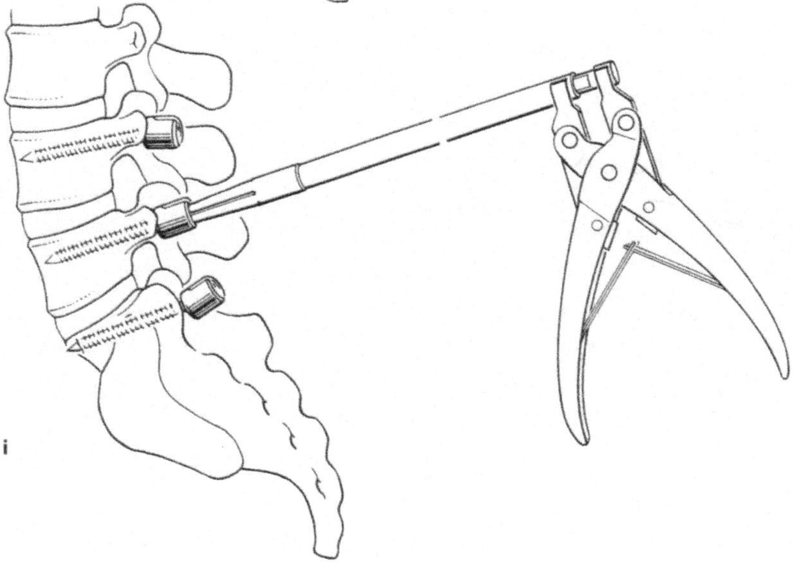

i

(Fig 8.129)

h compression or distraction can be applied as long as the set screw is loose (mobile 3D-head)

i The 3D-head can be remobilised by using the extraction forceps after having removed the rods

Compression/Distraction with Mobile 3D-Head

Compression or distraction with a mobile 3D-head can be carried out as long as the blue set screw of the pedicle screw to be moved has not been tightened.

Compress/distract using the compression/distraction forceps (Fig. 8.131h) and tighten the blue set screws as described.

Compression/Distraction with Fixed 3D Head

Tighten all blue set screws. Loosen the blue set screw of the pedicle screw to be moved using the hexagonal screwdriver. Thereby use the screwdriver to counteract the loosening moment on the locking cap. Compress/distract using the compression/distraction forceps and tighten the set screws as described above.

Remobilisation

The 3D-heads can be remobilised at any time using the extraction forceps (Fig. 8.129i). After having removed the rod, insert the working end of the forceps into the 3D head and press the handles.

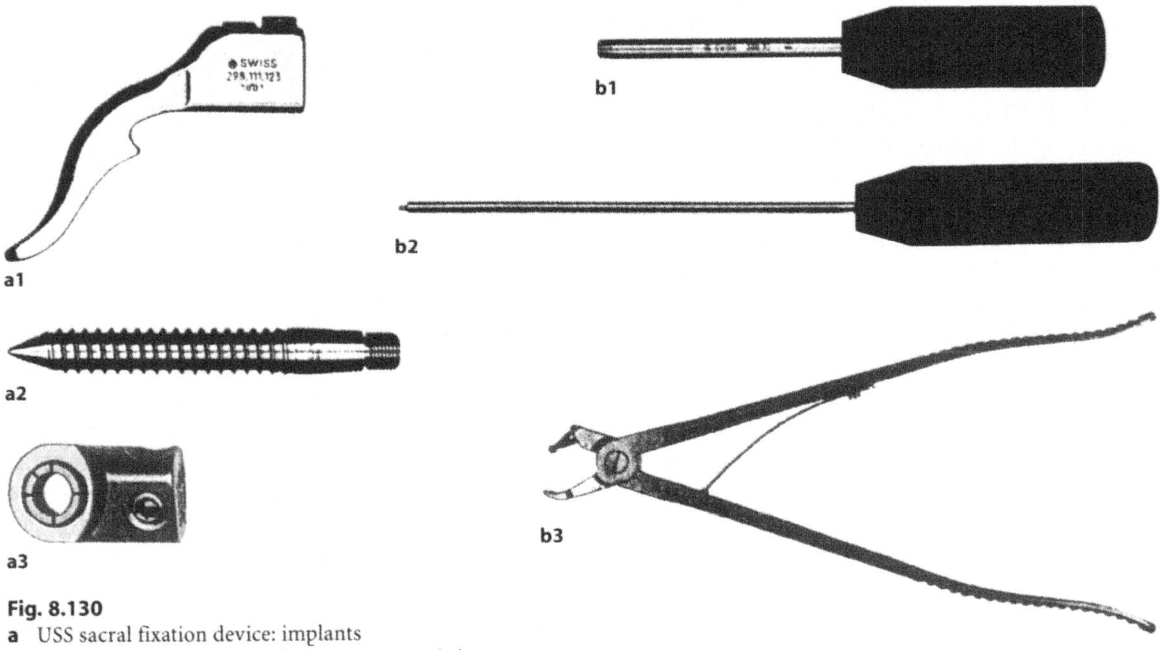

Fig. 8.130
a USS sacral fixation device: implants
a1 sacral clamp, **a2** sacral screw, **a3** sacral clamp
b USS sacral fixation device: instruments
b1 sacral threaded screw holder, **b2** sacral handle, **b3** removing forceps

8.2.3.2 Sacral Fixation

Implants (Fig. 8.130a)

Instruments (Fig. 8.130b)

Principle
Fixation to the sacrum is an essential part of any implant system. The failure of long constructs at the lumbosacral junction is well documented. The design of the system should allow attachment to the sacral pedicles, the alar and iliac wing. It should be low profile. The USS sacral system allows a variable angle screw to be inserted independent of the 6-mm rod, and it can be connected to the USS rod with variable-length plate-connectors (Fig. 8.130a). It is compatible with the standard USS system. The core of the system is a variable-angle screw which can be applied in different positions and create different assemblings of screw rod connections.

Position of Screws
S1–S2 Screws. The insertion of the screws is described in the section on Pedicle Screw Insertion.

Alar Screw
The ideal screw position is angled cranially 45° laterally 20° running parallel to the sacroiliac joint.

Iliac Wing Screw (Galveston Type Technique)
A long 90 to 100 mm screw is placed into the iliac wing, the direction being anterolateral in a 50–70° angulation from the sagittal plane. A small portion of the posterior iliac crest may need to be removed.

USS Technique: Sacral System Insertion
The entry point into the sacrum is identified. The appropriate length sacral clamp is placed loosely on the rod so that the opening of the clamp lies over the entry point into the bone. The screw can be angled up to 20° in the clamp; if a greater angulation is required then the 30° angle sacral clamp is used to increase the total angulation of the screw. The USS awl is passed through the clamp into the bone; depending on the direction of the screw it may be dangerous to penetrate the far cortex because of the close proximity of nerves and vessels. The mid-line is the only safe area to penetrate. The awl is removed and the depth measured.

The appropriate-length sacral screw is inserted into the sacral handle with the attached spanner. The screw is inserted and the clamp is then placed over the screw. Once the screw is in the clamp, the sacral handle is placed on the screw while the sacral threded screw is tightened. This mechanism pushes the slotted ball into the conically shaped end of the sacral screw causing it to be locked into the clamp.

The sacral 6-mm socket wrench is loaded with the locking screw and fixed to the thread protruding from the clamp. This locks the screw to the clamp. Finally the clamp is fixed to the USS 6-mm rod by tightening the hexagonal screw.

Sacral Clamp Removal
The locking screw is removed with the sacral 6-mm socket wrench (Fig. 8.130b). The sacral clamp removing forceps are placed underneath the clamp and closed (Fig. 8.130b). This disconnects the clamp from the screw (Fig. 8.130a2).

8.2.4 USS for Spondylolisthesis Reduction and Stabilization

8.2.4.1 Spondylolisthesis

The USS offers the scope to reduce and stabilize spondylolisthesis, if used with the addition of a few special devices, and at the same time allows a short fixation. We do not encourage surgeons to rely exclusively on posterior reduction and fixation in spondylolisthesis more severe than grade II. In these cases we recommend a 360° circumferential fusion, specifically after a significant reduction.

Principles
The pedicle screws are placed into the pedicle with the extension screw holders (sticks), which allows the screws to be used as Schanz screws with a significant lever arm. The L5 vertebra is rotated in the sagittal plane around the sacrum, eliminating the kyphotic deformity and at the same time performing a posteriorly directed translation. The final stabilization is performed using the tension band principle posteriorly and an anterior buttress graft, if necessary through a separate anterior interbody fusion (ALIF) or a posterior interbody fusion (PLIF).

Indications
- Spondylolisthesis L5/S1 (grade 0-V) combined with anterior surgery if necessary.
- Spondylolisthesis L4/L5.

Advantages
- *Reduction and stabilization with the same instrumentation.*

Disadvantages
- Technically demanding.
- Visualization of the L5 and S1 nerve roots is necessary when a relevant reduction is planned.
- L5 nerve root injury.

Techniques

Spondylolisthesis Grade II-IV. In the case of isthmic spondylolisthesis grade II, the loose arch of L5 is removed and the roots of L5 and at times S1 are identified and decompressed, this allowing visualization of the roots during reduction in order to avoid any traction on the roots. A complete posterior release of the posterior annulus and disc is helpful to facilitate the reduction procedure. Special Schanz screws with a machine thread along one shaft and with a 6 mm diameter in the threaded part (occasionally 5 mm if the pedicles are small) are inserted in the pedicles of L5 and lateral opening screws are inserted in the S1 pedicles (Fig. 8.131a). These latter screws are preferably 7-mm-diameter screws but the load during the reduction maneuver may be so significant that a second screw may be placed in the lateral sacral mass. The Schanz screws have a maximum thread of 3 cm length at the top for the reduction maneuver.

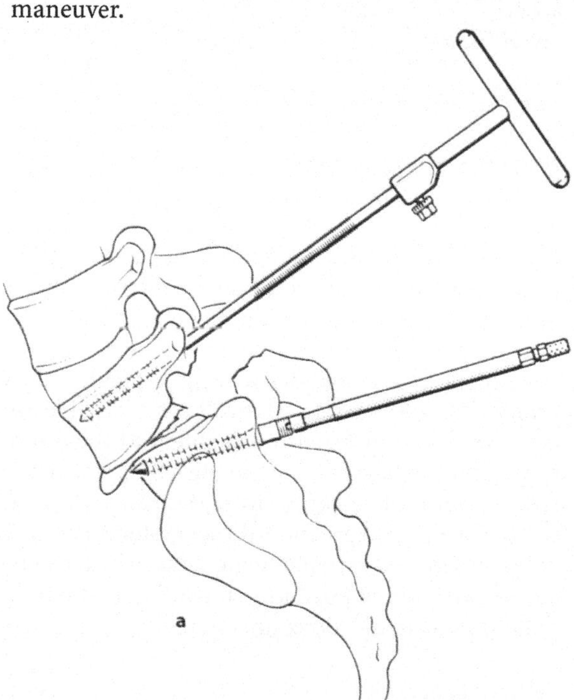

Fig. 8.131
a Special Schanz screws with a 6-mm threaded part are inserted in the L5 pedicle on each side and lateral-opening USS preferentially 7-mm screws are inserted in each S1 pedicle. The Schanz screws have a machine thread of 3 cm in length at the top of the shaft

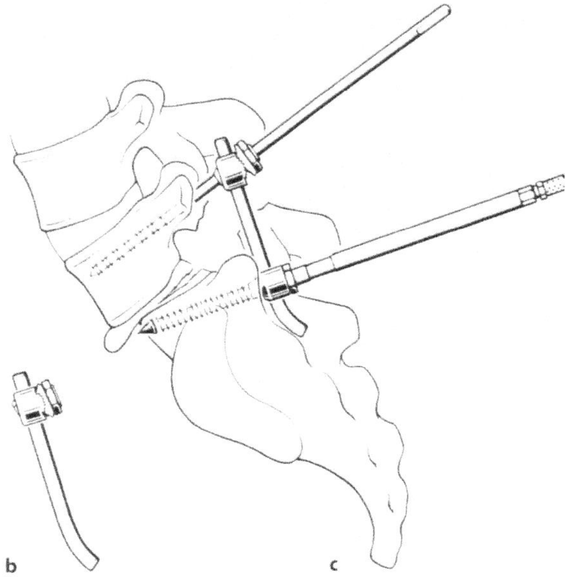
b
c

(Fig. 8.131)
b Two USS rods about 8 cm in length are contoured to the desired lumbosacral lordosis and implemented with a clamp of the internal fixator component of the USS
c The rods are mounted to the Schanz screws in L5 and the lateral opening screws in the sacrum

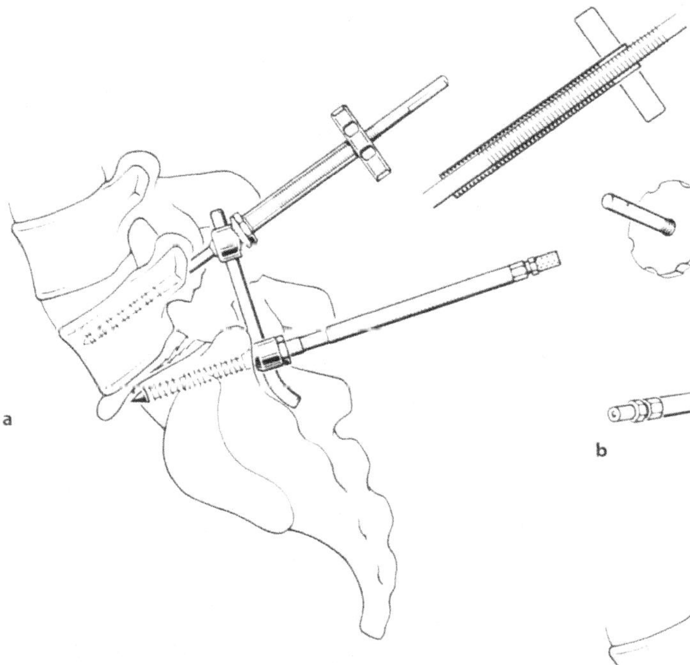
a

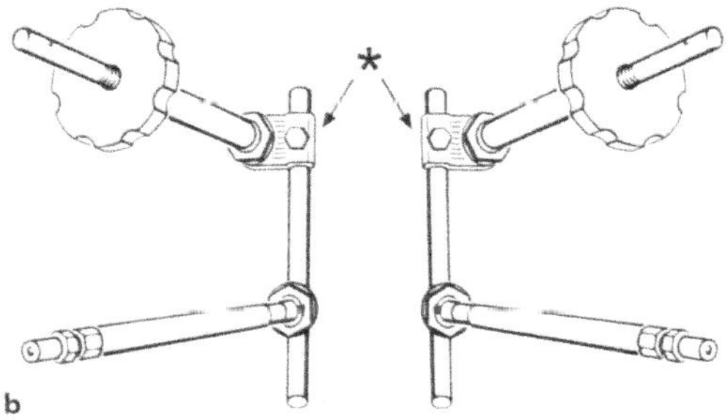
b

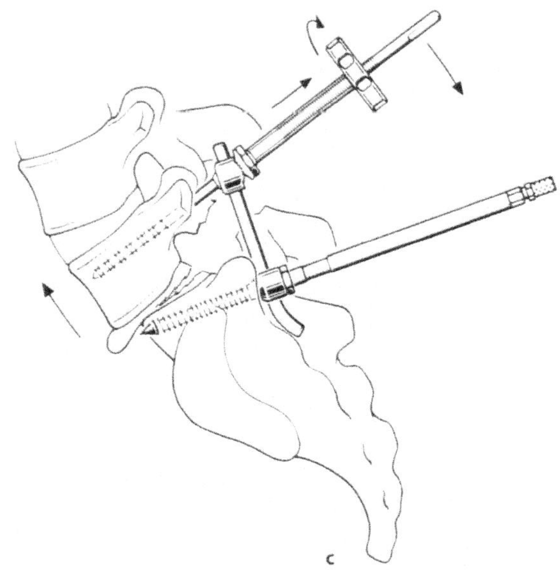
c

Fig. 8.132
a Two internally threaded tubes 5,5 mm in diameter and 6 cm in length are now sleeved over the Schanz screws. Big handy nuts are mounted at the hexagonal end of the tubes allowing the tightening of the tube along the threaded part of the Schanz screws, therefore gradually pulling back the vertebra of L5
b The external fixator clamps glide loosely on the rod. The small 6-mm hexagonal set screws of the internal fixator clamps are left loose
c The Schanz screws are compressed against the sacral screws, thus creating a lordosis of the original kyphotic deformity at L5 – S1

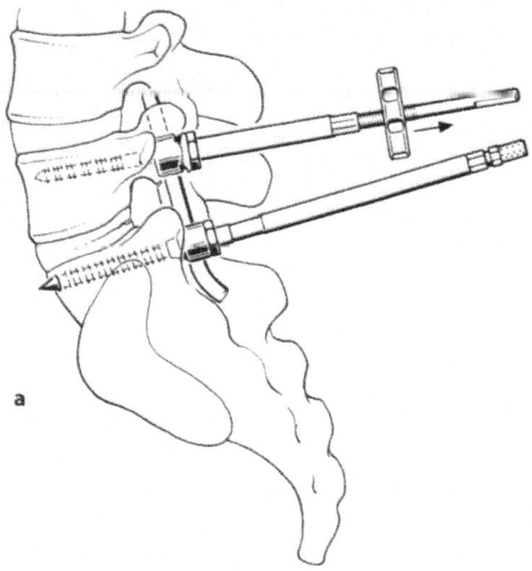

a

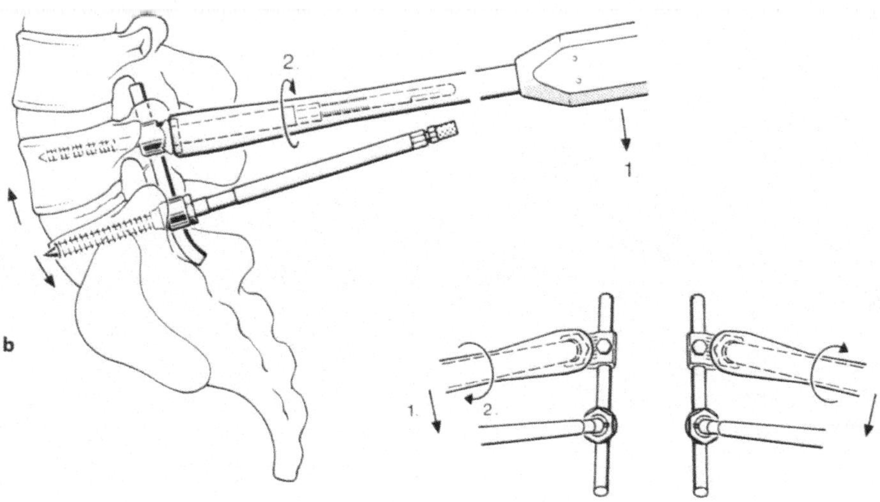

b

Fig. 8.133
a The large nut on the Schanz screw is removed
b The socket wrench is slipped over the Schanz screw on each side at the same time and by compressing the shaft of the Schanz screws against the S1 screw with extension sticks, the hexagonal nut of the clamp is tightened

Two rods each about 8 cm in length (if the montage is taken to L4, the rod needs to be longer) are contoured to the desired lumbosacral lordosis and implemented at the cranial end with a posterior opening clamp from the internal fixator component of the USS (Fig. 8.131b) is attached. The rods are mounted with the posterior-opening clamp to the Schanz screws at L5 and inserted caudally into the heads of the lateral-opening pedicle screws in the sacrum (Fig. 8.131c). The rods are locked in place by adding the sleeve and nut to the screw heads of the sacrum. The nuts are tightened completely. The posterior opening clamp is kept loose on the rod as well as the Schanz screw in order to allow the clamp to glide on the rod during the reduction maneuver (Fig. 8.132c). Tubes of 5,5 mm in diameter and 6 cm in length are now sleeved over the Schanz screws (Fig. 8.132a). Large nuts are mounted at the hexagonal end of the tube and tightened against the threaded screw shaft, this leading to a gradual posterior reduction of the vertebra L5 with the Schanz screws (Fig. 8.132b). Before tightening the nuts of the posterior-opening clamps, the Schanz screws can be manipulated so that the original kyphotic deformity is reduced into lordosis (Fig. 8.123c). This can be achieved with a powerful handle which is linked to the two long tubes (Fig. 8.132b). However, care must be taken not to pull or tear out the screws, either in L5 or in the sacrum. During the reduction maneuver the roots of L5 and S1 need to be repeatedly checked in order to avoid squeezing or pulling them.

When the reduction is achieved, which can be checked by image intensifier, the big nut on the Schanz screw is first removed on one side (Fig. 133a), the socket wrench is slicked over the Schanz screw with the tube still in place and the hexagonal nut

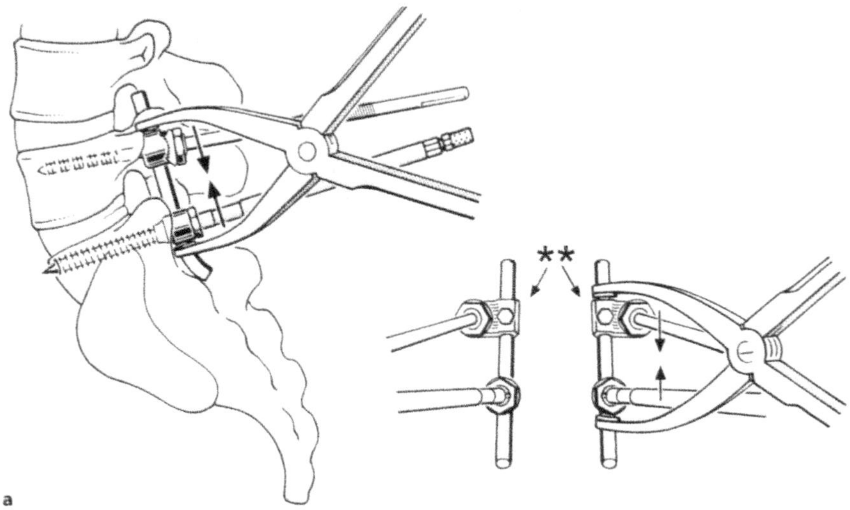

a

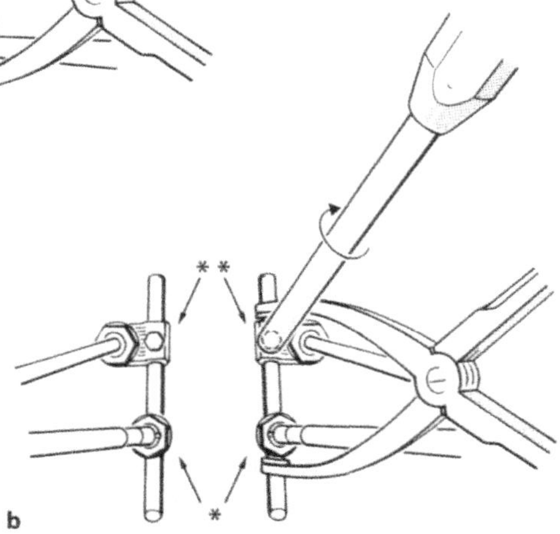

b

Fig. 8.134
a The screws may be compressed against each other to maintain the tension bandings system while the set screws of the fixator clamps are loose (*); however, the USS screws are securely tightened
b When the end position is reached, the set screw of the internal fixator clamp is tightened

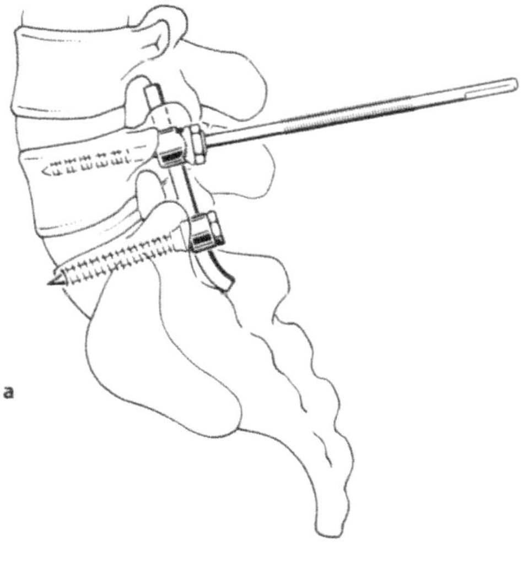

a

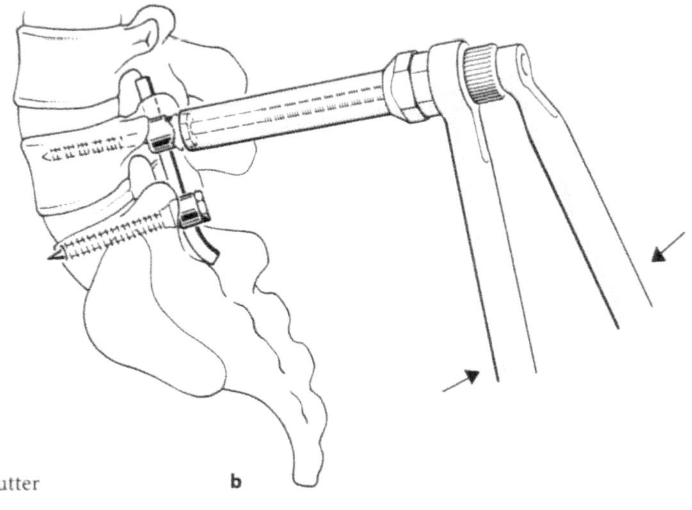

b

Fig. 8.135
a The extension sticks of the S1 screw are removed
b The Schanz screws are shortened with the bolt cutter

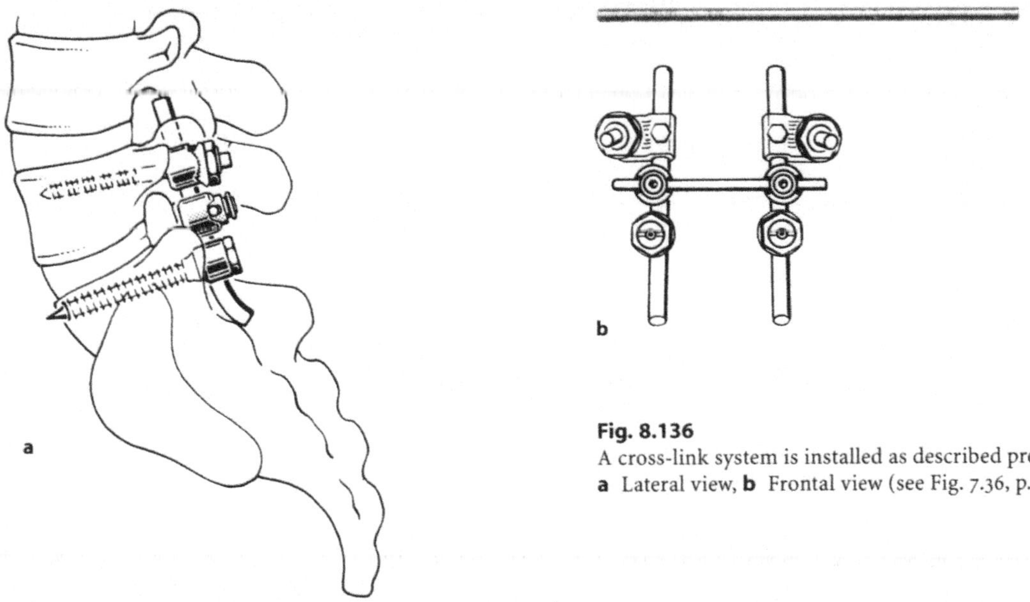

Fig. 8.136
A cross-link system is installed as described previously
a Lateral view, **b** Frontal view (see Fig. 7.36, p. 119 – 120)

of the clamp is tightened (Fig. 8.133b). The same procedure is then performed on the other side. Now the tubes are removed by untightening. With the USS compression clamp the head of the L5 screws and those from the S1 screws are compressed applying the tension-banding force (Fig. 8.134a). Then the small 6-mm hexagonal screws are tightened, in order to block the clamps on the rod (Fig. 8.133b). The extension sticks of the S1 screws are removed (Fig. 8.132a). The Schanz screws are cut over the clamp with the bolt cutter (Fig. 8.132b). The tightening of the sacral screw is checked. The two rods are connected with the cross-link (Fig. 8.133a, b). If there is not enough space between the L5 and S1 screw to place a cross-link clamp, a special cross-link is used. A posterolateral fusion is added and if there is any doubt about the maintenance of the reduction and the stability of the fixation, either a PLIF or an anterior interbody fusion needs to be added.

Spondylolisthesis IV – V. If it is anticipated that the reduction of a grade IV or V spondylolisthesis will be difficult to achieve, two-step surgery is an alternative. The first step consists of local posterior radical release of the lumbosacral junction and the percutaneous insertion of the external fixator (see Fig. 9.17, p. 209 – 210) with gradual reduction.

In a second surgical session a combined anterior posterior procedure is then performed. The patient will be positioned in the first stage with the external fixator in place and an anterior interbody fusion L5/S1 (L4/5) is performed and stabilized using a long 6.5-mm cancellous screw with mounted washer which acts as a compression screw (Fig. 9.17g, p. 204). In the second stage the patient is positioned prone, the external fixator is removed and replaced by a USS pedicular system from L4/L5 to S1 and is enhanced by a posterolateral fusion. If there is any concern regarding pin-track infection, the posterior procedure is delayed for 1 week.

CHAPTER 9

Other Fixation Systems

9.1
Hook-Screw System for Spondylolysis Treatment

Surgical Technique

A mid-line incision is made between the spinous processes of L4 and S1 (for spondylolysis L5 and S1). The soft tissues are dissected subperiostially on both sides, and the entire neural arch, the spondylolysis and the inferior circumference of the upper intervertebral joint are exposed. A clear exposure of these structures is mandatory to avoid technical faults (Fig. 9.1). The spondylolysis is cleared, the 'pseudoarthritic' connective tissue is removed and the spondylolysis is freshened (Fig. 9.2).

The joint capsule is then opened in its caudal circumference, and the tip of the inferior articular process of the vertebra above is resected according to Louis. The tips of the articular process press on the interarticular portion of the vetebral arch like a pair of pincers when lordosis takes place and are thought to play an important role in the pathogenesis of spondylolysis (Fig. 9.3). The ligamentum flavum is partially removed from the inferior surface of the neural arch and the caudal area of the neural arch is slightly notched using a Kerrison rongeur to prevent lateral slipping of the hook (Fig. 9.4). The spondylolysis hook is slid over the vertebral arch from the caudal end by means of the special holding

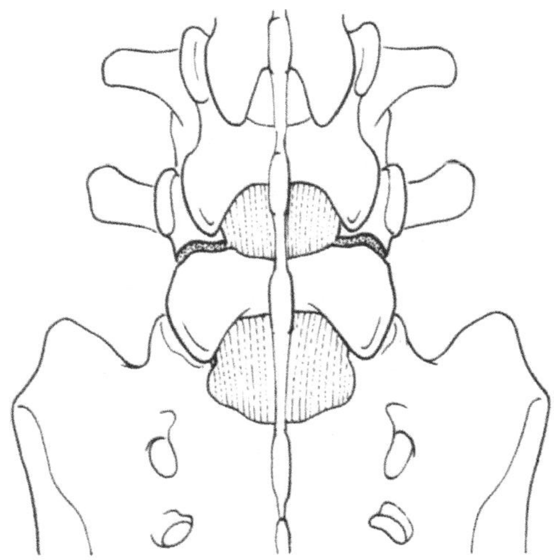

Fig. 9.1 The spondylolysis is exposed

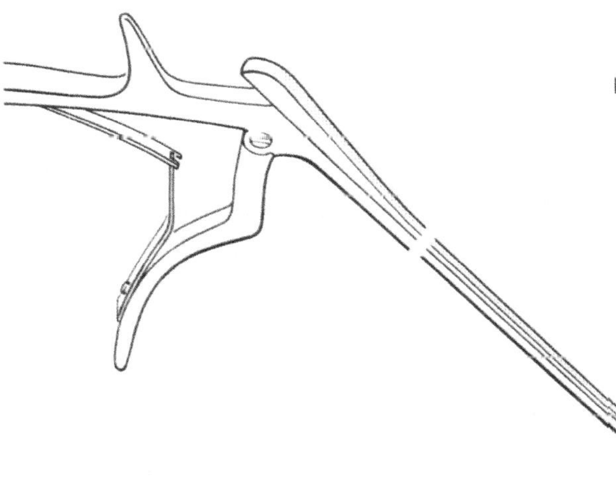

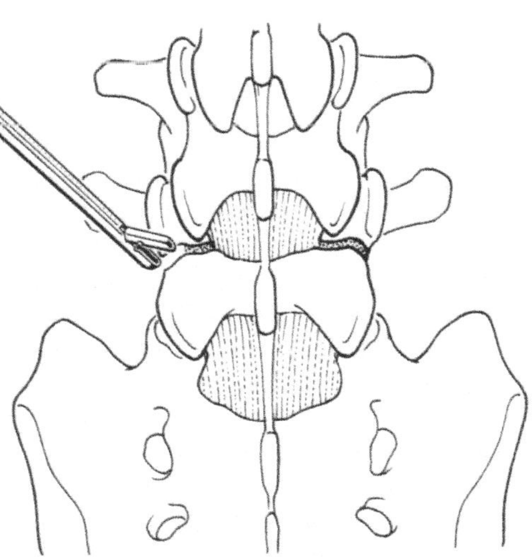

Fig. 9.2 The 'pseudoarthritic' connective tissue is removed with a rongeur

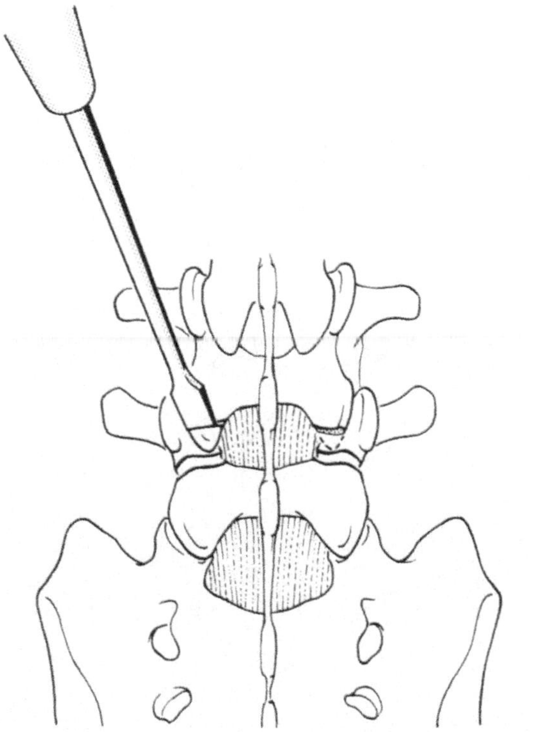

Fig. 9.3 The joint capsule of the facet joint is opened and an osteotomy of the tip of the inferior articular processes of the vertebra above is done

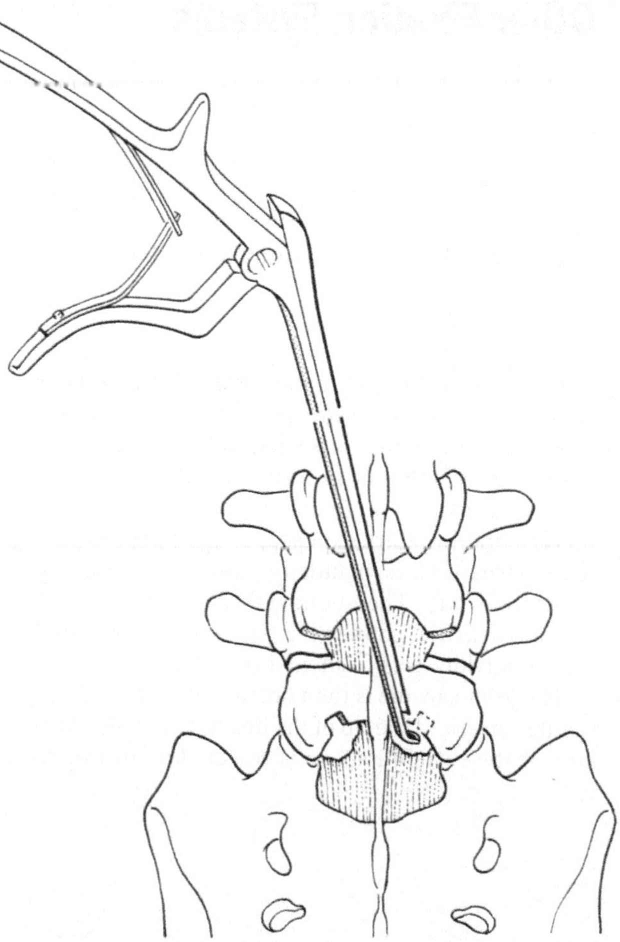

Fig. 9.4 The flavum must be removed from the inferior surface of the loose arch. A small notch is added at the caudal area of the arch by a Kerrison rongeur to keep the hook from sliding sidewards

forceps, with the screw directed towards the base of the superior articular process (Fig. 9.5a).

When the base of the superior articular process has been precisely identified by K-wires (Fig. 9.5b/b'), a hole for the hook screw is drilled in the base of this articular process with the 2.5-mm drill through the hole of the hook (Fig. 9.5c/c'). The drill is introduced through the hole of the hook, which ensures that the entry point of the screw will come to lie posteriorly outside the spondylolysis, directly at the base of the superior articular process of the spondylotic vertebra. The drill must penetrate the entire breadth of the base of the articular process.

The length of the drilled canal is measured and is normally approximately 18 mm. The thread length of all screws is uniformly 20 mm. Thus it is easy to determine how deep the screw is inserted. In every

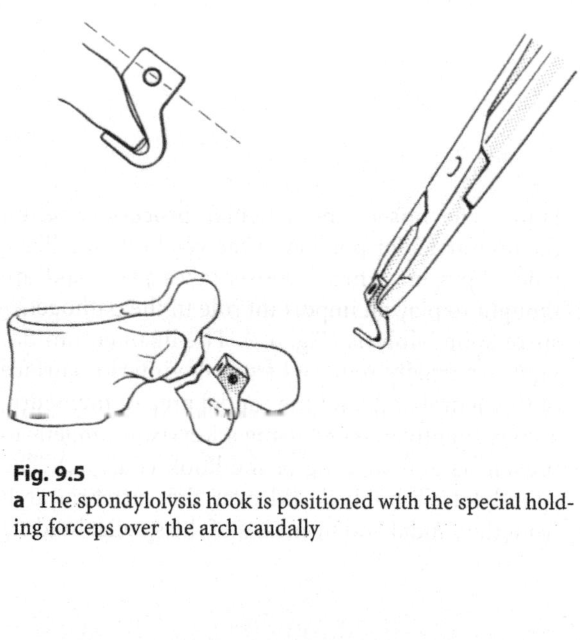

Fig. 9.5
a The spondylolysis hook is positioned with the special holding forceps over the arch caudally

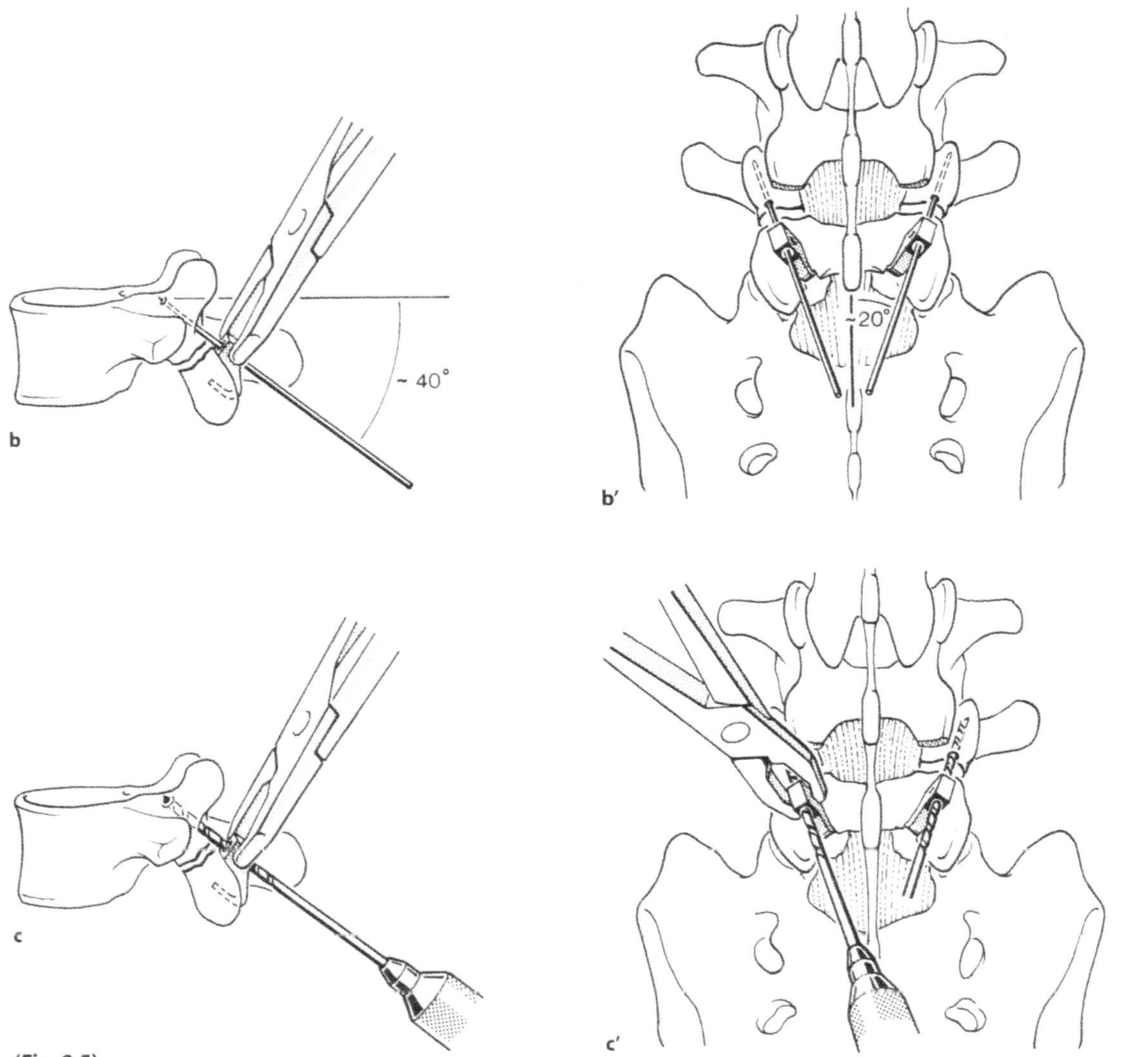

(Fig. 9.5)
b, b′ The screw or K-wire in the hook giving the direction for drilling in the superior articular-pedicle complex

c, c′ The drill must penetrate the entire breadth of the base of the superior articular-pedicle complex

case, the screw must penetrate the two cortices and project anteriorly by 1–2 mm over the circumference of the base of the articular process (Fig. 9.6a). Before the osteosynthesis is compressed by means of the compression spring and nuts, fresh cancellous bone, which can be taken from the iliac crest through the same incision, is inserted into and along the lateral side of the spondylolysis (Fig. 9.6c, d). Care must be taken to ensure that afterwards, when the hook is tightened and the cancellous bone is compressed in the spondylolysis, no bone fragments are pressed anteriorly against the nerve root or towards the spinal canal.

If a gap of the spondylolysis is relatively large, compression should be carried out by tightening the nuts on both sides after both implants are in situ. Thus a twisting of the vertebra is avoided. Direct repair and compression, allowing closure of the spondylolisthesis, may be at least partially achieved. Furthermore, care should be taken when the second nut is being tightened with the hexagonal wrench (Fig. 9.7) to avoid the screw from being inserted further, thus preventing excessive compression from taking place. The thread projecting over the nuts is cut off (Fig. 9.8a, b).

Postoperative Care
The patient can usually be mobilized the 2nd day after surgery. A lumbar corset (prepared preoperatively) may be worn for 3 months, i.e., until definite consolidation of the spondylolysis has taken place.

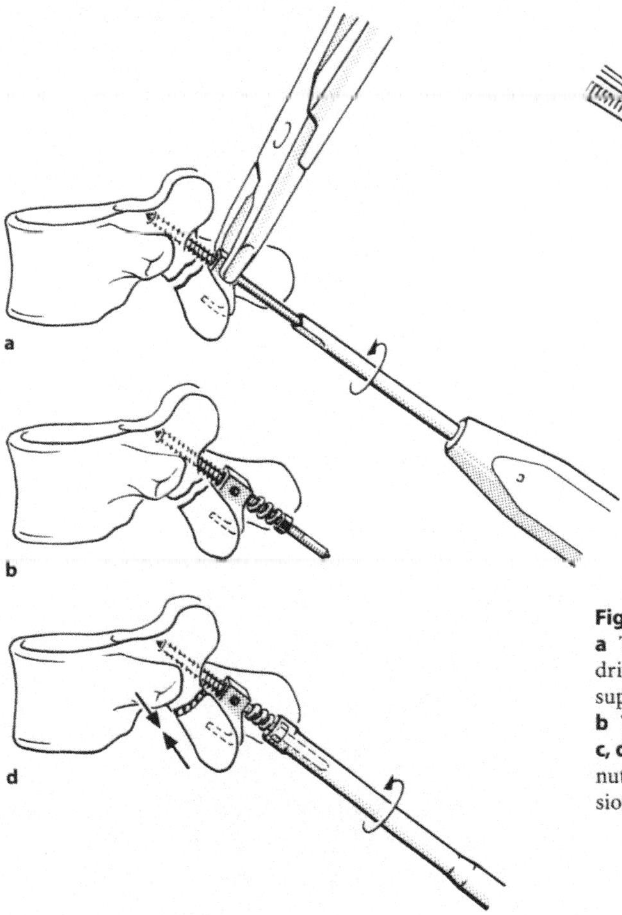

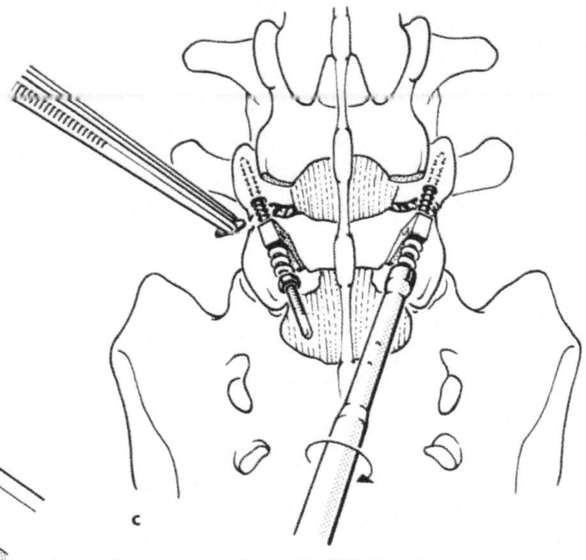

Fig. 9.6
a The screw is inserted through the hook with a special screwdriver. The screw should penetrate 1–2 mm at the base of the superior articular process
b The nut and spring are inserted over the screw
c, d Once the lytic gap is filled with cancellous bone graft, the nut is tightened, and the gap and graft are put under compression

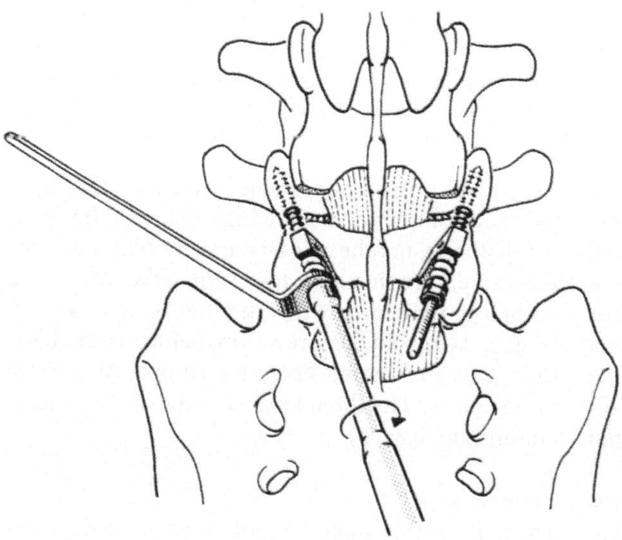

Fig. 9.7 To finish with, a second nut is inserted. In order to avoid further compression, the first nut needs to be withheld with the hexagonal key while the second nut is tightened with the hexagonal screwdriver

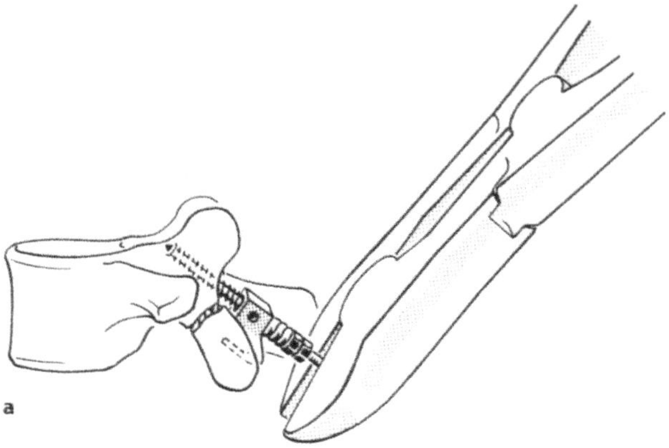

a

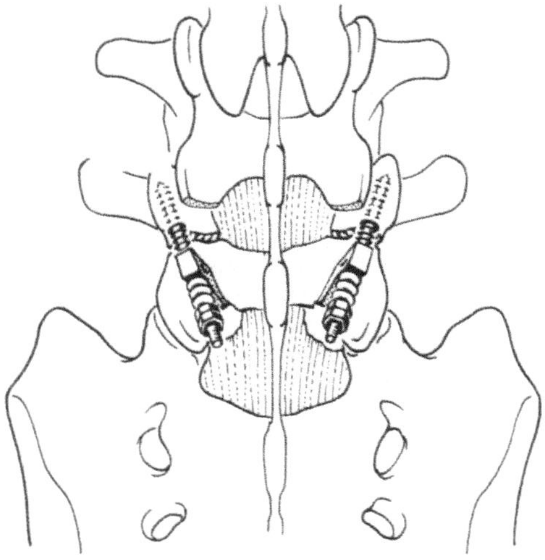

b

Fig. 9.8
a, b The protruding part of the spondylolysis screw is finally cut off

9.2 External Spinal Skeletal Fixation

9.2.1 Principles and Technique

External fixation of the spine was developed by Magerl in 1977 for the treatment of thoracolumbar and lumbar fractures. With external spinal skeletal fixation (ESSF), effective reduction and stabilization of comminuted fractures was possible immobilizing only two motion segments (Figs. 9.9, 9.10). Furthermore, both decompression and stabilization were feasible in one session from the less traumatic posterior approach and functional aftertreatment was possible. ESSF was used with success in more than 100 fractures. After the advent of the AO internal fixation device, ESSF was abandoned as a routine mode of treatment for spinal fractures because of the potential risk of infection and the demanding postoperative care required. Today, ESSF is primarily used as a diagnostic tool for chronic low-back pain, as a reduction tool in high-grade spondylolisthesis and as a treatment modality for spinal osteomyelitis. Exceptionally, it is used as a mode of treatment for spinal fractures or for posterior stabilization of unstable pelvic fractures of the Malgaigne type. Although originally inserted by open means for the treatment of spinal fractures, ESSF is nowadays exclusively inserted percutaneously. Entry points and optimal sites of the Schanz screws are identical to those for open insertion; the technique of percutaneous insertion, however, is different and will be discussed in this section.

9.2.1.1 Technique of Percutaneous Insertion of Schanz Screws

Antibiotics are administered preoperatively and during the entire duration of external fixation. The patient is intubated and placed prone on a radiotranslucent operating table which allows anteroposterior (AP) and lateral image intensifier control of the thoracic and lumbar spine, of the sacrum and of the ilium if necessary. No plastic drape is used to avoid subcutaneous penetration of plastic material. The technique of insertion is illustrated in Figs. 9.11–9.14.

9.2.1.2 Postoperative Care

Postoperatively and during the whole duration of treatment, a foam mattress is used to enable the patient to remain in the supine position while resting. A window is cut out of the mattress to accommodate the external fixator (Fig. 9.15). The dressing is changed daily (Fig. 9.16), and the skin and the Schanz screws are cleaned.

9.2.1.3 Insertion of Thoracic Screws

For insertion of Schanz screws in the thoracic spine (T2–T12), the technique of insertion is basically the same as described above with three important exceptions:

(contin. on p. 206)

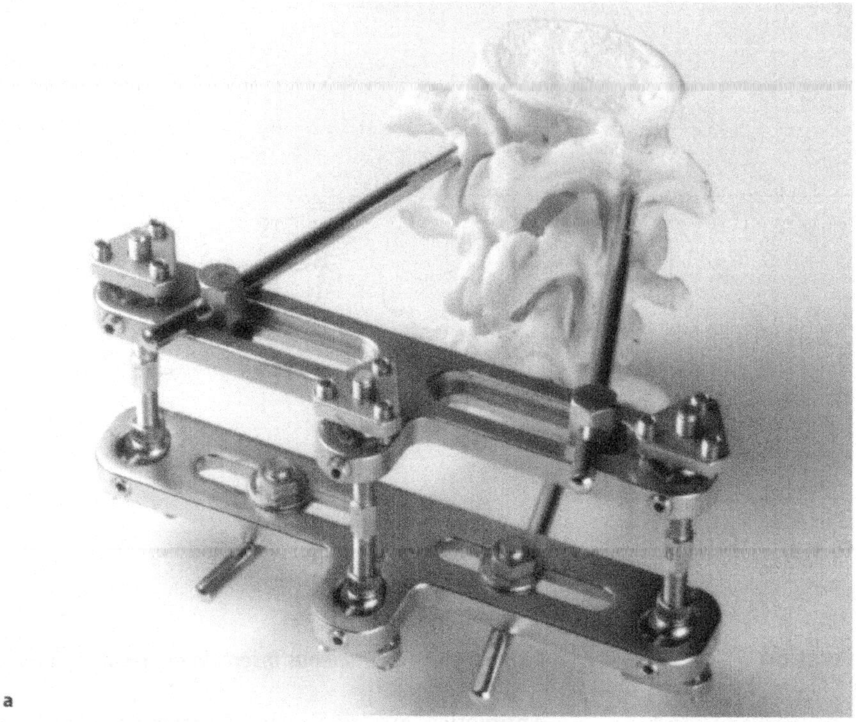

a

Fig. 9.9 AO external fixator. The AO external fixator consists of four Schanz screws and a fully adjustable frame

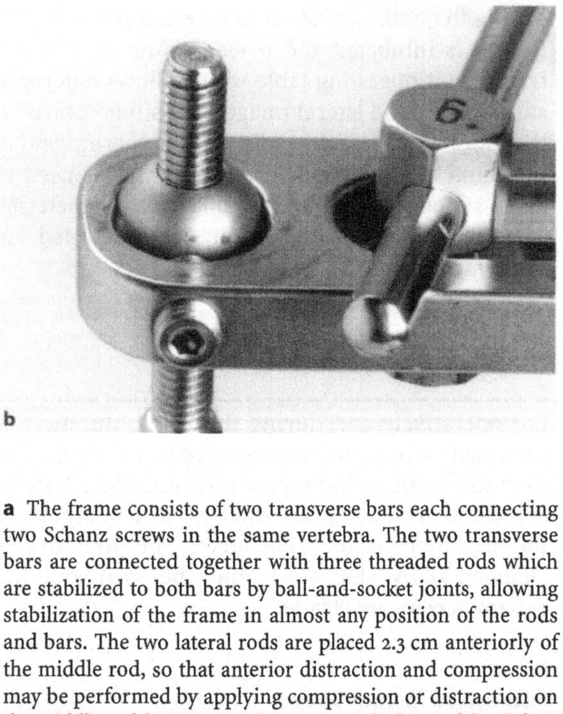

b

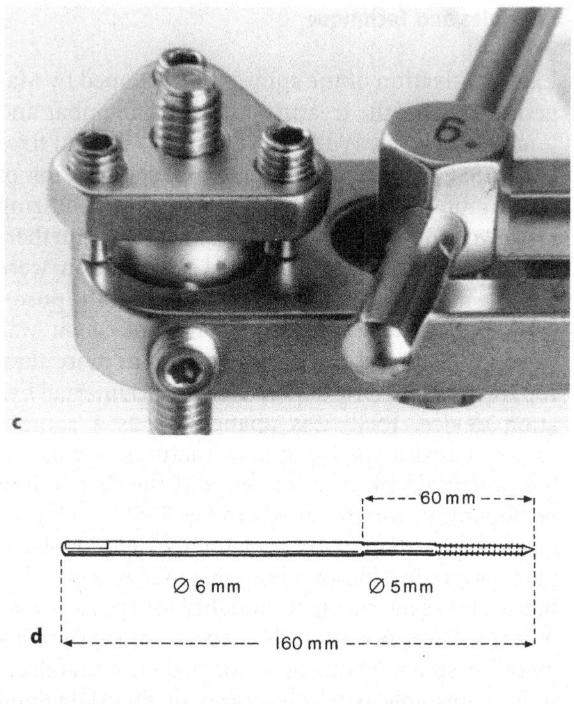

c

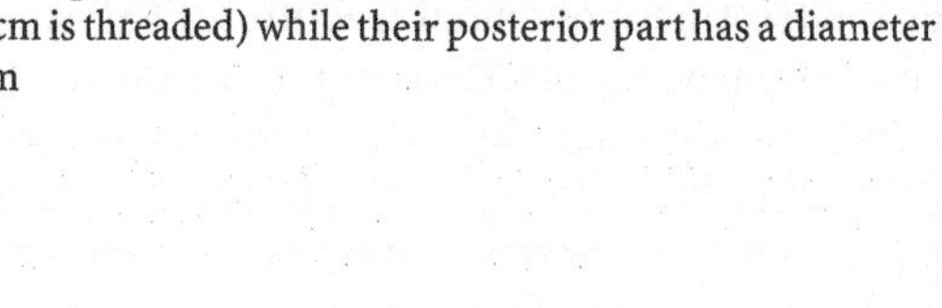

d

a The frame consists of two transverse bars each connecting two Schanz screws in the same vertebra. The two transverse bars are connected together with three threaded rods which are stabilized to both bars by ball-and-socket joints, allowing stabilization of the frame in almost any position of the rods and bars. The two lateral rods are placed 2.3 cm anteriorly of the middle rod, so that anterior distraction and compression may be performed by applying compression or distraction on the middle rod (see Fig. 9.10). For secure locking of the definitive position, triangular locking plates with three set screws are mounted at each end of the threaded rods. Varying sizes of bars and rods enhance the versatility of the system

b Ball-and-socket joint connecting the transverse bars with the threaded rods

c Locking plate

d The Schanz screws are 16 cm long and self tapping. Their anterior part has a diameter of 5 mm over a distance of 6 cm (3.5 cm is threaded) while their posterior part has a diameter of 6 mm

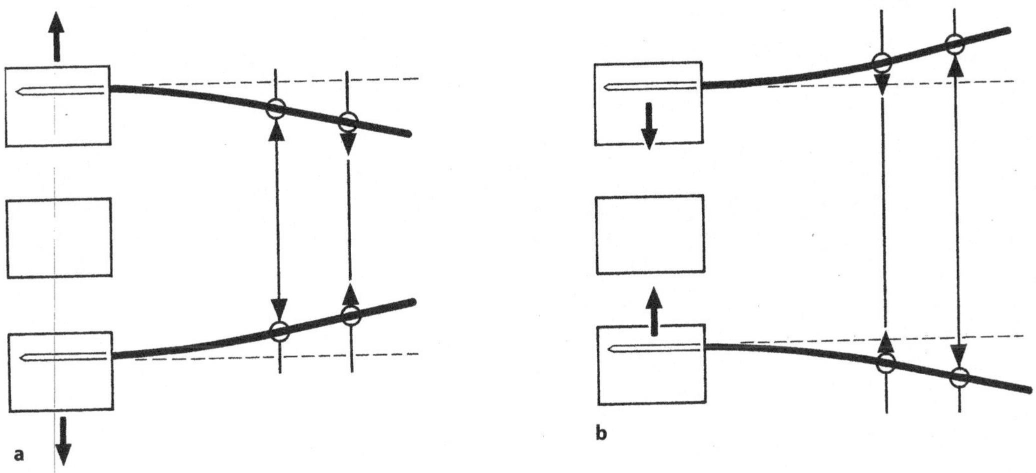

Fig. 9.10 Preloading. The ESSF is always applied with preload. This increases the stability of the construct
a Distractive preload is used for stabilization of painful motion segments during diagnostic stabilization, for reduction of spondylolisthesis or kyphotic deformities in osteomyelitis of the spine and for stabilization of compression injuries of the spine or Malgaigne fractures of the pelvis
b Compressive preload is only used in the treatment of osteomyelitis of the spine to enhance spontaneous fusion or for stabilization of pressure-resistant intervertebral fusions after additional anterior interbody fusion

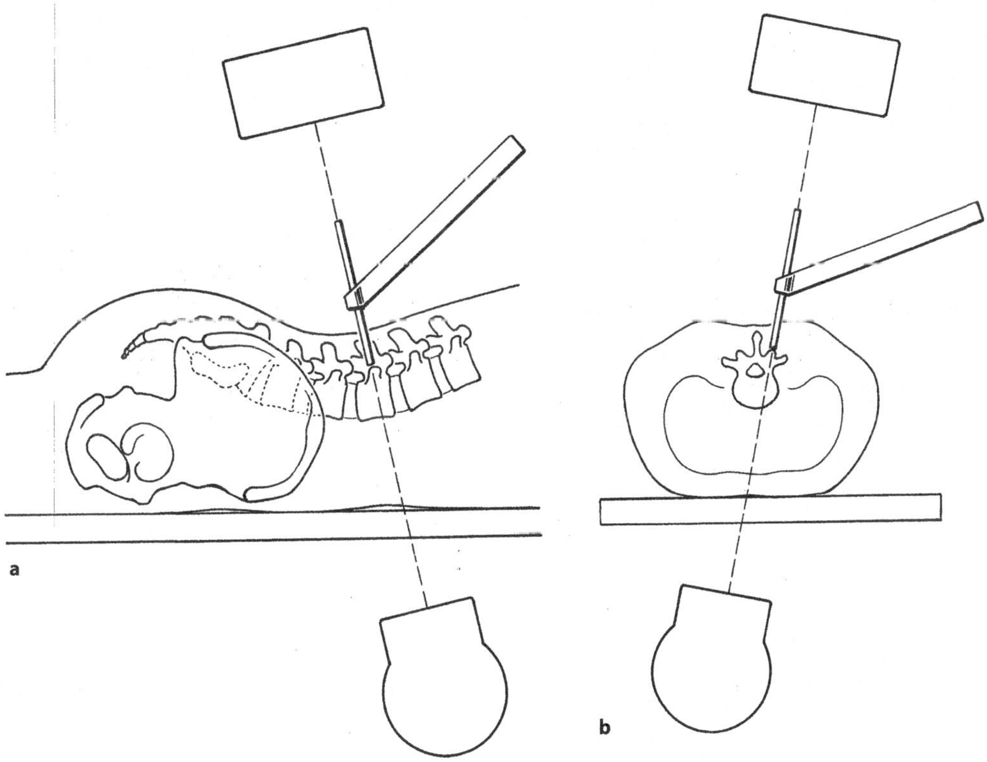

Fig. 9.11 a, b Installation of the image intensifier
For transpedicular insertion of Schanz screws, an AP view of the spine is obtained and the image intensifier tilted in the craniocaudal direction (a) so as to be parallel to the end plates and also tilted 5–20° laterally (b) according to the mediolateral inclination of the pedicles (the exact angle can be measured on a preoperative CT scan)
For insertion of screws into the sacrum, an AP projection of the sacrum is obtained, the image intensifier beam being tilted craniocaudally to be parallel to the end plate of S1. For insertion of Schanz screws into the iliac bone, iliac-oblique and obturator oblique views must be obtained (see Fig 9.13–9.14)

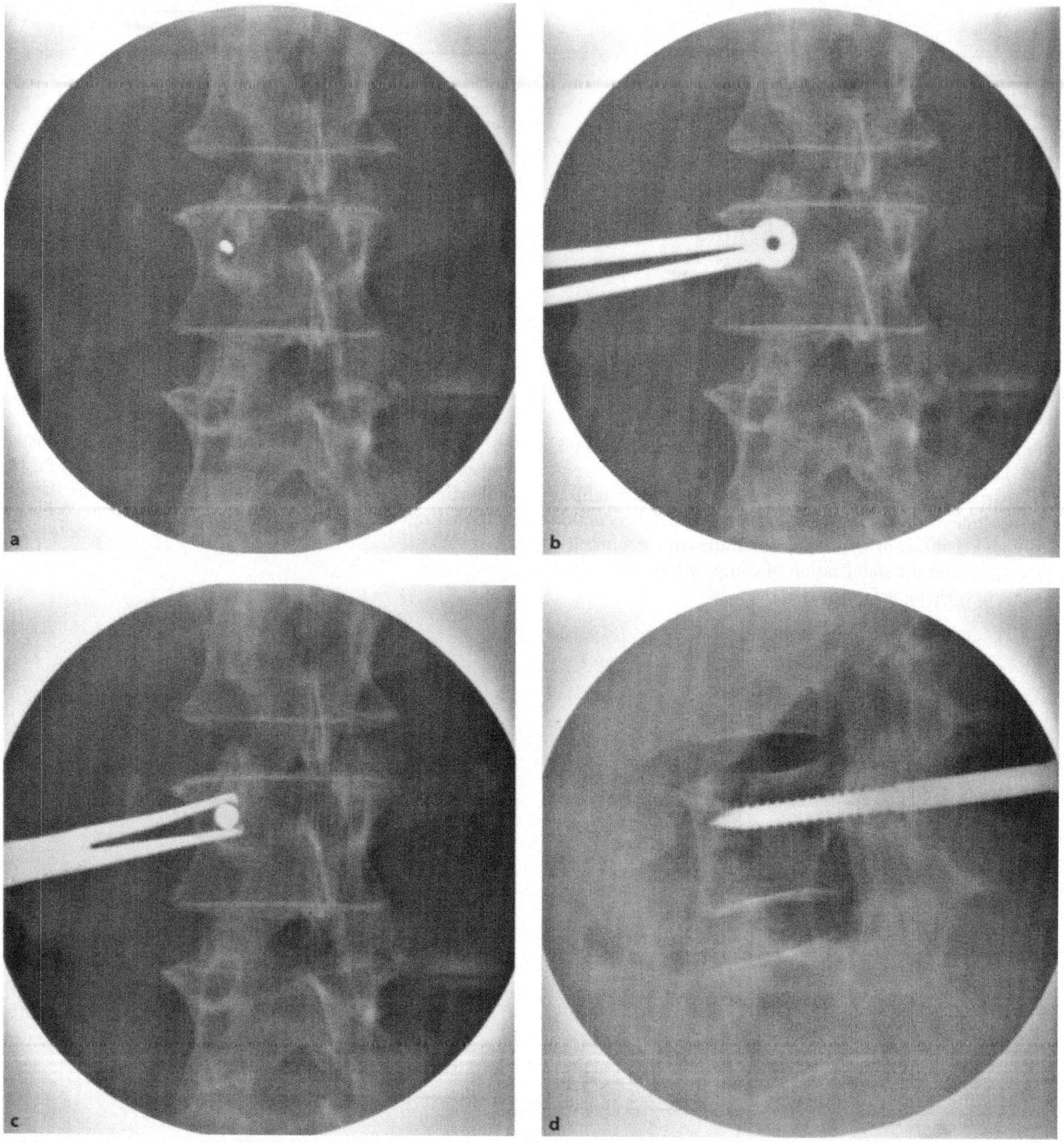

Fig. 9.12 Insertion of Schanz screws in the thoracic and lumbar spine

a A stab incision is made over the center of the pedicle's projection. 2.5-mm K-wire is brought to bony contact with the posterior elements, still in the center of the pedicle's projection. To prevent inadvertent slipping of the K-wire towards the nerve root, it should be directed slightly cranially before being lightly hammered in to stabilize it

b A drill sleeve with a denticulated end is inserted over the K-wire and hammered onto the bone. The K-wire is removed without moving the drill sleeve, the adequate site of which is controlled under the image intensifier

c A 0.5-cm-deep drill hole is made with a 3.2-mm drill and a K-wire is inserted in this hole to check its adequate placement in the pedicle after removing the drill sleeve. The K-wire is removed and replaced with a Schanz screw, which is slightly driven in.

d Once the Schanz screw has a good grip, a lateral projection is obtained and the screw is inserted under image intensifier control close to the anterior cortex, which should not be perforated

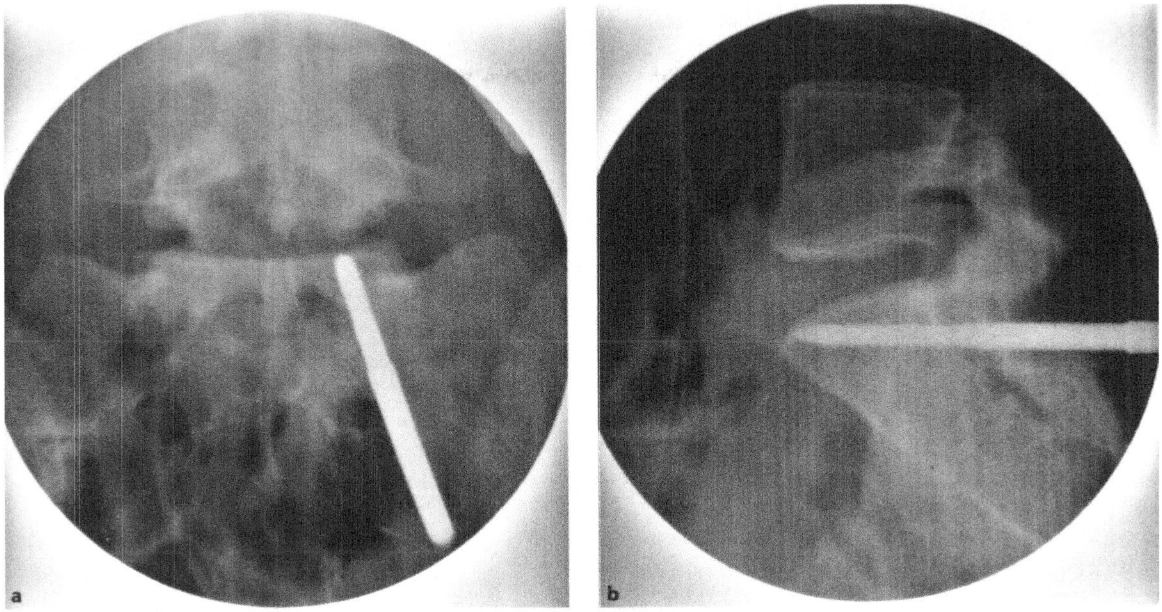

Fig. 9.13a, b Insertion of Schanz screws in the sacrum. Stab incision is performed and a Schanz screw is inserted without previous drilling. **(a)** The Schanz screw enters the sacrum midway between the lateral border of the posterior foramen of S1 and the lateral border of the superior articular process of S1 and converges 10–15° medially towards the promontorium **(b)**

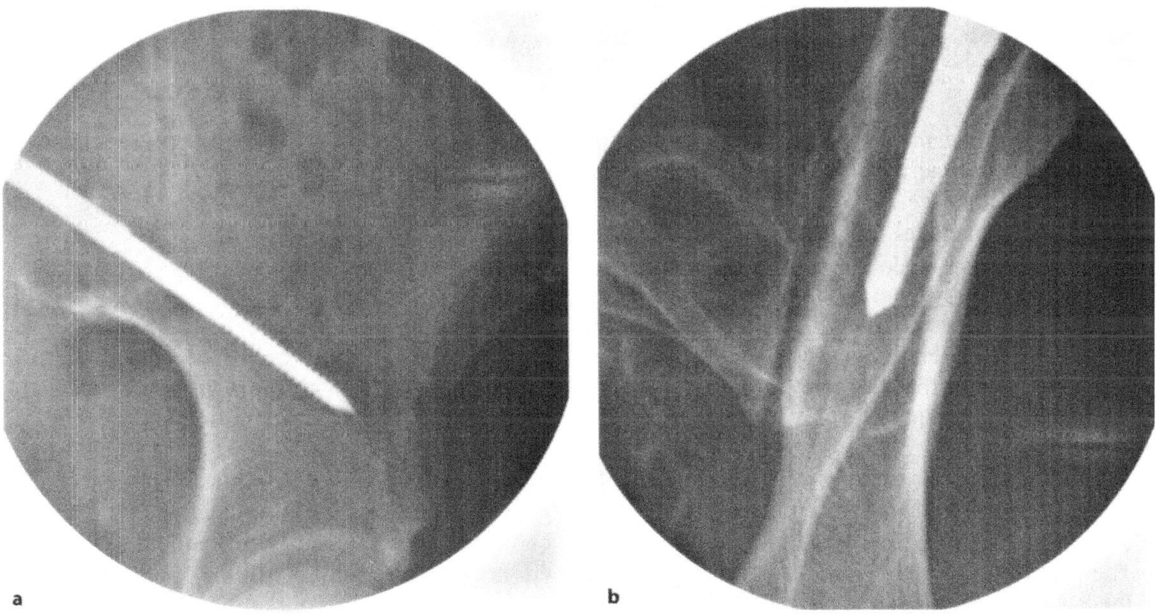

Fig. 9.14a, b Insertion of Schanz screws in the ilium. Entry point of the Schanz screws is the posterior superior iliac spine **(a)**. The screws diverge 15–25° from the sagittal plane according to the plane of the iliac wing and point towards the anterior inferior iliac spine, passing cranially to the greater sciatic notch **(b)**. The exact lateral deviation is parallel to the image intensifier beam when the iliac wing is seen tangentially as in the obturator-oblique view

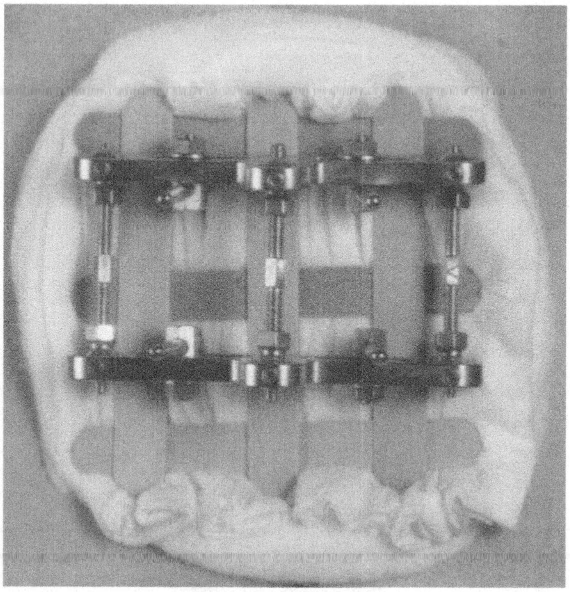

Fig. 9.16 Wound dressing
The wound dressing is made with sponges and a wooden tongue spatula is inserted under the frames of the fixator to prevent window edema developing in this area

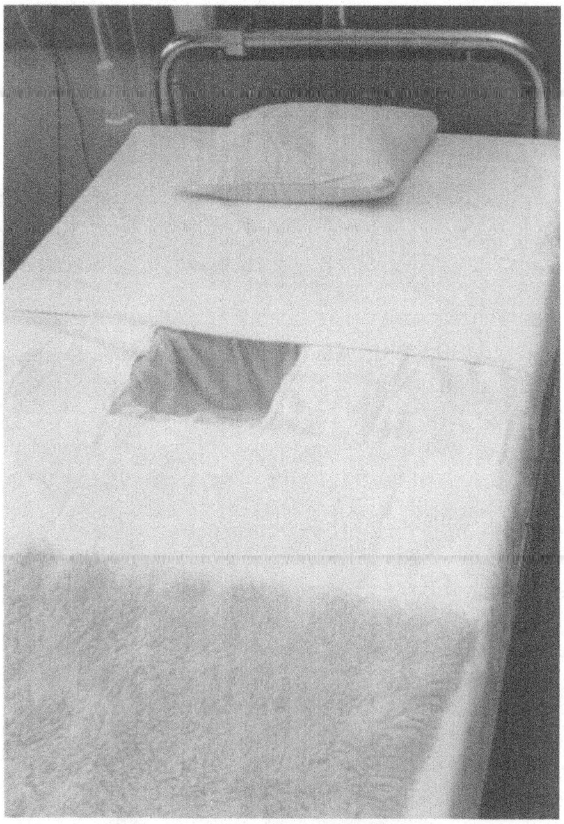

Fig. 9.15 A cut is made in the foam mattress to accommodate the external fixator

1. The screwhole must be predrilled in its entire length to make sure that the screw still follows the desired route.
2. Since the pedicles may be smaller than the Schanz screw, the entry point of the screw must be located in the lateral half of the pedicle's projection. The screw hole will therefore perforate the pedicle laterally, covered by the rib. Care must be taken that the screw reenters the bone and does not slip along the outer cortex of the vertebral body.
3. Since the thoracic pedicles are oriented caudally, the screws should aim 10–20° caudally.

The percutaneous stab wounds for the insertion of the Schanz screws must be cleaned daily with H_2o_2 and alcoholic antiseptic solution. The Schanz screws must be cleaned very carefully to prevent any retention of secretion by crust formation, which could be the cause of infection spreading along the Schanz screws. If the external fixator has to be left in place for several weeks or even months, a custom-made plastic corset with a rigid housing covering the assembly is worn to protect the external fixator and prevent screw penetration in case of a fall on the assembly. The patient is followed up biweekly for pin care control.

9.2.1.4
Treatment of Complications

Infection
Superficial infection is treated by removal of the infected Schanz screw, cleaning of the screw canal by irrigation with antiseptic solution and systemic antibiotic therapy. A deep infection is treated by removal of all Schanz screws while the patient is under general anesthesia as an emergency procedure, combined with extensive debridement of the infected screw canal including drilling out the canal in the vertebral body. Systemic antibiotic therapy is installed.

Screw Loosening
Any loose screw should be removed since this may cause infection.

9.2.1.5
Removal of Schanz Screws

Removal of the Schanz screws is performed without anaesthetics. Intramuscular administration of an analgesic 30 min before removal is usually sufficient. Prior to removal, all stresses within the assembly are released. After removal of the screws, the screw canals are irrigated with antibiotic solution using a long needle with a ball tip. The wounds are covered with a sterile dressing.

9.2.2
External Fixation as a Diagnostic Tool in Low-Back Pain

Principle
The sacroiliac joints and specific motion segments of the lumbar spine may be immobilized for several days or weeks to test the effect of stabilization on the patient's pain and therefore evaluate the potential benefit of a fusion operation.

Indications
Chronic, intractable low-back and/or referred pain due to degenerative disease or spondylolisthesis is present. Since percutaneous stabilization of the lumbar spine is an invasive diagnostic method with all the inherent risks both of the general anesthesia and of the surgical procedure itself, indications must be restricted. This method should only be used as a last diagnostic resource in chronic low-back pain, and only if facet blocks and diskography both failed to demonstrate the pain origin.

Technique

Operative Technique. The vertebrae to be instrumented are chosen based on plain and functional X-rays as well as on magnetic resonance imaging (MRI): the aim of the fixation is to stabilize the motion segments expected to be responsible for the pain. The screws are inserted percutaneously according to the technique described previously. Each lumbar vertebra can be instrumented and every motion segment may be examined sequentially. However, we usually only instrument the top and bottom vertebrae of the segment(s) expected to be responsible for the pain. If the segment L5/S1 has to be included in the stabilization in the presence of osteoporotic bone, it is advisable to insert the Schanz screws in the os ilium rather than in the sacrum, where the bone stock may be very poor. The transverse bars of the external fixator, each connecting the two Schanz screws of the same vertebra, are mounted. However, no stabilization is performed at that time: this is important in order to detect a placebo effect of the Schanz screw insertion itself. The patient is allowed to get up the 1st day after surgery.

Clinical Evaluation. As soon as the acute postoperative wound pain has disappeared, the patient is asked to do everything which was painful before surgery (e.g., sitting, standing, walking, bending, lifting). Usually, some of these exercises may provoke additional mild back pain due to interference of the Schanz screws with the muscles and the skin. However, the pain provoked by the Schanz screws can easily be differentiated by the patient from the original low-back pain itself. The original back pain will usually reappear within 4–5 days after surgery, after the acute postoperative pain has disappeared. The transverse bars of the external fixator are then connected together with the threaded rods and the fixator frame is stabilized in distractive preload, which stabilizes the corresponding motion segment(s). All manipulations are performed without anesthetics while the patient is awake. Too much anterior distraction must be avoided, since this may cause severe back pain. If the painful motion segment has been stabilized, this stabilization should lead to immediate relief of the original pain, which should reappear as soon as the frame is destabilized 1 or 2 days later. This procedure must be repeated several times without the patient knowing in which state of stability the frame is in. This is very important in order to detect a placebo effect. Furthermore, the patient's responses to these changes must always be concordant in order to allow a reliable statement of the pain origin. If Schanz screws have been inserted in more than two levels, e.g., in L2, L3, L5 and S1, then the stabilization and destabilization is performed stepwise, e.g., L2/3, L2/5, L5/S1 and L2/S1, but again always without the patient knowing which segments have been stabilized and what is expected to happen with the pain. The patient's response to the direct manipulation of the nonstabilized horizontal bars may also be recorded. In this manner, specific motion segments may be manipulated and pain reproduced.

Therapeutic Consequences of the Percutaneous Stabilization

- If reliable pain responses are obtained by the stabilization and destabilization of one or more motion segments of the lumbar spine, a definitive fusion of this (these) segment(s) may be performed. The Schanz screws are removed and the fusion operation is performed several weeks later, after complete healing of the stab wounds.

- If stabilization does not relieve the patient's pain or even worsens the pain, then the pain is not likely to be relieved by a fusion operation of the motion segments examined. No fusion operation should be performed.
- If the pain is relieved by insertion of the Schanz screws alone and does not reappear even after 7 days, then a placebo effect must be postulated. No fusion operation should be performed.

9.2.2.1
Gradual Reduction of Severe Spondylolisthesis L5

Principle
Gradual closed reduction of severe spondylolisthesis while patient is awake. This allows exact neurological monitoring and therefore early detection and treatment of neurological complications.

Indication
- Grade III and IV spondylolisthesis L5/S1
- Spondyloptosis

Advantages
- Neurological monitoring possible during the entire period of reduction
- Early detection and treatment of neurological complications possible
- Facilitates anterior interbody fusion

Disadvantages
- Technically demanding

Technique
Schanz screws are inserted percutaneously into L4 and the iliac bone. The transverse bars and the longitudinal connecting threaded rods are inserted intraoperatively and slight anterior distraction is applied to distract the soft tissues. Once the acute wound pain has disappeared (4–5 days after surgery), gradual anterior distraction is started without anaesthesia by applying as much anterior distraction as is tolerated by the patient. Once the intervertebral disc hight has increased (in a grade III and IV spondylolisthesis) or the lower posterior edge of L5 has reached a position cranial to the anterior edge of S1 (in a spondyloptosis), the lordosis is gradually increased by decreasing the distance between both transverse bars, while maintaining distractive preload. During this maneuvre, all ball-and-socket joints must be loose to permit rotational movements in these joints. As reduction is accomplished and kyphosis reduced, the longitudinal threaded rods may have to be exchanged and shorter ones inserted. Otherwise, the cranial end of the rods would impinge on the skin. During the whole procedure, the neurological status of the legs (especially of the nerve roots L5) is watched very carefully. If any neurological disturbance is encountered, reduction is discontinued. This maneuvre alone is usually sufficient to allow reduction to a grade I-II.

If adequate reduction is not possible with this maneuver, gradual posterior traction may also be applied on the transverse bar mounted on L4. Today, no marketed device is available for this purpose. However, a simple traction device mounted at the top of the Schanz screws in the os ilium and pulling the transverse bar in L4 backwards may be manufactured locally by any mechanic. If the kyphotic deformity of L5 cannot be corrected as desired, additional correction may be obtained with Schanz screws implanted in L5, after maximal correction has been obtained with the Schanz screws inserted in L4.

Once adequate reduction has been obtained, anterior interbody fusion is performed and the external fixator is removed (Fig. 9.17). It is advisable to prevent postoperative extrusion of the grafts by using a cancellous screw inserted into the sacrum and acting as a buttress maintaining the anterior grafts in place. Posterior stabilization with internal fixation of L5/S1 or L4/S1 (depending on whether the intervertebral disk L4/L5 is intact or degenerated as seen in the MRI) is added after complete healing of the posterior stab incisions. After posterior stabilization and fusion, the patient is allowed to get up with a lumbar corset for 3 months.

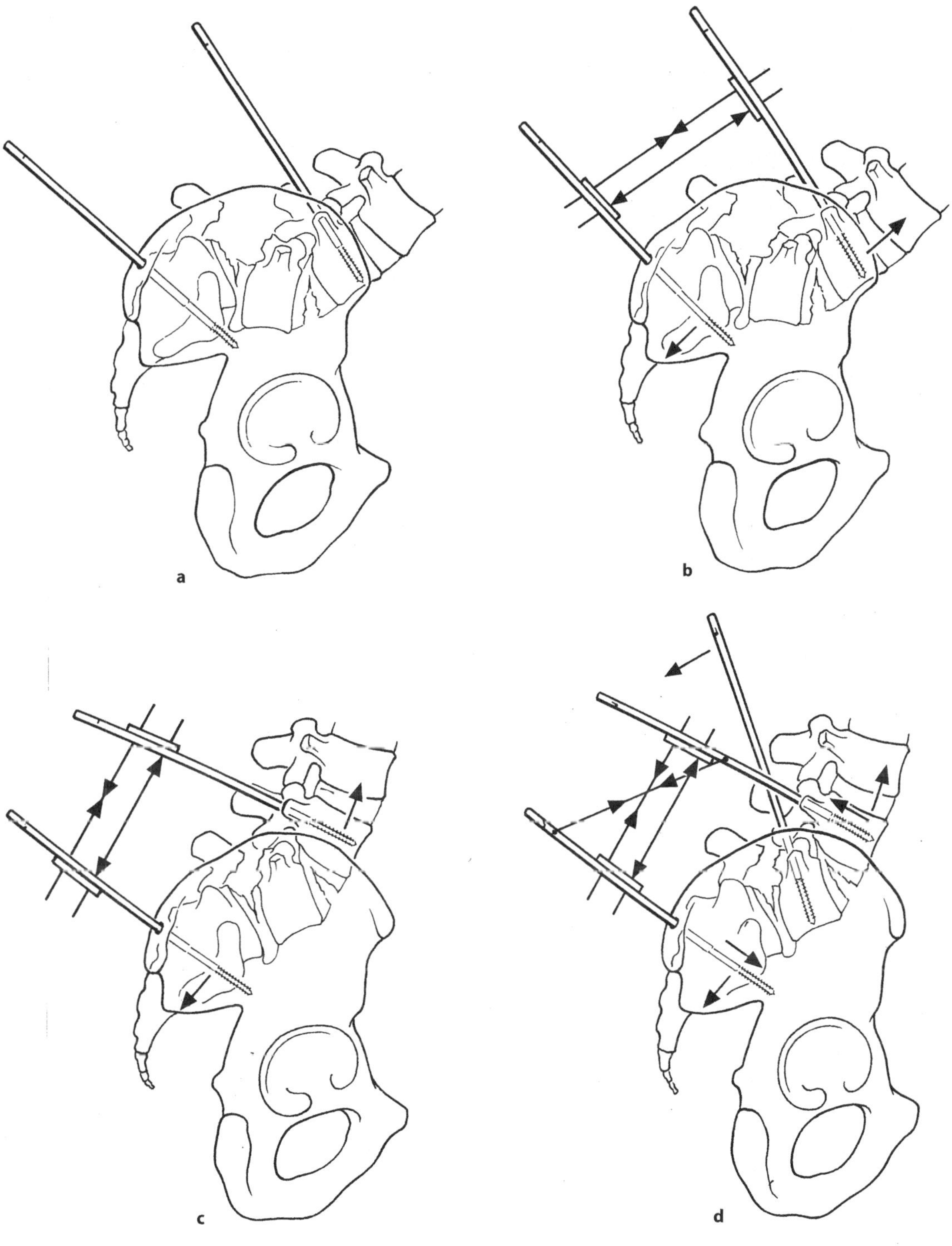

Fig. 9.17
a Schanz screws are inserted into L4 and the iliac bone
b Slight anterior distraction is applied to screch the soft tissues
c Once the acute wound pain has subsided, gradual closed reduction ist started by increasing anterior distraction and lordosis
d If increasing lordosis alone is not sufficient to reduce L5 to a grade I–II slip, L4 may additionaly be pulled backwards or

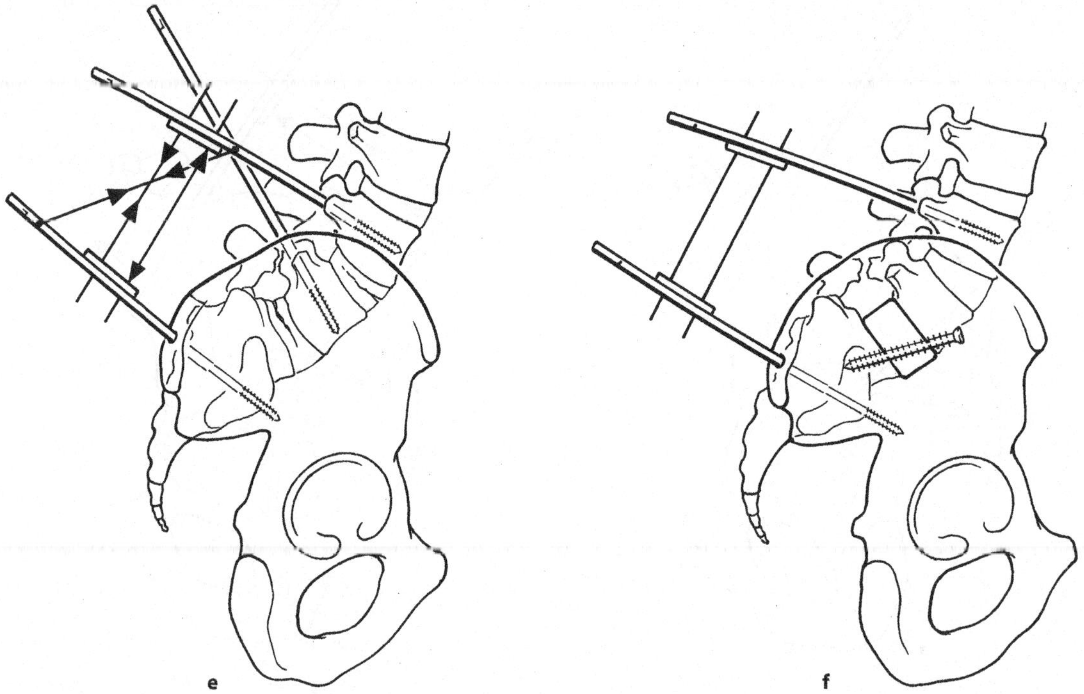

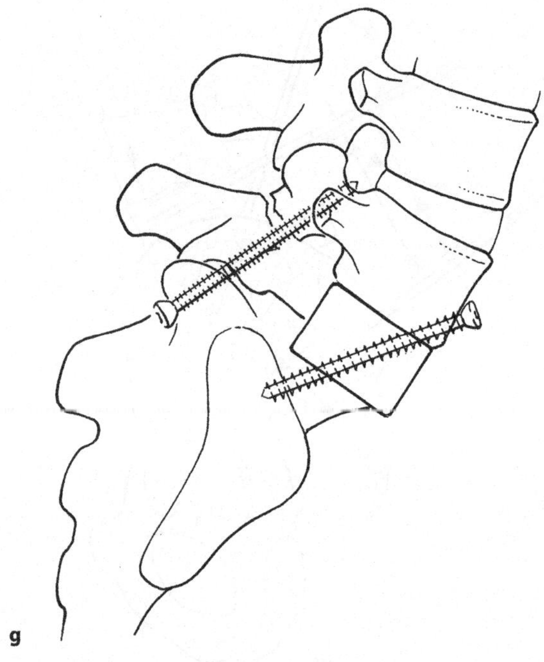

(Fig. 9.17)
e L5 itself may be instumented and manipulated
f After reduction to grade I–II, anterior interbody fusion is performed in situ without adding any distraction. The grafts are secured with a buttress screw (with a washer, if necessary)
g After healing of the stab incisions, posterior stabilization is performed using a pedicle device or this 'paralaminar screw fixation' S1/L5. The screws are anchored in the articular process of S1 and aim towards the pedicle of L5. They enter its pedicle at the level of the lysis and cross the pedicle in a caudocranial direction

9.2.3
Percutaneous Treatment of Osteomyelitis of the Spine

Principle

Treatment of osteomyelitis of the spine using percutaneous reduction of kyphotic deformity and decompression of the spinal cord, percutaneous drainage of the abscess with suction/irrigation and percutaneous stabilization of the unstable spine.

Indications

- Osteomyelitis of the spine from T3 to S1, when emergency decompression of the spinal cord is mandatory, but anterior decompression is not suitable.
- Pyogenic osteomyelitis of L5/S1, when surgical treatment is indicated.
- Painful lesions of the spine (even with minimal destruction) not amenable to efficient orthotic stabilization (T3–T9, L5/S1, elderly patients).
- Infected wounds making open surgery unsuitable.

Advantages

- Minimal invasive treatment.
- No emergency anterior approach is needed.
- Anterior interbody fusion possible later on if necessary.
- Mobilization of the patient possible soon after surgery.

Disadvantages

- Technically demanding.
- Anterior bone loss is not replaced.
- Inconvenience for the patient (external fixator).
- Demanding postoperative care.
- Potential risk of infection (not seen so far).

Technique

The patient is placed prone on a radiolucent operating table. A needle biopsy of the infected intervertebral disk space is performed with a biopsy needle with a 3.5 mm core diameter (Fig. 9.18a). The biopsy needle is introduced through the pedicle of the lower vertebra involved. Once material has been aspirated for bacteriological examination, wide-spectrum antibiotics are administered and the extent of the abscess cavity is demonstrated with contrast medium injected through the biopsy needle. Through the same biopsy needle, a drain is inserted into the disk space and secured in its position with a skin suture. A second drain is inserted into the disk space through the opposite pedicle (Fig. 9.18b). Schanz screws are inserted one level above and one level below the two affected vertebrae. The frame is mounted and the kyphosis reduced by applying lordosis and anterior distraction on the destroyed motion segment. The reduction is monitored with lateral image intensifier control (Fig 19.18c). This maneuver not only reduces the kyphosis, but also stretches the posterior part of the annulus fibrosus

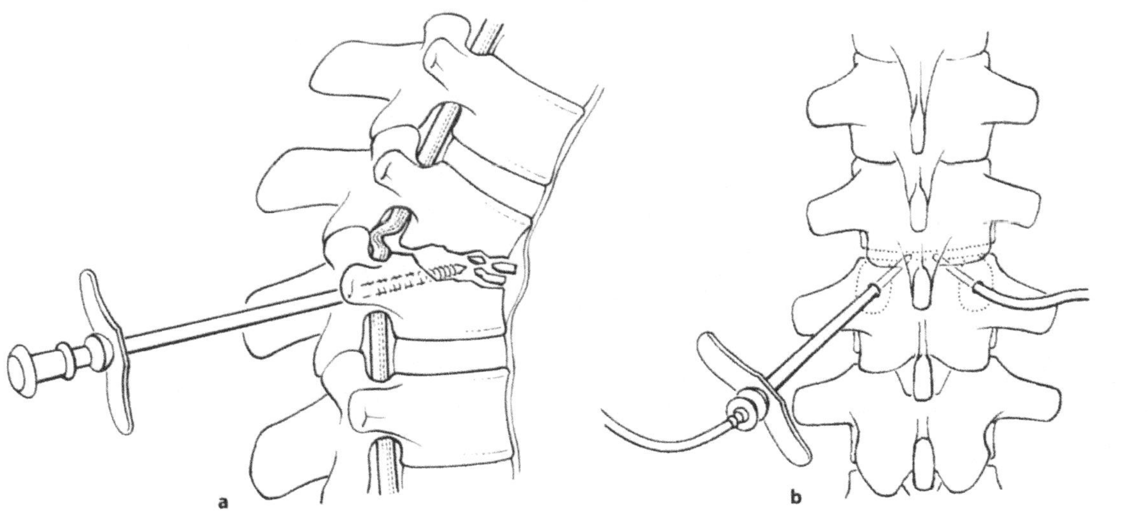

Fig. 9.18
a Needle biopsy is performed through the pedicle of the lower vertebra involved
b A drain is inserted on both sides into the intervertebral disk space for suction/irrigation

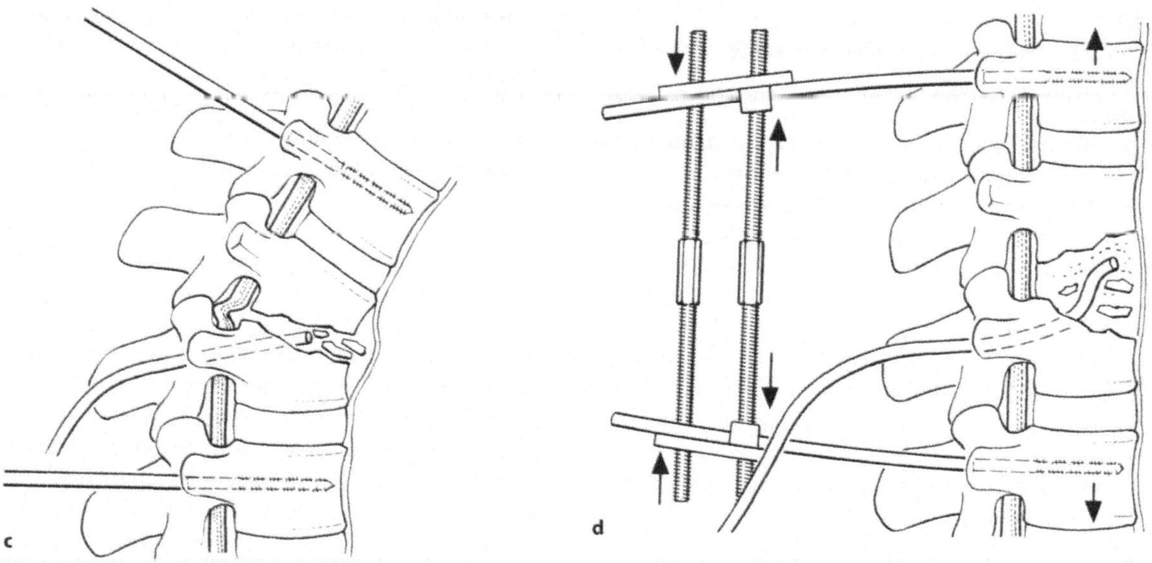

(Fig. 9.18)
c Schanz screws are inserted into the vertebra above and below the affected vertebrae

d Anterior distraction and lordosis are applied to restore lordosis, stretch the posterior annulus fibrosus, decompress the spinal cord and stabilize the spine

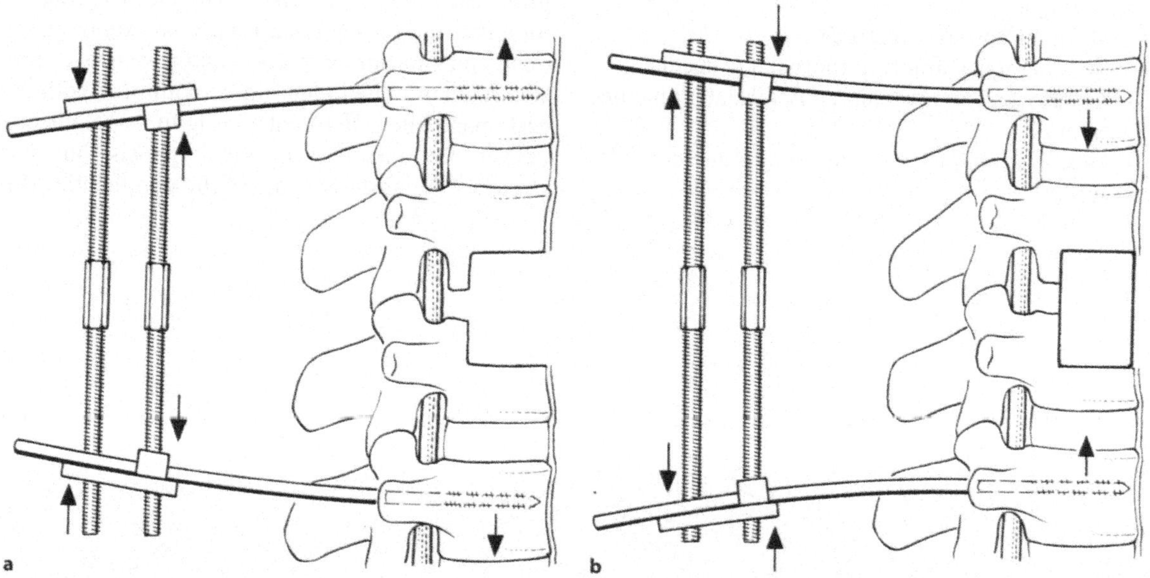

Fig. 9.19a, b In cases with severe bone defect, debridement and anterior interbody fusion using tricortical autologous bone grafts from the iliac crest may be performed later on to prevent secondary kyphotic deformity after removal of the external fixator. In this case, anterior compression is applied with the external fixator to stabilize the bone graft and enhance healing **(b)**

and decompresses the spinal cord, which is usually compressed by the retropulsed annulus fibrosus, by the apical part of the lower vertebra and by a possible epidural abscess. Irrigation of the intervertebral disk space and of the abscess is started by introducing alternately H_2O_2 and isotonic solution through one drain and aspirating it through the other one. Irrigation with isotonic solution is performed for 7 days.

In cases with severe bone defect or large abscess formation, anterior debridement and interbody fu-

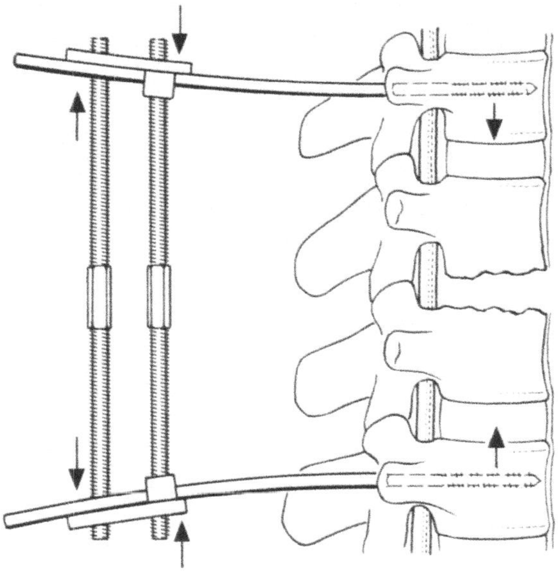

Fig. 9.20 In cases with small bony defects, anterior compression may be applied after several weeks to enhance spontaneous anterior bony fusion

sion with stable corticocancellous bone grafts is performed 3–4 weeks after initial surgery (Fig. 9.19). At this time, sterile conditions may be anticipated. To enhance healing of the bone grafts, anterior compression is now applied with the external fixator, which, up to that time, was applied with anterior distraction. The external fixator is left in place until healing of the anterior interbody fusion has been demonstrated in lateral tomograms usually after 3 months. At the thoracolumbar junction, the external fixator may also be removed after the anterior procedure and replaced by a corset.

When the external fixator is used for stabilization in patients with small and painful lesions not amenable to orthotic stabilization (especially upper thoracic spine and lumbosacral junction), distractive preload is slowly diminished after 4 weeks under constant neurological observation and changed to compressive preload to enhance spontaneous bony healing of the lesion (Fig. 9.20). After 3 months, the fixator is destabilized and removed even if no anterior bony bridging has occurred.

9.2.4 External Fixation for Spinal Fractures

Principle

Reduction and stabilization of fractures of the thoracic and lumbar spine using percutaneous external skeletal fixation.

Indications

- Thoracic, thoracolumbar and lumbar fractures with acute cord compression associated with:
- Deleterious general conditions making open surgical procedure unsuitable (e.g., coagulopathy, which cannot be corrected within 1 or 2 h, associated brain contusion with edema, which makes prolonged prone position and/or unsteady blood pressure undesirable, unstable angina pectoris).
- Open, contaminated or infected wounds.

Advantages

- Possible even when open surgical procedures are impossible (quick procedure, no blood loss).

Disadvantages

- No bone grafting possible.
- No open decompression or spinal canal possible.

Technique

Immediately after positioning the patient, closed longitudinal traction and lordosis is applied to the patient to partially reduce the fracture (Fig. 9.21). Schanz screws are inserted percutaneously in the two vertebrae immediately adjacent to the injured vertebra. Compressional rotational injuries are reduced by applying anterior distraction. Reduction is supervised under lateral image intensifer control. The correct reduction is obtained when the vertebral end plates adjacent to the fractured vertebra are parallel to each other. In this position, anterior distration is increased for optimal reduction of the posterior wall fragment and preloading of the system. Care must be taken not to overdistract a distraction injury. If performed during the first 24 hrs after injury, this closed maneuver is almost always sufficient to reduce compression-burst fractures with even large and massively retropulsed bone fragments. If spinal canal compromise persists (postoperative CT scan), open decompression and internal stabilization are performed as soon as general conditions allow.

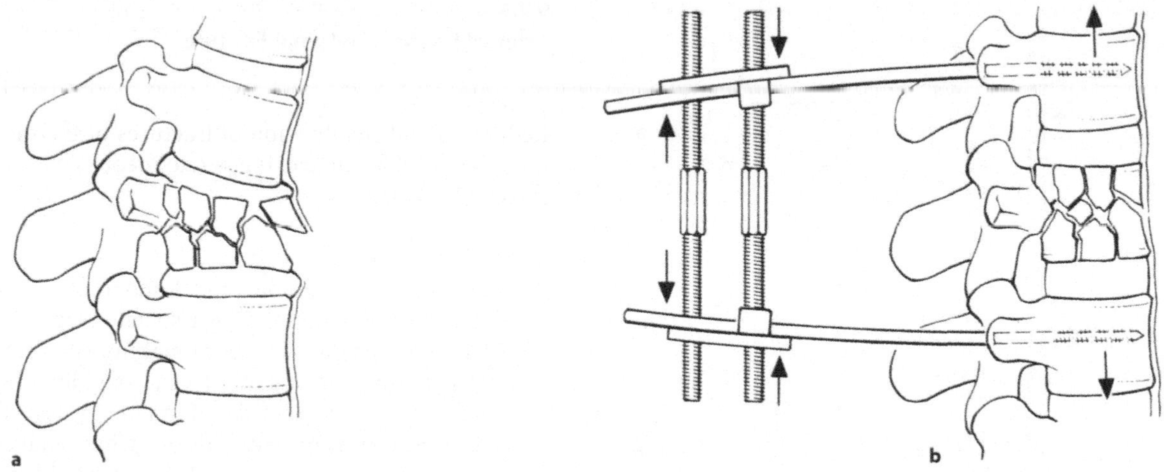

Fig. 9.21 Reduction of burst fracture
a Complete burst fracture (A3.3)
b Reduction under distraction+lordosizing

Postoperative Care
If adequate spinal canal decompression has been achieved by closed reduction, external fixation may be left in place until fracture healing has occurred. Since no bone grafting is possible, external fixation should be left in place for 4 months. An alternative is to replace ESSF after 2 months with a cast which is worn for another 2 months. At that time, the posterior vertebral elements are sufficiently consolidated to prevent displacement of the posterior wall fragment during application of the cast. However, we recommend removing and replacing ESSF by an internal fixation device a few days after surgery, once the general conditions of the patient have improved and allow open surgery. Secondary internal fixation should not be delayed for more than 1 week because of the possibility of contamination of the stab incisions.

9.2.5 Stabilization of Unstable Malgaigne Fractures

Principle
Stabilization of Malgaigne fractures by inserting Schanz screws into L4 and the iliac bones.

Indications
Unstable pelvic fractures of the Malgaigne type in the presence of skin lesions, making open surgical procdures impossible.

Advantages
- Percutaneous reduction and stabilization possible even in the presence of deleterious skin lesions.
- No blood loss, quick procedure.

Disadvantages
- Difficult control of reduction.
- Demanding postoperative care.

Technique
Schanz screws are inserted into L4 and the iliac bones on both sides (Fig. 9.22). Reduction of a cranial dislocation is achieved by applying distraction between L4 and the dislocated iliac bone. A lateral displacement is reduced by applying compression between both iliac bones.

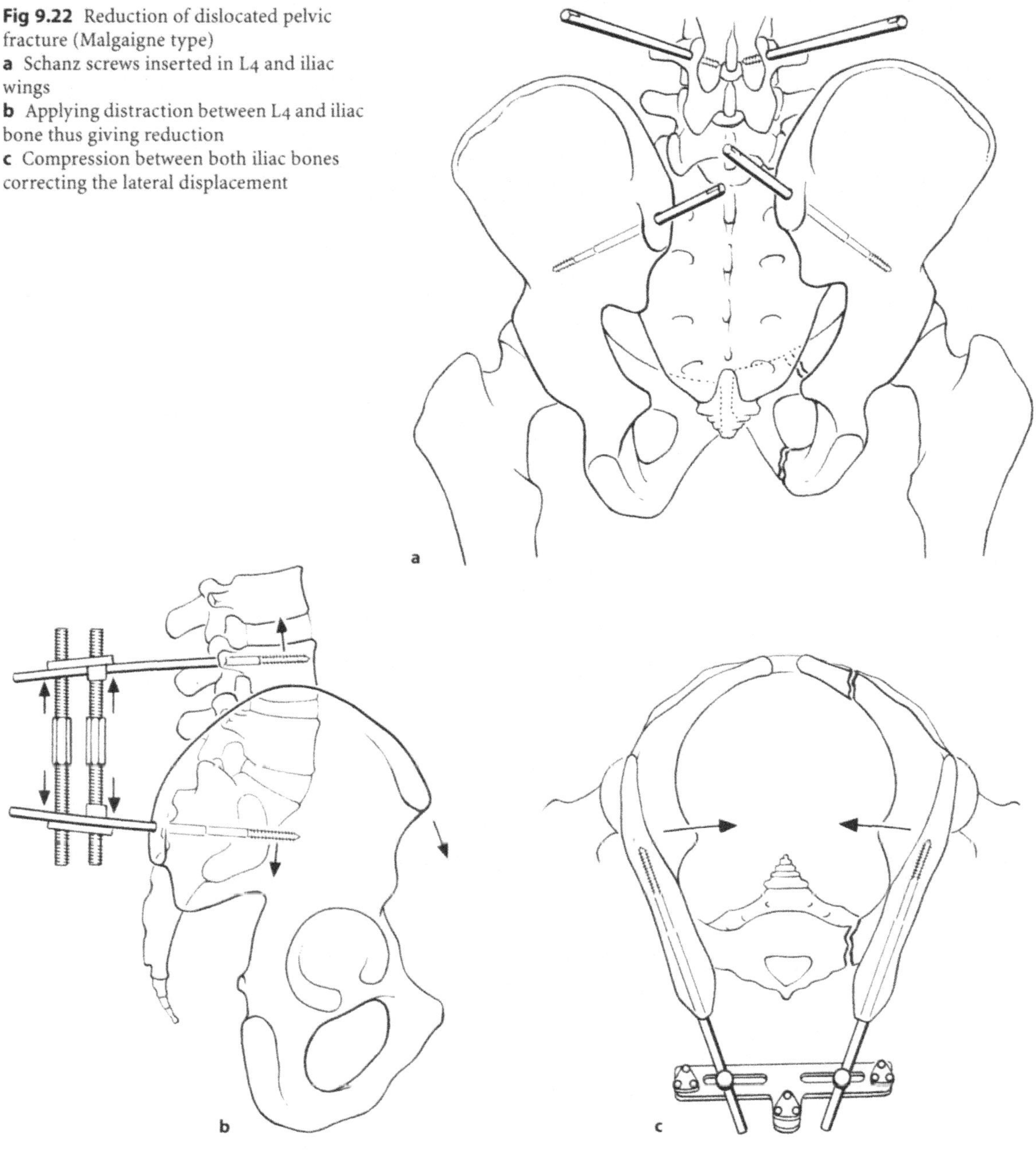

Fig 9.22 Reduction of dislocated pelvic fracture (Malgaigne type)
a Schanz screws inserted in L4 and iliac wings
b Applying distraction between L4 and iliac bone thus giving reduction
c Compression between both iliac bones correcting the lateral displacement

9.3 Cage Systems

9.3.1 Fixation with the Titanium Interbody Spacer

Principle

The titanium interbody spacer (TIS) is a titanium ring which provides immediate structural stability and reproduces the natural lordosis of the lumbar spine. The spacer is wedge shaped and has a secondary arc curvature which mirrors the dome of the vertebral end plate in the lumbar spine. The spacer has teeth on both sides which allows fixation into the end plate and prevents migration. The spacer is designed in an oval fashion to follow the anatomy of the end plate (Fig 9.23). The large hollow, center space allows for autograft or allograft. The spacer may also be used with coralline hydroxyapatite, which allows osteoconduction to occur at the end

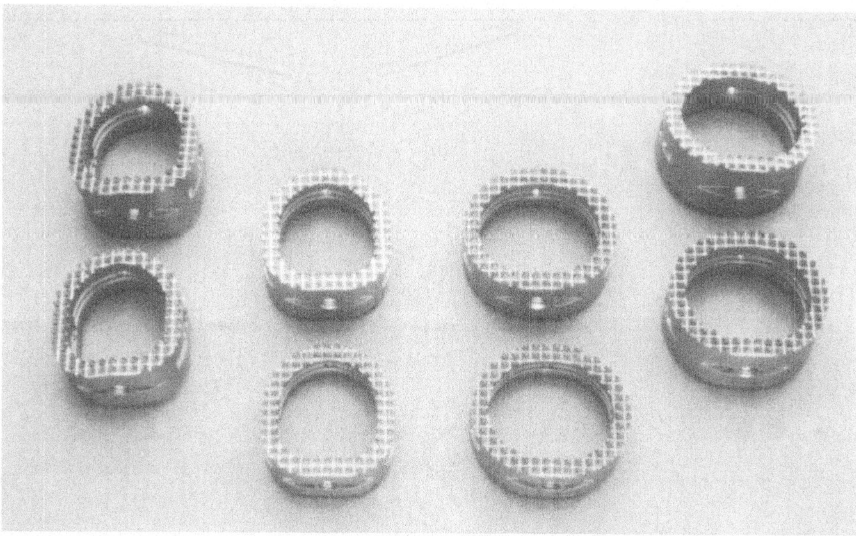

Fig. 9.23 Different sizes of titanium interbody spacers (TIS)

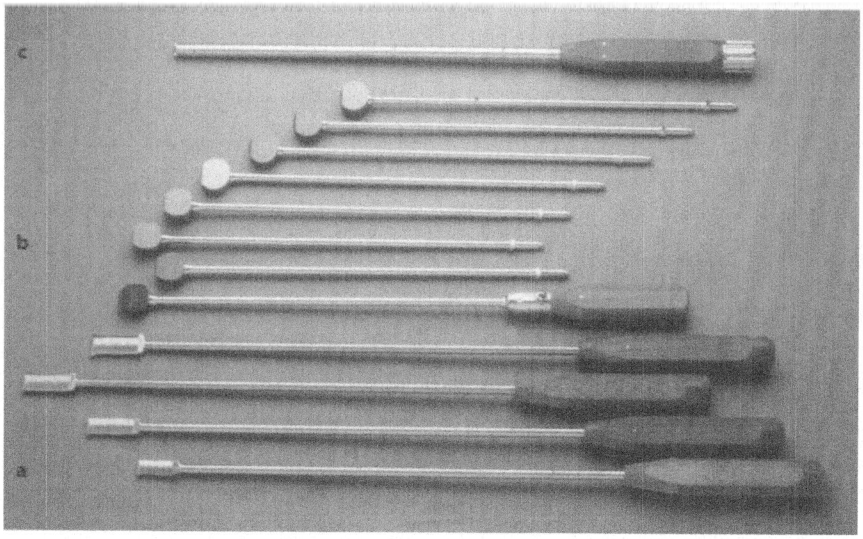

Fig. 9.24 Instruments: Different size templates to open the disc space **(a)** and to test the size and position of the cage **(b)**. Instrument to deliver the cage **(c)**

plate-coralline hydroxyapatite interface (Fig 9.25). This may be used in conjunction with posterior instrumentation.

Indications
- For anterior lumbar interbody fusions from L1–L2 to L5/S1. It may be used for degenerative disk disease, spondylolisthesis, failed lumbar laminectomy syndrome, pseudoarthrosis and internal disk disruption.

Advantages
- Due to its wedge shape, it recreates the lumbar lordosis within the disk segment. It allows distraction and maintenance of the intervertebral disk space height.
- Provides immediate, secure anterior lumbar support.
- When used with coralline hydroxyapatite it eliminates the need for bone graft to obtain fusion.

Disadvantages
- Difficult to assess radiographic fusion at the titanium-bone interface.
- Requires an intact end plate to prevent subsidence into the vertebral body.
- Does not have expansion capabilities for vertebrectomy.
- May require an additional posterior fixation in case of an unstable motion segment which cannot be immobilized enough with the anterior spacer alone.

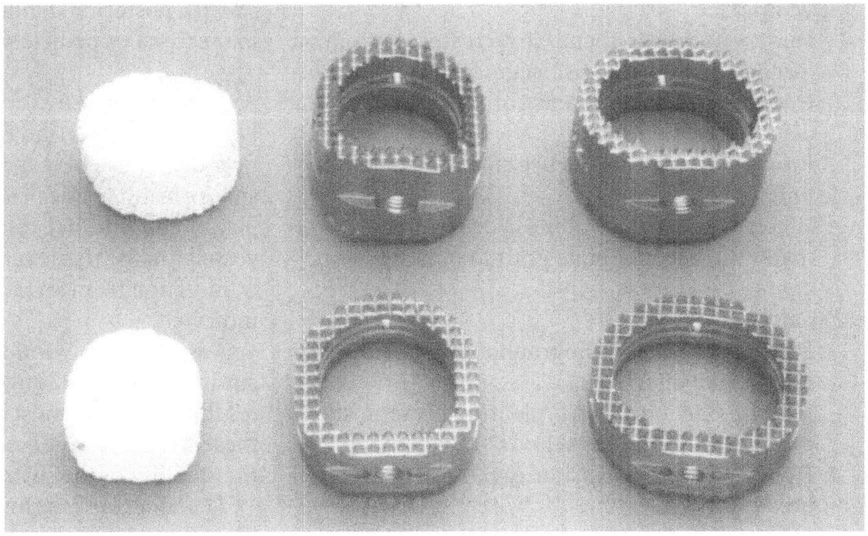

(Fig. 9.24d)
Different size of T15 with possible Coralline inserts

Instruments and Implants (Fig. 9.24d)

Surgical Technique
A standard anterior retroperitoneal or transperitoneal approach is made to expose the anterior lumbar spine. The anterior annulus is opened with the scalpel and the disk is separated from the end plates with an end plate cutting tool. The disk is then removed with a curette and rongeur down to the posterior annulus. The posterior annulus is left intact. The cartilage is removed from the end plate preferentially with a ring curette. This is done carefully to maintain the structural integrity of the vertebral end plate. Once this is completed the disk space is sized with the spacers by placing the spacers into the disk space horizontally and then turning them vertically to distract the disk space (Fig. 9.24a/b). Once the appropriate size has been determined, the titanium interbody cage is selected and filled with bone graft or coralline hydroxyapatite (Fig. 9.24d). Using special introduction device (Fig 9.24c) the spacer is placed into the disk space and hammered into position, while the template or intervertebral body spreader are in place, still allowing the cage to be in the midline put in the optimal position (Fig. 9.25c). The spacer is designed to stay within the disk space. It should be midline and to the anterior aspect of the vertebral body to cover the exposed teeth of the spacer. This is done to prevent vascular injury.

Alternative Surgical Technique

BERG Approach. The balloon-assisted endoscopic retroperitoneal gasless (BERG) approach involves an endoscopic minimally invasive approach to the spine. This approach decreases operative morbidity and is done through a balloon dissection of the retroperitoneum. The operative field is maintained by a series of special balloon retractors as well as standard anterior operative instruments. The gasless minimally invasive approach allows tract access to the anterior aspect of the spine and the use of standard anterior instruments to perform the anterior diskectomy and placement of the TIS.

Postoperative Care
The patient is mobilized in a lumbosacral orthosis for 12 weeks, and in the hospital, on the first postoperative day. If the minimally invasive BERG approach is utilized, the patient is mobilized immediately.

9.3.2 Anterior Titanium Interbody Spacer (SynCage)

Surgical Technique

Principles
The anterior titanium interbody spacer (SynCage) is a titanium spacer which provides immediate structural stability and reproduces the normal lordosis. The spacer is designed to fit between the endplates.

Indications
- For anterior lumbar interbody fusions from L1/L2 to L5/S1. It may be used for degenerative disc disease, spondylolisthesis, failed lumbar laminectomy syndrome, pseudoarthrosis and internal disc disruption.

Advantages

- Due to its wedge shape, it recreates the lumbar lordosis within the disc segment. It allows distraction and maintenance ot the intervertebral disc space height.
- Provides immediate, secure anterior lumbar support.
- When used with a coralline hydroxyapatite it estimates the need for bone graft to obtain fusion.

Disadvantages

- Difficult to assess radiographic fusion at the titanium-bone interface.
- Requires an intact end plate to prevent subsidence into the vertebral body.
- Does not have expansion capabilities for vertebrectomy.
- May require an additional posterior fixation in case of an unstable motion segment which cannot be immobilised enough with the anterior spacer alone.

Instruments and Implants (Fig. 9.25)

Surgical Technique

Implantation of the spacer is performed in three stages. First preoperative planning; second the surgical approach and finally, insertion of the spacer.

Preoperative Planning

Prior to surgery, the desired surgical approach and an estimation of the appropriate spacer height should be determined. The desired surgical approach is dependent on the level to be treated and the surgeon's preference. As the spacer can be inserted either from the anterior, antero-lateral or lateral direction, the surgeon is free to use the approach of choice. The technique for insertion of the spacer varies slightly depending on the direction chosen.

An initial estimate of the spacer size can be determined by comparing the Radiographic Template with the adjacent intervertebral discs on a lateral radiograph. The height of the template is 1-mm (half the height of the two sets of teeth) shorter than that of the respective spacer to account for penetration of the teeth into the vertebral bone.

The spacer must fit firmly with a tight press-fit between the endplates with the segment fully distracted. It is essential that the tallest possible spacer be used so as to minimise the stability of the segment resulting from tension in the ligament and annulus fibrosus.

It is recommended that the spacer is supplemented with posterior stabilisation either with translaminar screws or pedicle fixation.

Anterior Approach

For anterior insertion the midline of the intervertebral disc must be exposed so that there is a clear space on either side of the vertebral midline (sagittal plane) equal to half the width of the spacer. If the vessels and/or tissues cannot be retracted sufficiently, insertion from an antero-lateral direction may be indicated.

A rectangular window the width of the spacer is cut in the anterior longitudinal ligament and annulus fibrosus. Care must be taken to retain as much of these structures as possible as they are important for the stability of the instrumented segment.

The anterior longitudinal ligament and annulus fibrosus, the disc material is excised and the superficial layers of the cartilaginous endplates are removed to create a bleeding bone surface. Adequate cleaning of the endplate is important for vascular supply to the bone graft, however, exessive cleaning may weaken the endplate due to removal of the denser bone of the endplate.

Once the endplates have been prepared and any additional surgical procedures completed, the spacer is introduced into the intervertebral space as follows:

Distraction of the segment is essential for restoration of disc height, opening of the neural foramen and stability of the spacer. Distraction is achieved prior to insertion of the spacer with the distractor and distractor blades.

The distractor blades are placed into the disc space. To ensure that the spacer is inserted symmetrically in the disc space, place the line on the blades in the midline (Fig. 9.26a).

Compressing the distractor handle opens the disc space.

Once desired level of distraction is achieved, the required spacer size is determined using the trial implants as follows:

Select the trial implant which corresponds with the spacer size determined during the pre-operative planning. Slide the trial implant over the distractor blades into the disc space (Fig. 9.26 b,b'). If a tight fit is not achieved, try the next larger trial implant size; or if the trial implant cannot be inserted, try the next smaller trial implant size. With the segment fully distracted, the spacer/trial implant must fit firmly with a tight pressfit between the endplates such that the disc height is not lost once the distractor is removed. It is essential that the tallest possible spacer be used so as to maximise the stability of the segment resulting from tension in the ligament and annulus fibrosus.

Fig 9.25 Instruments and Implants for the anterior titanium interbody spacer (SynCage)
a Trial implant holder, straigt and angled
b Trial implants
c Anterior interbody spacer holders
d Disc space distractor
e Lateral distractor
f Packing block
g Graft punch
h Anterior titanium interbody spacers – four sizes

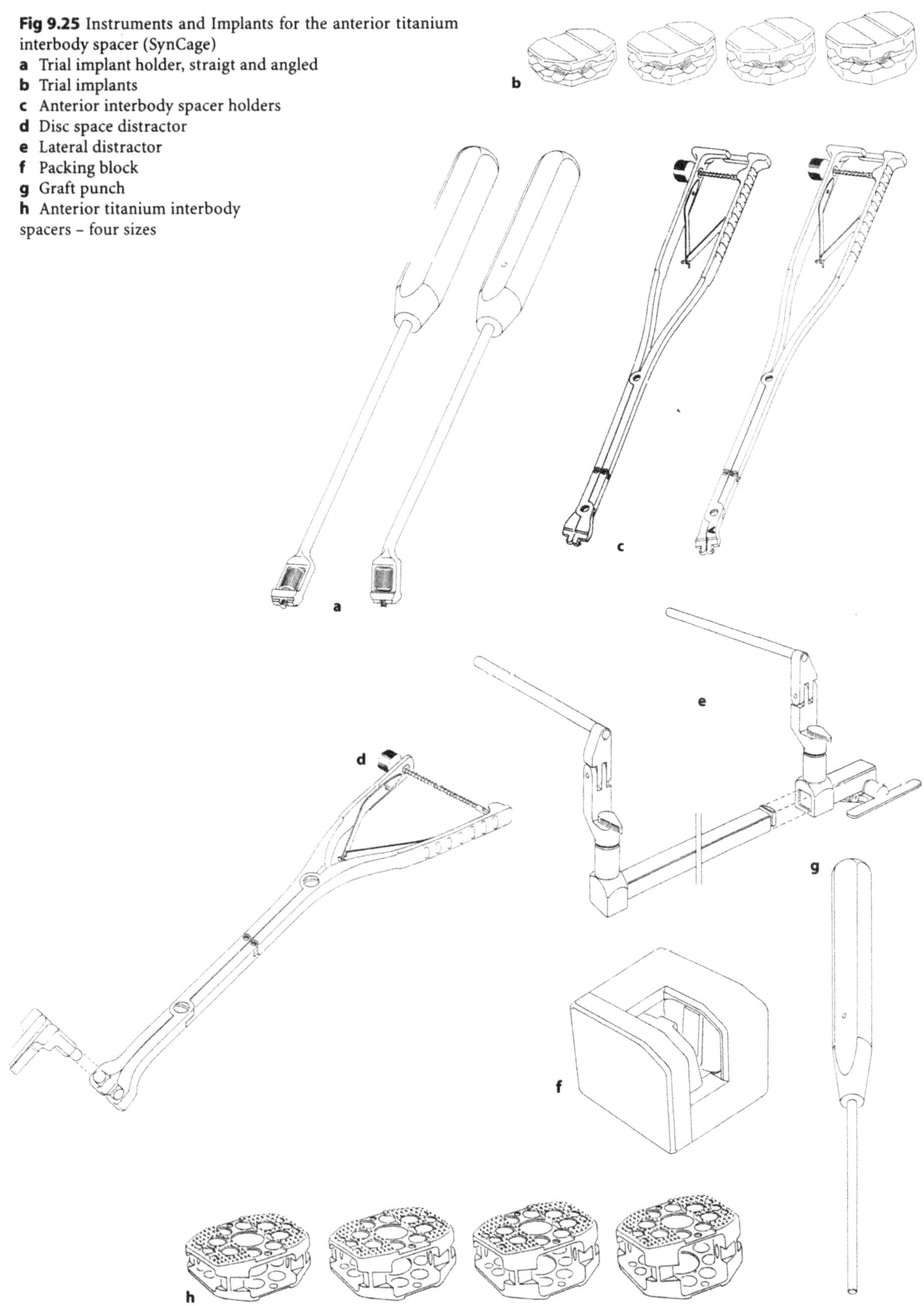

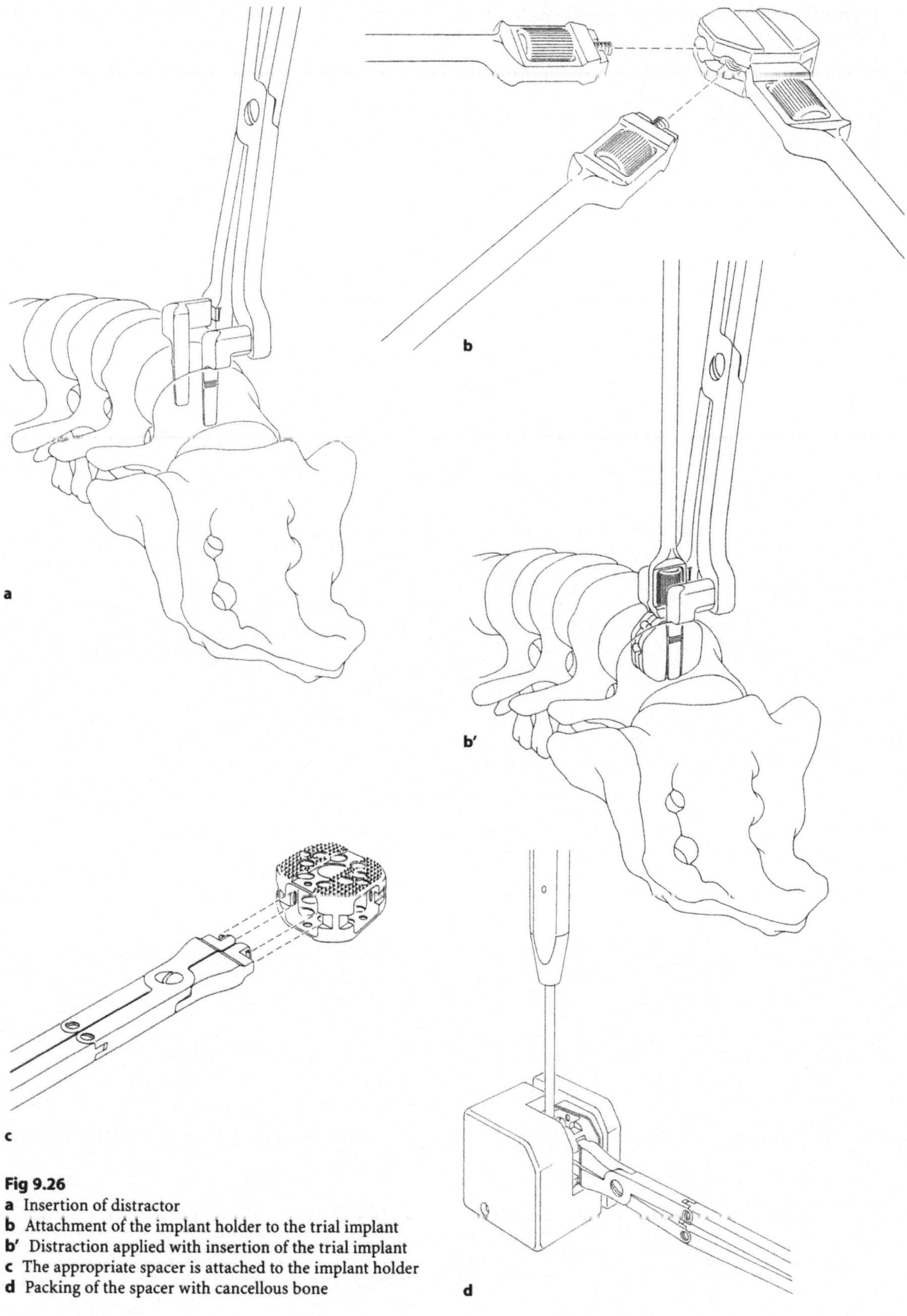

Fig 9.26
a Insertion of distractor
b Attachment of the implant holder to the trial implant
b' Distraction applied with insertion of the trial implant
c The appropriate spacer is attached to the implant holder
d Packing of the spacer with cancellous bone

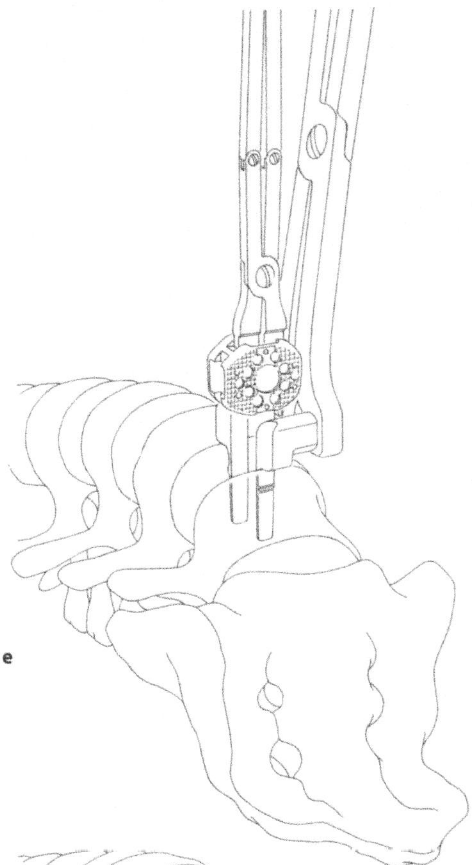

e

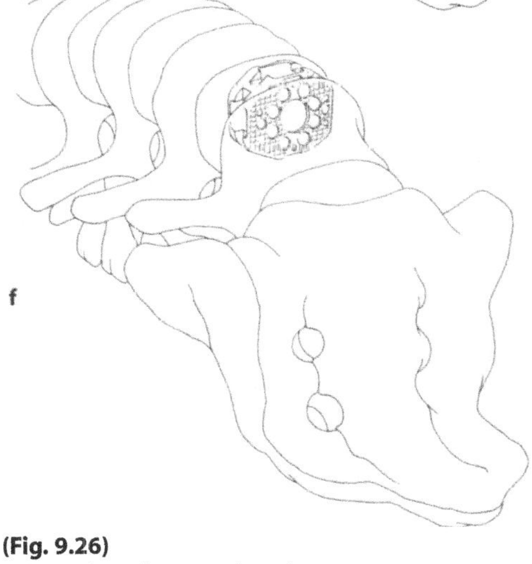

f

(Fig. 9.26)
e Insertion of appropriate size spacer
f Spacer inserted

Once the size of spacer has been selected the distraction can be temporarily relaxed.

The spacer corresponding to the trial implant is then selected. The spacers are colour coded by height (extra small – yellow; small – blue; medium – violet and large – green). With the spacer of the correct height chosen, it is secured on the straight implant holder (Fig. 9.26c).

The cancellous graft is morsellised for ease of packing into the interior of the spacer. To assist packing the graft, the spacer with the implant holder attached can be set into the packing block. The bone graft impacter can be used to firmly pack the graft material (Fig. 9.26d).

In order to optimise blood supply to the graft, it is important that the spacer is completely filled such that the graft protrudes from the holes in the spacer.

With the spacer ready for insertion, the segment is again distracted. The distraction is fixed by lightening the locking screw on the handle.

The spacer is then introduced into the disc space by placing it between the blades of the distractor such that the slots on the superior and inferior surfaces on the spacer fit over the blades of the distractor (Fig. 9.26e).

The spacer usually requires light hammering to introduce it into the disc space. The distractor should be withdrawn once the spacer is inserted but not fully seated in the disc space and prior to the final insertion by hammering. Once the spacer is in the correct position, the locking screw on the distractor's handle is loosened and the distraction released. The distractor is gently removed while the spacer is maintained in position by the implant holder.

The optimal position for the spacer is such that it is centred within the middle of the vertebral endplate.

Depending on the size of the vertebrae, the anterior edge of the spacer will be approximately 3-5 mm posterior from the anterior edge of the adjacent vertebvrae. The location of the space relative to the vertebral bodies in the AP direction should be verified using an image intensifier (Fig. 9.26)f.

Any additional bone graft may be packed in spaces remaining around the spacer, in particular into the anterior slot of the spacer.

Antero-Lateral and Lateral Approach

Once exposure of the intervertebral disc is attained and the surrounding tissues and vessels retracted, a special screw is inserted into each of the vertebral bodies adjacent to the disc to be treated. These screws should be introduced parallel to each other.

Care must be taken to ensure that these screws are not inserted too deeply.

The tubular extensions of the lateral distractor are then slid over the screws (Fig. 9.27a).

The vertebral segment is distracted by turning the knob of the distractor.

If neccessary, additional distraction may be achieved using a vertebral spreader to open the space using the lateral distractor to hold the distraction. The trial implants may also be used to help open the segment.

To determine the correct size of spacer, the trial implant is slid into the disc space (Fig. 9.27b).

If a tight fit is not achieved, try the next larger trial implant size, or if the trial implant cannot be inserted, try the next smaller trial implant size. With the segment fully distracted, the spacer must fit firmly with a tight press-fit between the endplates such that the disc height is not lost once the distractor is removed. It is essential that the tallest possible spacer be used in order to maximise the stability of the segment resulting from tension in the ligament and annulus fibrosus.

Once the spacer has been selected the distraction can be temporarily relaxed.

The appropriate spacer chosen, it is secured on to the implant holder (Fig. 9.27c).

Depending on the angle of the approach the spacer will be introduced from an offset direction or 90° offset. The former is achieved using the offset implant holder which grips the spacer on its lateral edge.

If the spacer is to be introduced perpendicular to the vertebral midline (90° offset) the straight implant holder is used to grasp the spacer on its lateral side.

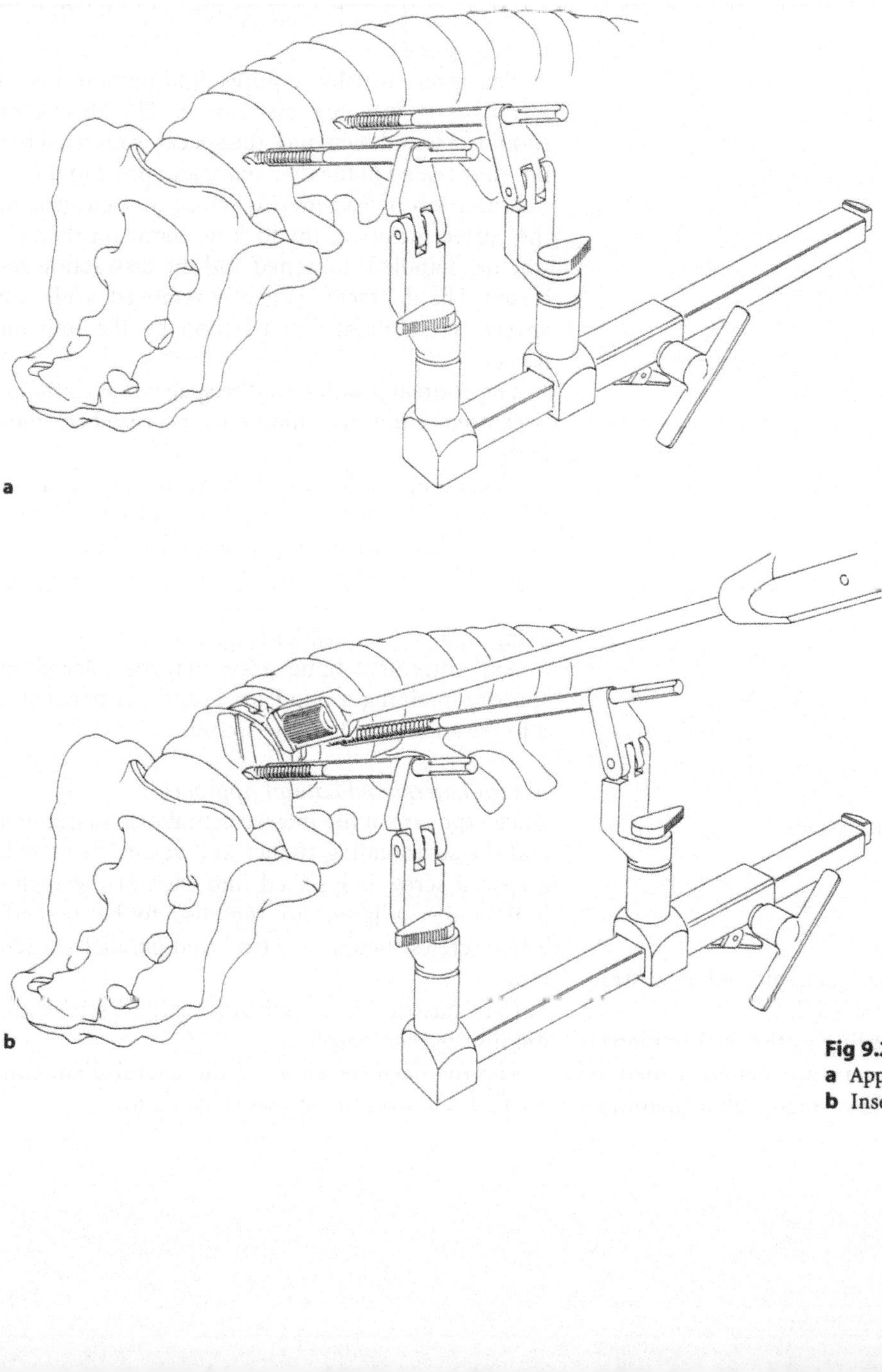

a

b

Fig 9.27
a Application of lateral distraction
b Insertion of trial implant

(Fig. 9.27)
c Attachment of angled implant holder to the titanium spacer
d Insertion of spacer with cancellous graft

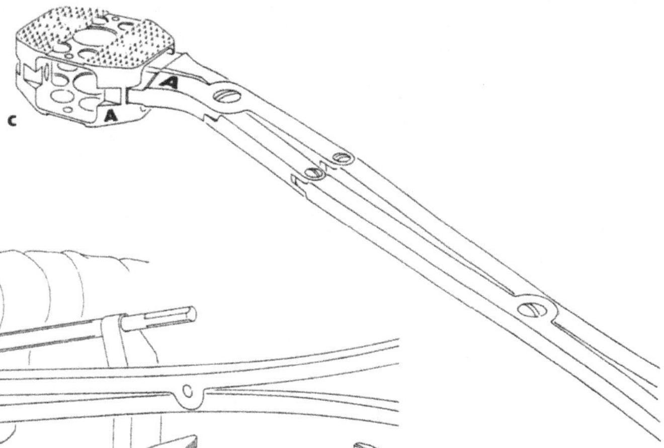

c

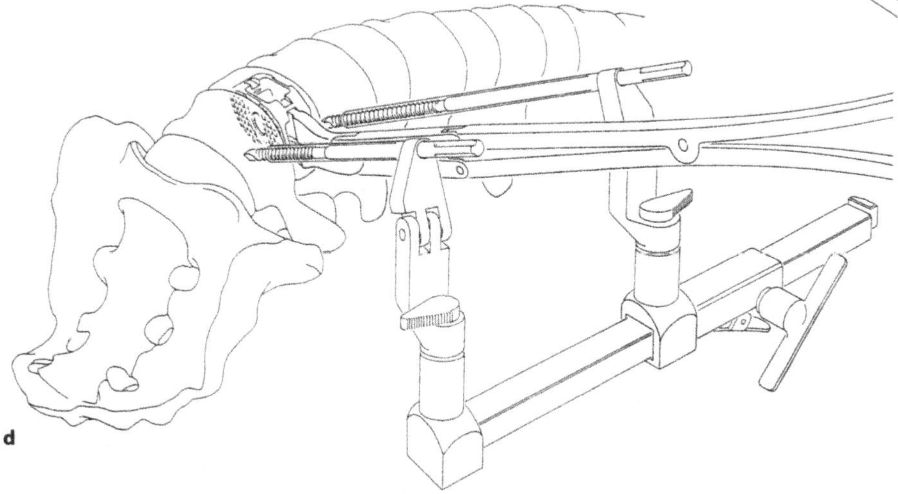

d

With the spacer packed with cancellous bone ready for insertion, the segment is again distracted.

The spacer is then introduced into the disc space. The spacer may require light hammering to introduce it into the space (Fig. 9.27d).

The optimal position for the spacer is centred within the middle of the vertebral endplate. Depending on the size of the vertebrae, the anterior edge of the spacer will be approximately 3-5 mm posterior from the edge of the adjacent vertebrae. The location of the spacer relative to the vertebral bodies in the AP direction should be verified using an image intensifier.

Once the spacer is in position, the distraction is released and lateral distractor is removed. The two special screws are then removed.

Supplemental posterior procedure
Translaminar screws have been shown to significantly improve the biomechanical stability of the motion segment regardless of the design of ALIF implant. Therefore, the use of this simple and safe procedure is recommended to supplement the stability provided by the spacer. The procedure is performed after implantation of the spacer. For treatment of spondylolisthesis the use of supplemental pedicle screw construct is indicated. In such cases the posterior procedure may be performed first.

Postoperative care
The patients can be mobilised the day after surgery. A brace (T.L.S.O. or L.S.O.) should be worn for the first three months postoperatively. The patients should be cautioned against activities which place unreasonable stress on the region. Excessive physical activity and trauma affecting the involved vertebrae may cause premature failure through loosening and/or wear of the spacer.

9.3.3 Contact Fusion Cage

Principle
The contact fusion cage is an implant system for posterior lumbar interbody fusion (PLIF).
It was designed:

- To fuse the adjacent vertebral bodies in an optimal anatomic position.
- To allow distraction of the disk space to be bridged resulting in restoration of disk height, lordosis and widening of the foramen.
- To avoid penetration of the end plates by the cage.
- To support bone growth through the cage.

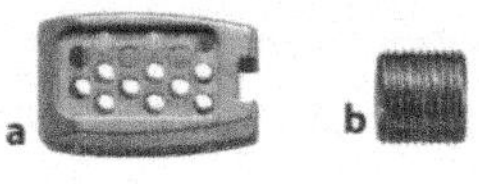

Fig. 9.28 Implants
CONTACT fusion cage, open at the top and the bottom, where the bone graft packed in the cage comes into contact with the adjacent vertebral end plates
b Bone compression screw

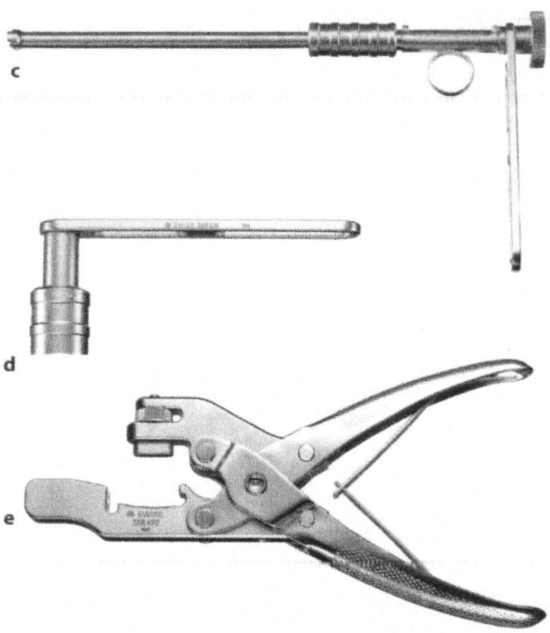

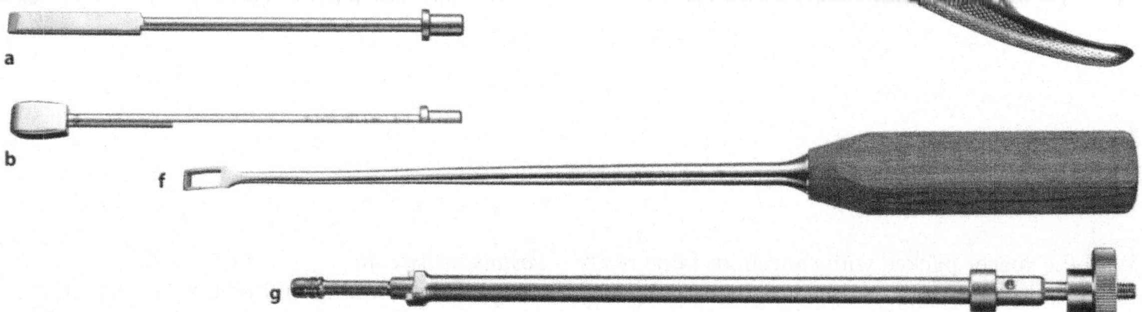

Fig. 9.29 Instruments
a Disc space opener
b Vertebral body spreader
c CONTACT fusion cage holder
d L-handle with quick coupling
e Bone compression forceps
f Bone curette, rectangular
g Emergency holder

Implants (Fig. 9.28)
The cages have a rectangular cross-section. They are introduced on the flat side and turned clockwise in order to spread the disk space and to bring the cage into its final vertical position. When viewed from the side, the cages have rounded superior and inferior edges, giving them a 'compact' lenticular form that conforms to the average form of the sagittal section of the lumbar disks (L4–L5, L5–S1). Thus, the posterior edge of the end plates is left intact and prevents the cages from migration posteriorly. Choosing the best-fitting cage from a range of seven sizes, the optimal disk height and the natural lordosis can be restored without having to cut an implant site into the end plates.

The superior and inferior surfaces of the cage are open, in order to receive the milled bone that is compressed inside the cages. The bone is pressed firmly against the end plates by a compression screw which is advanced into the middle of the cage after implantation. The autologous bone supports bone growth through the cages themselves and the bony fusion of the adjacent vertebral bodies. The cages are manufactured from strong titanium alloy (TAN), which provides MRI/CT compatibility.

Instruments (see Fig. 9.29)
The handling of the instruments needs to follow the instructions strictly, otherwise the system may fail and a proper application of the PLIF-contact fusion cages may be compromised.

Indications
Painful lumbar and lumbo-sacro pathologies indicated for segmental arthrodesis including:
- Degenerative disk disease and instability.
- Primary surgery for certain advanced disk diseases or extensive decompression.
- Laminectomy, facetectomy, foraminotomy.
- Revision surgery for failed disk surgery, recurrence of disk herniation, postoperative instability.
- Pseudoarthrosis of a posterolateral fusion.
- Degenerative spondylolisthesis grade I or II.
- Isthmic spondylolisthesis grade I or II.

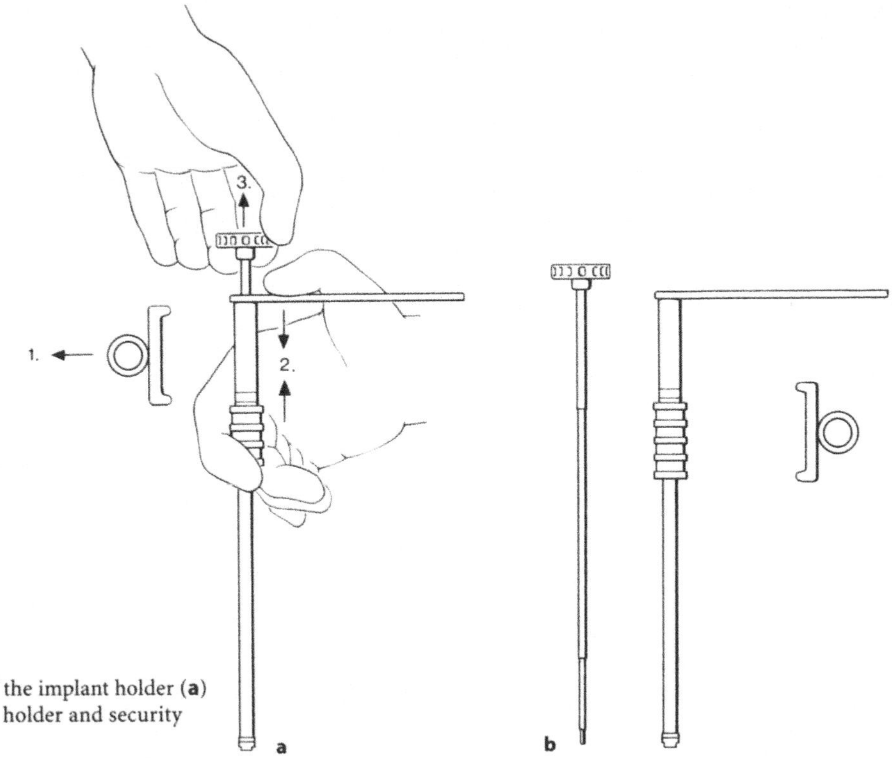

Fig. 9.30a Disassembling of the implant holder (**a**) into the screwdriver, implant holder and security sleeve (**b**)

It is recommended to use PLIF preferentially with an additional posterior instrumentation, putting the cages under compression and restoring the posterior tension banding system (load-sharing concept).

Contraindications

- Severe osteoporosis.
- Unstable burst fractures and compression fractures.
- Active infections.
- Destructive tumors.
- Involvement of three or more levels.
- Grade III or greater spondylolisthesis.

9.3.2.1
Mounting the Cage on the Implant Holder

First the screwdriver is taken out of the implant holder (Fig. 9.30a, b). This is placed on the bone compression screw, which is stored in the implant box and the upper end of the shaft slightly pressed. Its anterior telescopic shaft will click-couple inside the bone compression screw and enable it to be picked up (Fig. 9.31). The hexagonal screwdriver is inserted and slightly turned in the implant holder$_{(2)}$, pressing the telescopic shaft down to the second mark$_{(1)}$: The hexagonal screwdriver will snap in and

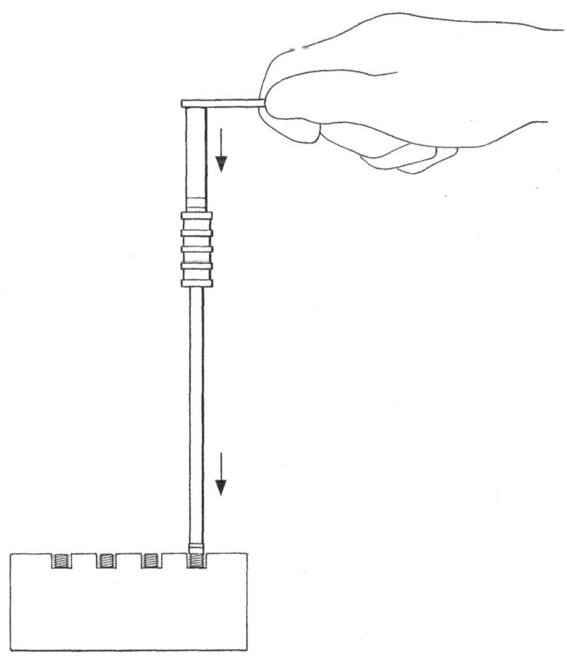

Fig. 9.31 Picking up the bone compression screw from the implant box

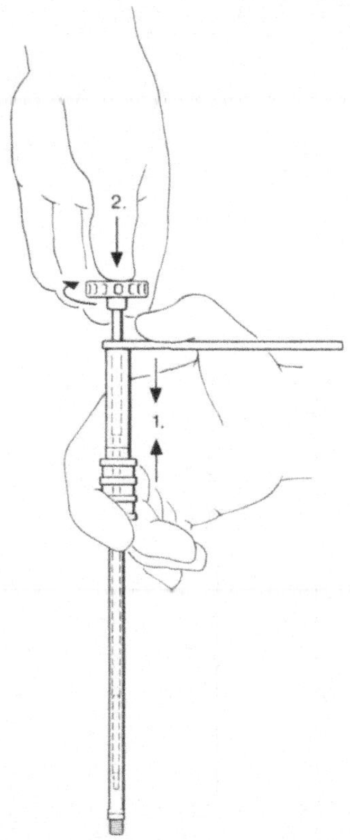

Fig. 9.32 Insertion of the screwdriver

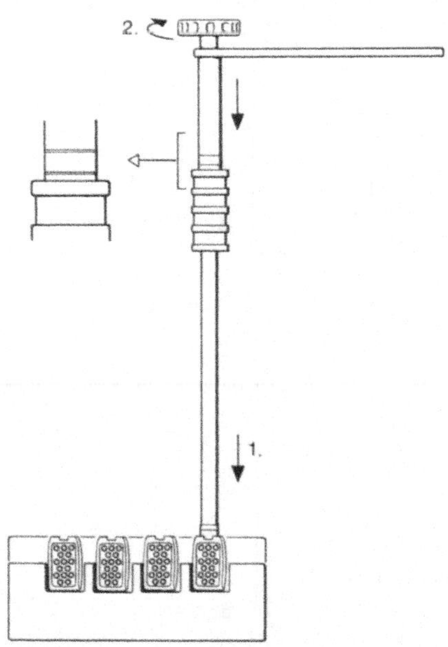

Fig. 9.33 Picking up the cage

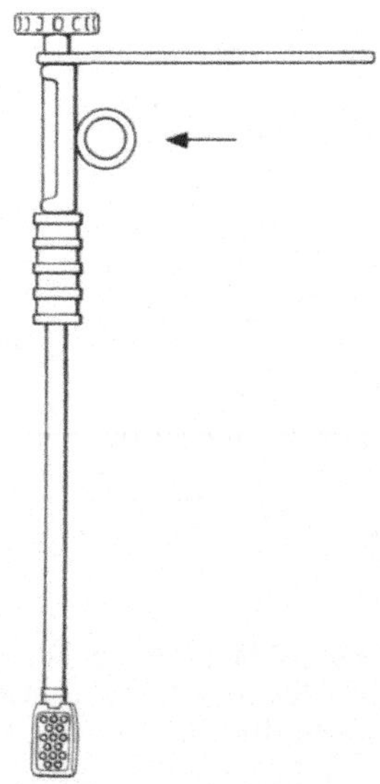

Fig. 9.34 Mounting the security sleeve

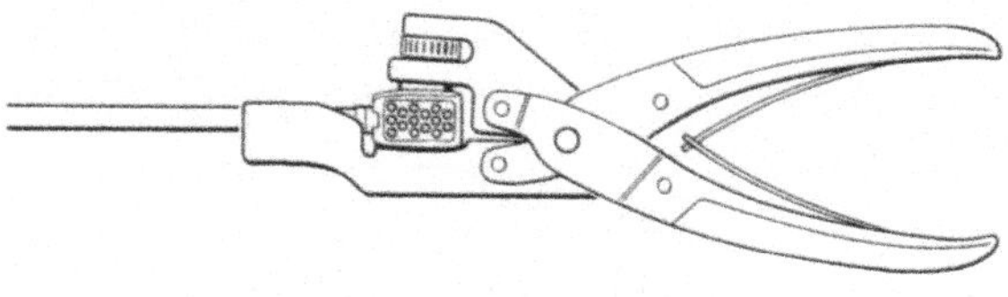

Fig. 9.35 Filling the case with bone graft

lock the screw to the tip of the inner shaft (Fig. 9.32). The assembled implant holder is then positioned on the cage (1) and the screwdriver is turned until the compression screw has engaged the thread. The small screw is advanced to the required depth when the first circular marking on the shaft is flush with the proximal end of the casing (2) (Fig. 9.33). The security sleeve is clipped over the telescopic shaft and the turning knob is tightened. As the security sleeve blocks the telescopic shaft the implant holder and the cage now form a 'continuous rod'. This step is very important since it blocks the telescopic action of the handle. Only then can the connection of the cage to the handle withstand the stresses that occur by introducing the cage into the disk space (Fig. 9.34). A second cage is mounted on the other implant holder in the same way.

9.3.2.2
Filling the Cage with Bone Graft

The cages are filled with finely milled autologous bone (the resected bone from the spinous processes and the facet joints will generally be sufficient). If more bone is needed, it can be harvested from the posterior iliac crest with the smallest size of hip reamer, generating in one working step 'milled' bone. The bone compression forceps are used to compress the bone in the cages (Fig. 9.35).

9.3.3.3
Removal of the Cage

If for any reason, retrieval of the cage should be necessary, a special handle, (Fig. 9.29), is provided. The bone compression screw is first removed with the hexagonal screwdriver and with the aid of tweezers (Fig. 9.36). Subsequently, the inner shaft of the emergency holder is inserted into the thread of the cage (Fig. 9.37), the sleeve of the emergency holder is mounted on the shaft and it is ensured that the coupling fits well into the slot of the cage (Fig. 9.38). The L-handle is mounted on the sleeve of the emergency holder by pressing the coupling a little bit forward (Fig. 9.39). The threaded turning knob is fixed on the threaded end of the shaft and firmly tightens it (Fig. 9.40). The cage is finally turned counterclockwise and taken out carefully (Fig. 9.41).

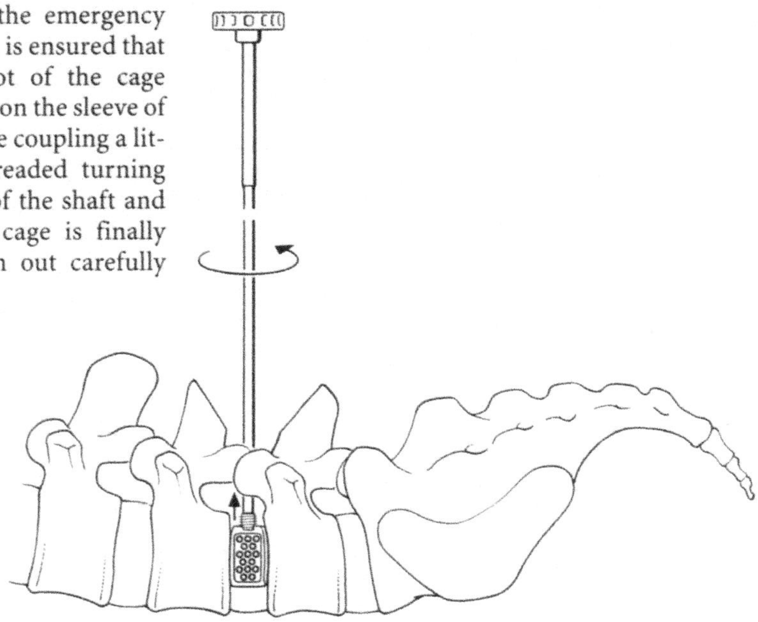

Fig. 9.36 Removal of the compression screw

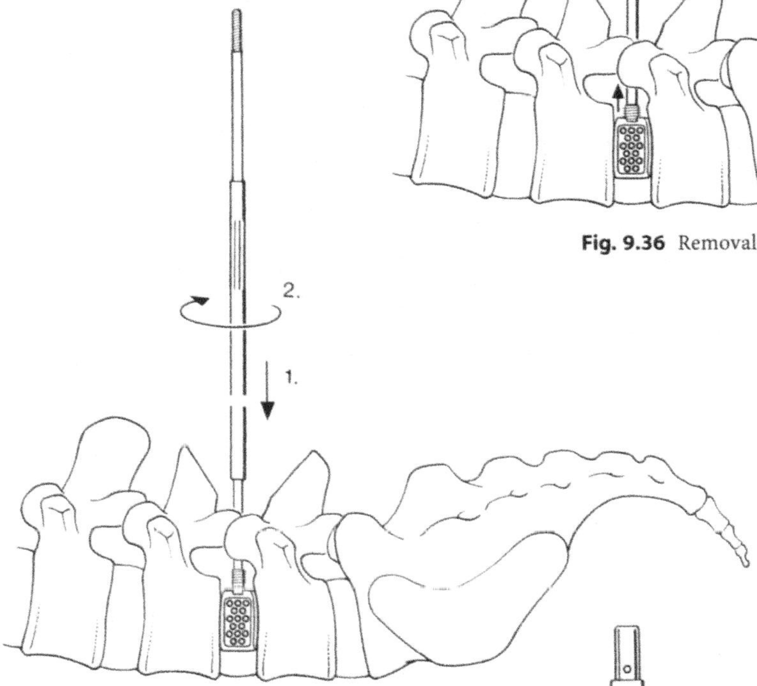

Fig. 9.37 Insertion of the inner shaft

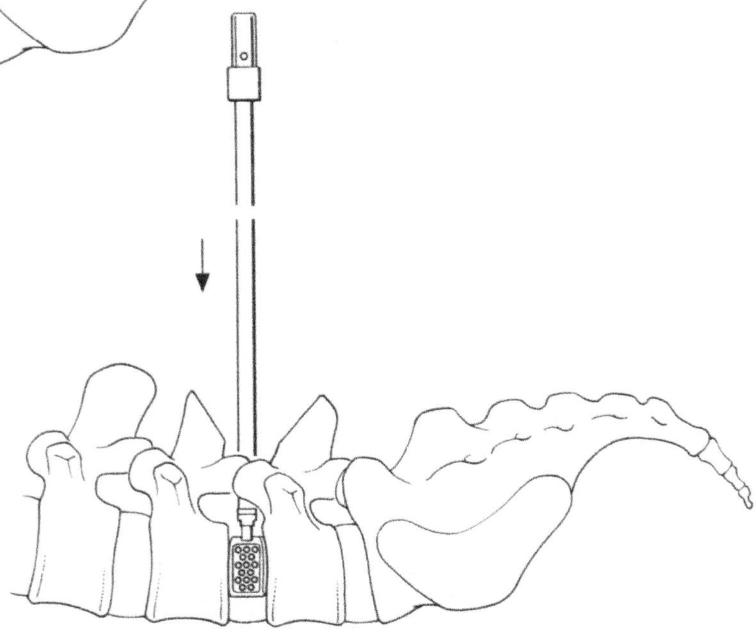

Fig. 9.38 Mounting the sleeve

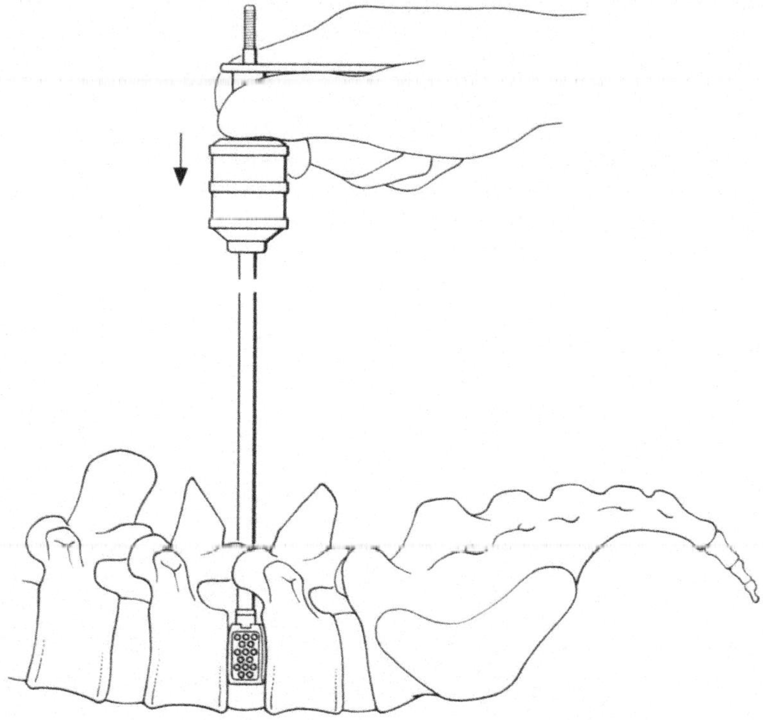

Fig. 9.39 Mounting the L-handle

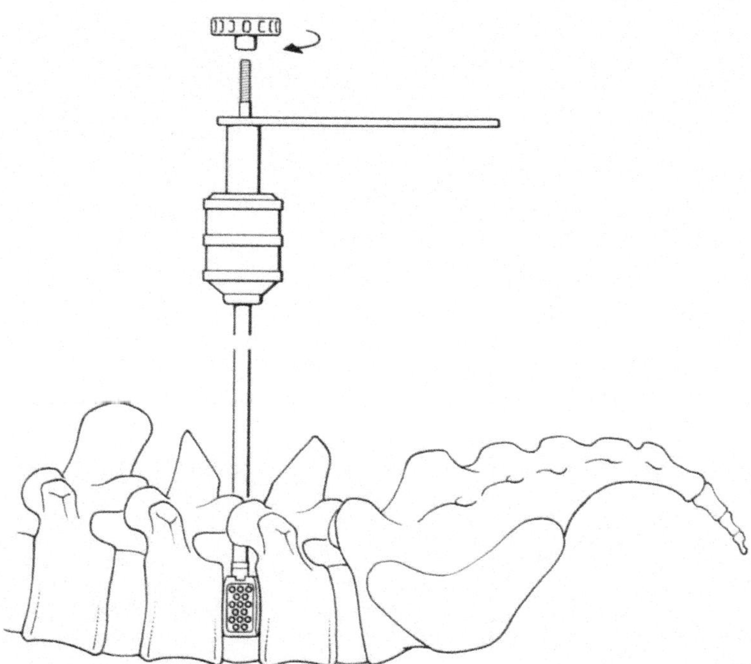

Fig. 9.40 Mounting the knob

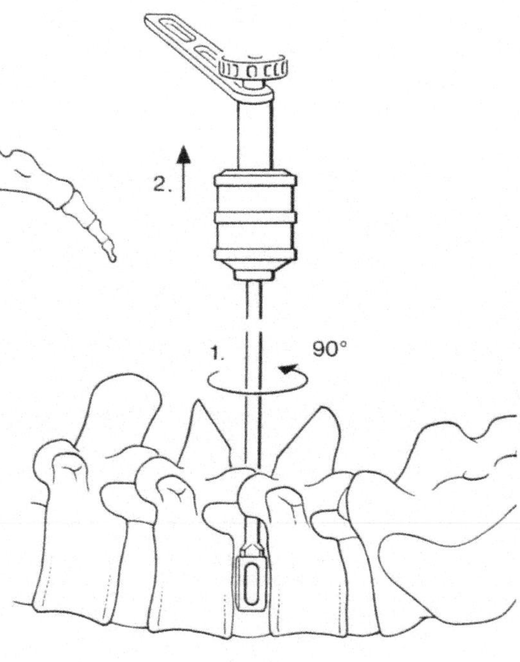

Fig. 9.41 Removal of the cage

Surgical Technique
A midline incision over the levels to be instrumented is performed. The muscles should not be stripped farther laterally than the lateral aspect of the facet joints unless a posterolateral fusion between the transverse processes is planned. Pedicle screws for additional posterior instrumentation can be inserted now or after having implanted the cages. The rod, however, is mounted on the screws only after the cages have been inserted.

In the case of intact posterior elements the lamina of the cephalad vertebra can be used for the application of translaminar screws. Pedicle screws for additional posterior instrumentation can be inserted now or after the cages have been implanted. The rod, however, is mounted on the screws only after the cages have been inserted. In case of intact posterior elements the lamina of the cephalad vertebra can be used for the application of translaminar screws.

The epidural space is now exposed: The spinous processes of the vertebrae to be fused are freed from all soft tissue. They are shortened in order to gain wider access to the interlaminar space (Fig. 9.42a). The removed bone is stored in a container under a moistened gauze, to serve as graft material. In order to allow as free access as possible to the dural sac and roots, a partial inferior laminotomy (one-third) of the upper adjacent vertebra is performed. The medial half of the facet joints is removed. A 10- or 15-mm gouge is used and a partial resection of the overlying inferior facet and lateral part of the laminar edge is performed (Fig. 9.42b).

At the L5–S1 level, usually the distal half of the lamina of L5 needs to be removed in order to ensure instrument access to the disk space. The underlying superior facet of S1 is then nibbled away to the level of the medial aspect of the pedicle. (It is essential to make sufficient room laterally to avoid excessive retraction on the neural tissue, but great care should be taken to protect the nerve root inside the foramen.) The next step is to evacuate the disk space by a bilateral diskectomy.

The posterior annulus is opened and resected to allow the introduction of the appropriate cage probes. The nucleus has to be cleaned out as completely as possible and the end plates need to be freed from the cartilage without, however, perforating the bone. A good instrument to prepare the end plates is the ring curette in different sizes (Fig. 9.43). Great care should be taken to protect the nerve root and the dura, with the appropriate nerve root retractor.

Once the disk space is prepared, a small disk space opener (4/8 or 5/9 mm) is introduced into the disk space on the right $_{(1)}$ (if you are standing left of the patient) (Fig. 9.44): distract the disk space by turning the instrument 90°$_{(2)}$. This will definitely open the posterior entrance into the disk space. While protecting the nerve root and dura with a root retractor, the smallest vertebral body spreader (7/9)

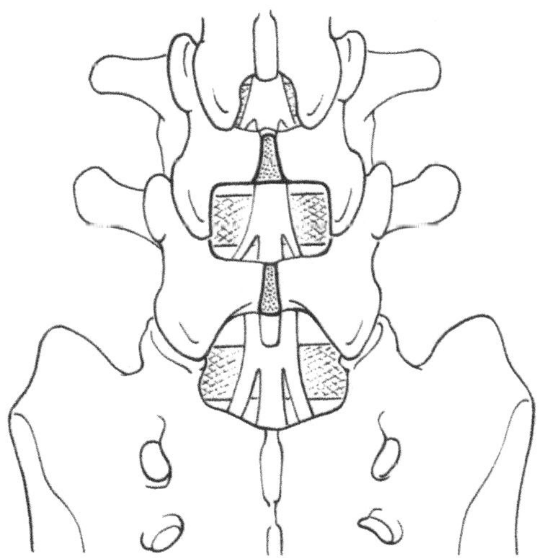

b

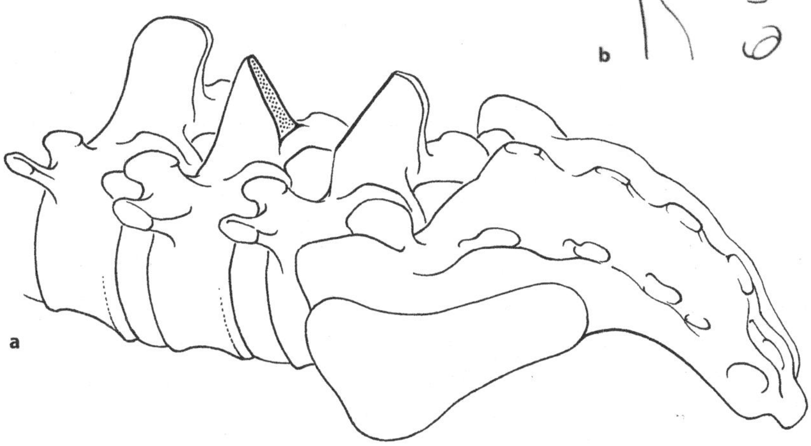

a

Fig. 9.41 Exposure of epidural space
a Partial resection of spinous processes
b Lateral enlargement of the access into the spinal canal

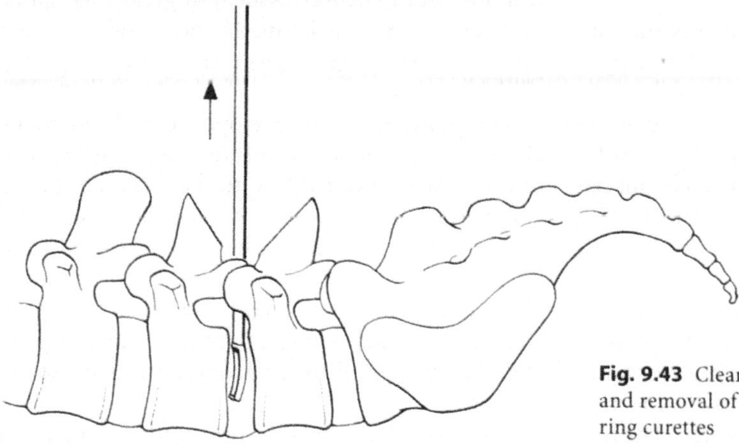

Fig. 9.43 Cleaning of the intradiskal space and removal of the end plate cartilage with ring curettes

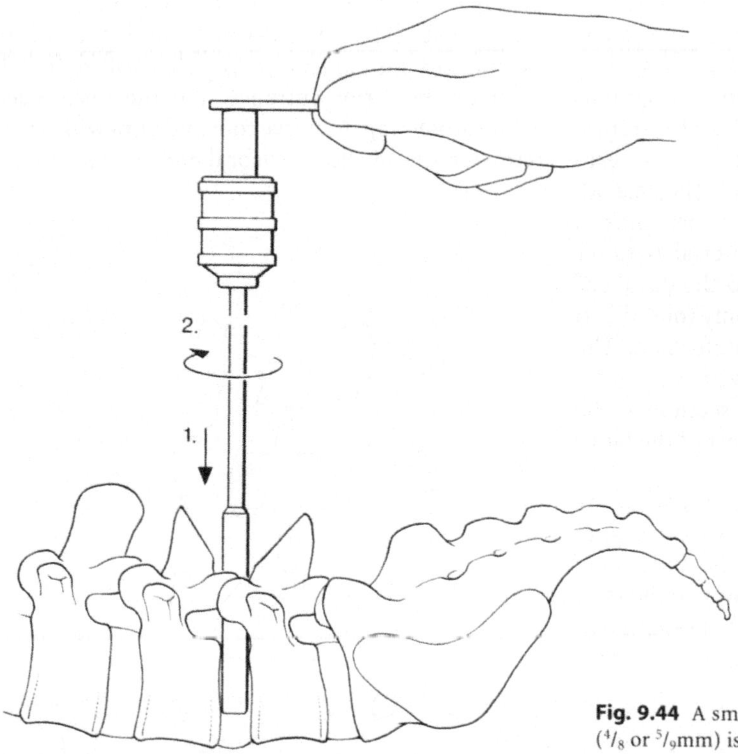

Fig. 9.44 A small disk space opener ($^4/_8$ or $^5/_9$mm) is introduced into the disk space

is introduced on the left side (Fig. 9.45) until the laser marks behind the head of the spreader are flush with the posterior edge of the vertebral body, and it is turned 90° in order to spread the disk space further. Then the 7/9 vertebral body spreader is removed and replaced with the next larger vertebral body spreader (8/10) and turned up 90° (Fig. 9.46). Spreading the disk is now repeated by introducing the next larger spreaders until resistance of the tense annulus is felt, indicating that the disk has been enlarged to its natural height. This last spreader should remain in place until the first cage is introduced on the other side, where the disk opener can now be removed.

A contact fusion cage of the same height as the largest accepted vertebral body spreader is now chosen. The cage previously prepared and filled with milled bone is now introduced into the disk (Fig. 9.47) by small gentle blows of a mallet, the root and dura being protected by a 'retractor.' The cage is introduced with the flat side top and bottom and to the appropriate depth, 3–4 mm inwards from the

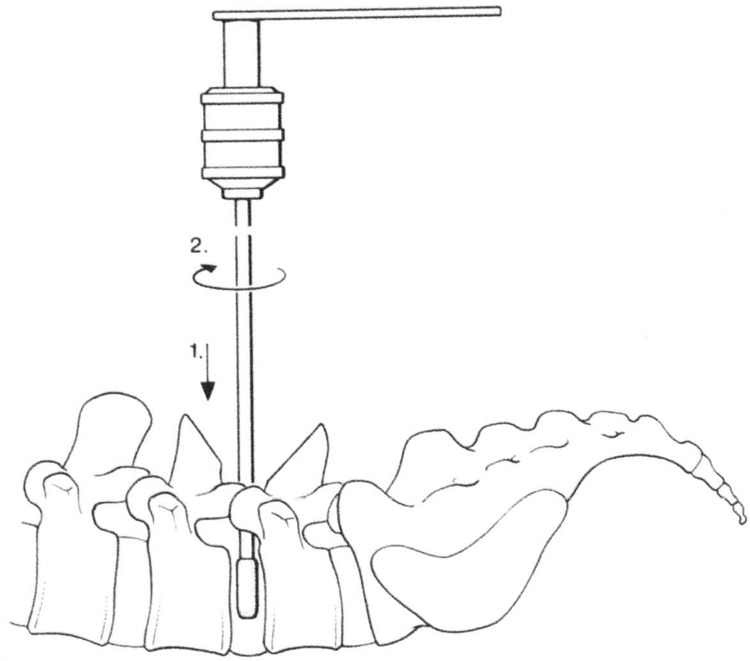

Fig. 9.45 Progressively different sizes of vertebral body spreaders are introduced until the natural height of the disk space is about to be restored

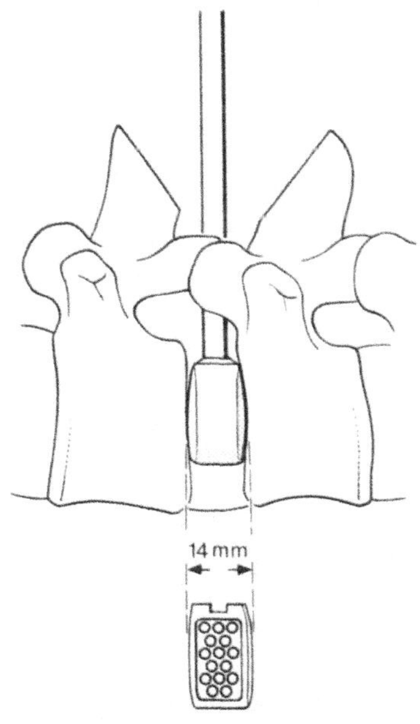

Fig. 9.46 A contact fusion cage of the same height as the largest accepted vertebral body spreader is chosen

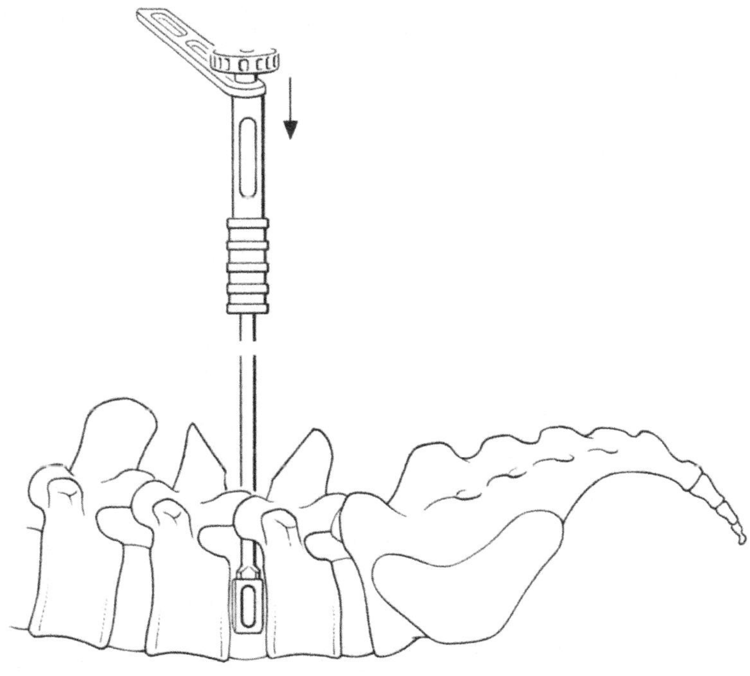

Fig. 9.47 The chosen contact fusion cage is now introduced into the disk space

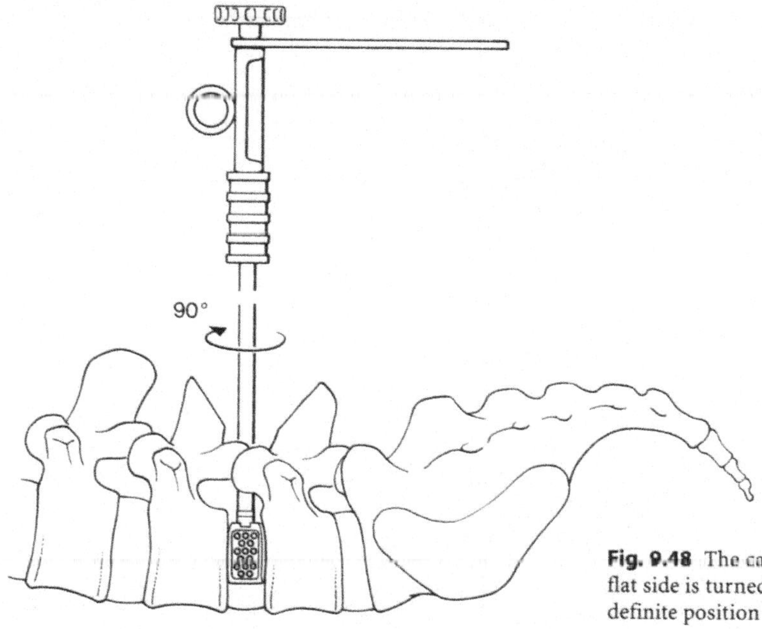

Fig. 9.48 The cage introduced with its flat side is turned 90° to the vertical, definite position

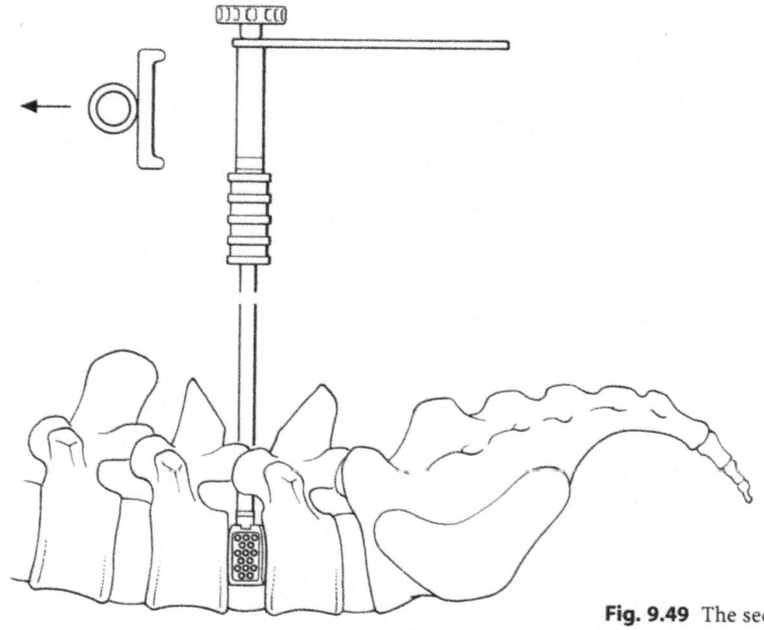

Fig. 9.49 The security sleeve is removed

posterior edge of the body (Fig. 9.48). When the heel of the implant holder tip is flush with the posterior edge of the vertebral body, the cage is in the right position (Fig. 9.47). Although the anterior annulus is resistant in most patients, keep in mind that the resistance of the anterior annulus can be lost in a very degenerated disk. If in doubt control the optimal position of the cage with a lateral X-ray.

Once the cage is introduced to the exact depth, it is turned *clockwise* (Fig. 9.48). The blade of the L-handle is in the vertical axis of the cage. When the blade is parallel to the body axis, the cage is also in the vertical position. If for some reason the cage has to be turned back on its side again, a *counterclockwise* turn is done. The security sleeve is removed by turning the screwdriver at the upper extremity of the introducer backward one or two full turns, thus disengaging the security sleeve (Fig. 9.49).

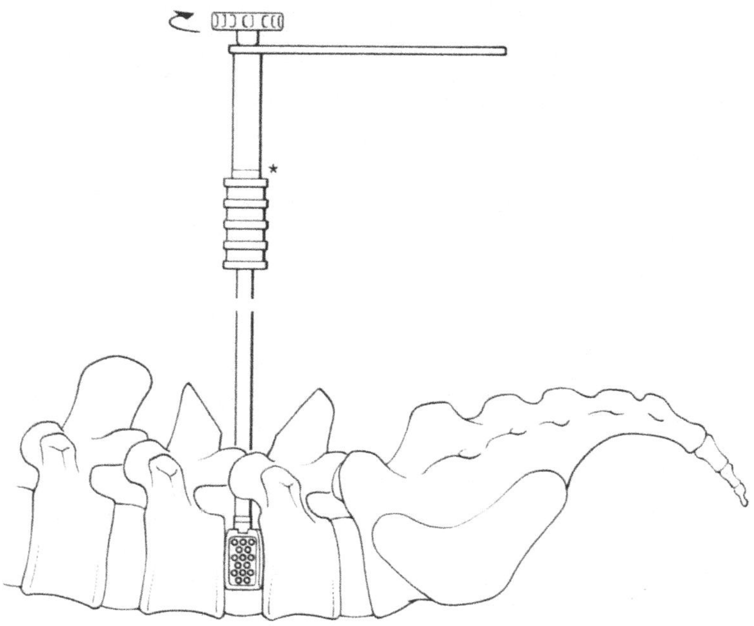

Fig. 9.50 The screwdriver is turned clockwise until the second circular notch on the shaft is flush with the proximal end of the cage (*)

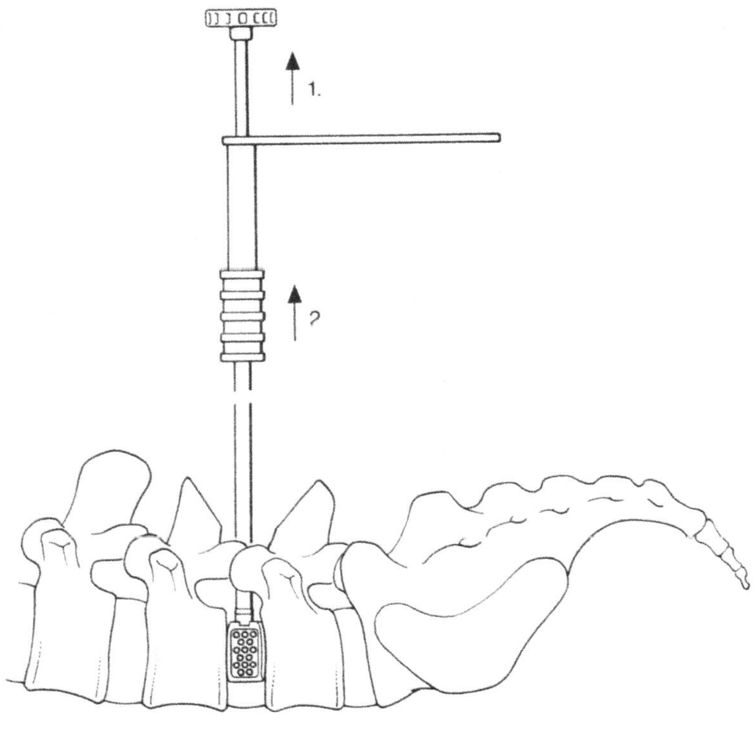

Fig. 9.51 After releasing the internal lokking mechanism of the screwdriver, the screwdriver is pulled out of the shaft (1) and the L-handle is removed (2)

The screwdriver is turned clockwise until the second circular mark on the shaft is flush with the proximal end of the cage (Fig. 9.48). When it is turned downwards, the internal locking mechanism of the screwdriver is released. Then the screwdriver is pulled out of the shaft(1). This automatically disconnects the implant holder from the cage at the slightest movement of the L-handle(2). (If the screwdriver should block, it can be disengaged by unscrewing the outer casing of the shaft.) (Fig. 9.51) The same steps are now repeated on the contralateral side.

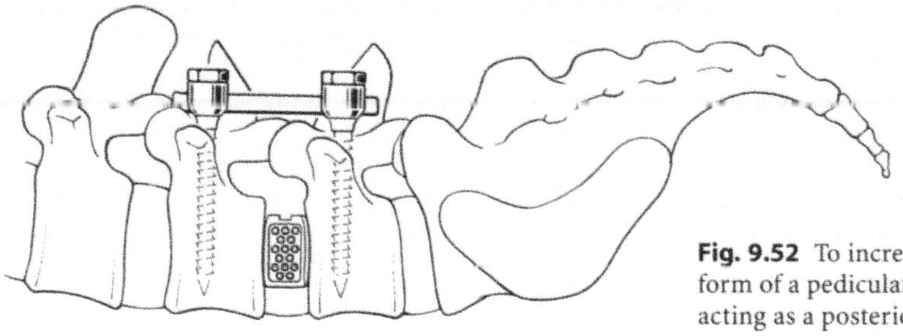

Fig. 9.52 To increase the stability, a posterior fixation in the form of a pedicular system or translaminar screws are added, acting as a posterior tension band system.

Care has to be taken that the second cage does not displace the first one on being introduced. It should be introduced well clear from the first one, and hammered down in a direction that is as sagittal as possible. Alternatively, if there is ample space on both sides of the neural tube, the handle on the first one may be left firmly connected until the second one is in place. A pedicular fixation system is now completed or translaminar screws are applied while maintaining a posterior tension/band force with a towel clamp set onto the two adjacent laminae in order to support the restoration of the lordosis (Fig. 9.52).

Postoperative Care

Postoperative X-rays should be taken to control the correct position of the cages and the pedicle screws before mobilization of the patient is started. The patient should be mobilized on the first postoperative day to the edge of the bed and then progressively the following days. A soft lumbar brace with a lordotic reinforcement in the back is given for the first 8–12 weeks postoperatively. Isometric exercises are started immediately postoperatively for the abdominal and back muscles, and rotation and flexion are avoided during this period.

Suggested Reading

Aebi M, Mohler J, Zäch G, Morscher E (1986) Indication, surgical technique and results of 100 surgically treated fractures and fracture-dislocations of the cervical spine. Clin Orthop 203: 244–257

Aebi M, Etter C, Coscia M (1989) Fractures of the odontoid process. Treatment with anterior screw fixation. Spine 14: 1065–1070

Aebi M, Zuber K, Marchesi D (1991) The treatment of cervical spine injuries by anterior plating. Spine 16: 38–45

Aebi M, Webb J (1991) The spine. In: Müller ME, Allgöwer M, Schneider R, Willenegger H: Manual of Internal Fixation, 3rd ed. Springer Berlin

Anderson PA, Henley MB, Grady M S, Montesano PX, Winn HR (1991) Posterior cervical arthrodesis with AO reconstruction plates + bone grafts. Spine 16: 72–79

Böhler J, Gaudernak T (1980) Anterior plate Stabilization for fracture - dislocation of the lower cervical spine. J Trauma 20: 203–205

Böhler J (1981) Schraubenosteosynthese von Frakturen des Dens axis. Unfallheilkunde 84: 221–223

Dick W (1987) „The fixateur interne" as a versatile implant for spine surgery. Spine 12: 882–900

Grob D, Jeanneret B, Aebi M, Markwalder TM (1991) Atlanto-axial fusion with transarticular screw fixation. J Bone Joint Surg 73-B: 972–976

Jeanneret B, Magerl F, Ward EH, Ward J-CH (1991) Posterior stabilization of the cervical spine (C 2–7) with hook plates. Spine 16: 56–63

Jeanneret B, Magerl F (1992) Primary posterior fusion C_1/C_2 in odontoid fractures: indications, technique and results of transarticular screw fixation. J Spin Disord 5: 464–475

Jeanneret B, Jovanovic M, Magerl F (1994) Percutaneous diagnostic stabilization for low back pain: correlation with results after fusion operations. Clin Orthop 304: 130–138

Jeanneret B, Magerl F (1994) Treatment of osteomyelitis of the spine using percutaneous suction/irrigation and percutaneous external skeletal fixation. Spinal Disord 7: 185–205

Laxer (1994) Eur Spine J 3

Magerl F (1984) Stabilization of the lower thoracic and lumbar spine with external skeletal fixation. Clin Orthop 189: 125–141

Magerl F, Aebi M, Gertzbein SD, Harms J, Nazarian S (1994) A comprehensive classification of thoracic and lumbar injuries. Eur Spine J 3: 184–201

Morscher E, Sutter F, Jenny H, Olernel S (1986) Die vordere Versplattung der Halswirbelsäule mit dem Hohlschrauben-Plattensystem aus Titanium. Chirurg 57: 702–707

Orozco Delclos R, Llovet TJ (1970) Osteosinthesis en las fracturas de raguis cervical: nota de technica. Rev Ortop Traumatol 14: 285–288

Subject Index

SPRINGER NATURE

GPSR Compliance

The European Union's (EU) General Product Safety Regulation (GPSR) is a set of rules that requires consumer products to be safe and our obligations to ensure this.

If you have any concerns about our products, you can contact us on ProductSafety@springernature.com

In case Publisher is established outside the EU, the EU authorized representative is:

Springer Nature Customer Service Center GmbH
Europaplatz 3
69115 Heidelberg, Germany

The manufacturer's authorised representative in the EU is Springer
Nature Customer Service Centre GmbH, Europaplatz 3, 69115 Heidelberg,
Germany. If you have any concerns regarding our products, please
contact ProductSafety@springernature.com

Printed and bound by CPI Group (UK) Ltd, Croydon, CR0 4YY
25/09/2026
02222905-0002